T0294796

ESSENTIALS OF

ESTHETIC
DENTISTRY

MINIMALLY INVASIVE ESTHETICS

VOLUME THREE

ESSENTIALS OF

ESTHETIC DENTISTRY

MINIMALLY INVASIVE ESTHETICS

VOLUME THREE

Edited by

Avijit Banerjee BDS MSc PhD (Lond) LDS FDS (Rest Dent) FDS RCS (Eng) FHEA

Professor of Cariology and Operative Dentistry
Honorary Consultant/Clinical Lead, Restorative Dentistry
Head, Conservative and MI Dentistry
King's College London Dental Institute at Guy's Hospital
King's Health Partners
London, UK

Series Editor

Brian J. Millar BDS FDSRCS PhD FHEA

Professor of Blended Learning in Dentistry;
Consultant in Restorative Dentistry; Specialist Practitioner, King's College London Dental Institute
London, UK

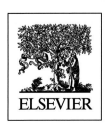

ELSEVIER

Edinburgh London New York Oxford Philadelphia St Louis Sydney Toronto 2015

ELSEVIER

ISBN: 978-0-7234-5556-1

Notices
Knowledge and best practice in this field are constantly changing. As new research and experience broaden our understanding, changes in research methods, professional practices, or medical treatment may become necessary.

Practitioners and researchers must always rely on their own experience and knowledge in evaluating and using any information, methods, compounds, or experiments described herein. In using such information or methods they should be mindful of their own safety and the safety of others, including parties for whom they have a professional responsibility.

With respect to any drug or pharmaceutical products identified, readers are advised to check the most current information provided (i) on procedures featured or (ii) by the manufacturer of each product to be administered, to verify the recommended dose or formula, the method and duration of administration, and contraindications. It is the responsibility of practitioners, relying on their own experience and knowledge of their patients, to make diagnoses, to determine dosages and the best treatment for each individual patient, and to take all appropriate safety precautions.

To the fullest extent of the law, neither the Publisher nor the authors, contributors, or editors, assume any liability for any injury and/or damage to persons or property as a matter of products liability, negligence or otherwise, or from any use or operation of any methods, products, instructions, or ideas contained in the material herein.

Printed in Great Britain
Last digit is the print number: 10   9   8   7   6   5   4   3

ELSEVIER your source for books, journals and multimedia in the health sciences

www.elsevierhealth.com

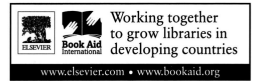

Working together to grow libraries in developing countries

www.elsevier.com • www.bookaid.org

The publisher's policy is to use paper manufactured from sustainable forests

For Elsevier:
Content Strategist: Alison Taylor
Content Development Specialist: Clive Hewat
Project Manager: Anne Collett
Designer/Design Direction: Miles Hitchen
Illustrator: AEGIS Media

CONTENTS

CONTRIBUTORS

Alma Dozic PhD DDS MSD
Specialist in Esthetic Composite Dentistry and Sleep
Apnoea Treatment
Department of Dental Material Sciences
Academic Centre for Dentistry Amsterdam (ACTA)
Amsterdam
The Netherlands

Jorien Hamburger DDS
Department of Dentistry
Radboud University Medical Center
Radboud Institute for Health Sciences
Nijmegen
The Netherlands

**Martin G D Kelleher BDS (Hons) MSc FDSRCPS
FDSRCS**
Consultant in Restorative Dentistry
King's College Dental Hospital
London, UK

Hein de Kloet DDS MSD
Specialist in Esthetic Composite Dentistry
Private Practice: Arnhem;
Department of Cariology, Academic Centre for
Dentistry Amsterdam (ACTA)
Amsterdam
The Netherlands

Bas A C Loomans DDS PhD
Assistant Professor
Department of Dentistry
Radboud University Medical Center
Radboud Institute for Health Sciences
Nijmegen
The Netherlands

Louis Mackenzie BDS
General Dental Practitioner
Selly Park Dental Centre;
Clinical Lecturer
University of Birmingham
Birmingham, UK

Niek J M Opdam DDS PhD
Associate Professor
Department of Dentistry
Radboud University Medical Center
Radboud Institute for Health Sciences
Nijmegen
The Netherlands

**Michael Thomas BDS MSc MRD RCSEng
DGDP(UK) LDS RCSEng**
Senior Teaching Fellow; Registered Specialist in
Prosthodontics
King's College London Dental Institute at Guy's
Hospital
London, UK

PREFACE FROM THE SERIES EDITOR

Esthetic dentistry is a complex subject. In many ways it requires different skills from those required for disease-focussed clinical care. Yet in other ways esthetic dentistry is part of everyday dentistry. The team which has created this series shares the view that success in esthetic dentistry requires a broad range of additional skills. Dentistry can now offer improved shade matching through to smile design to reorganising the smile zone.

The first volume provided useful, readily applicable information for those wishing to develop further their practice of esthetic dentistry. The provision of esthetic dentistry requires a different philosophy in the dental clinic and the in minds of the clinical team, a greater awareness of the aspirations of patients and a solid ethical footing. It also requires an ability to carry out a detailed assessment of dental and psychological factors, offer methods to show the patient the available options and, in some cases, be able to offer a range of treatments.

The second book in the series focussed on smile design techniques and some of the smile changing techniques particularly where tooth preparation is acceptable. However there is an increasing concern amongst clinicians and patients about the amount of tooth reduction – some would say destruction, carried out to enhance esthetics, while healthcare in general moves towards minimal intervention (MI). I believe patients should receive the best possible care, with the options not being limited by the clinician's skill (or lack of skills). Hence, the vision for this *Essentials* series and this third volume.

The single biggest task the team faced in putting this series together was to create information for dentists across the world: recognising that there are differing views on esthetics, MI, essential understanding and skills – and patients with different attitudes and budgets. The specific challenge was creating a series of books which addresses these diverse opinions, ranging from the view that tooth reduction is acceptable and inevitable in producing beautiful smiles – thinking reflected in Volume 2 – to the view that such tooth reduction is abhorrent and unacceptable and that the MI approach is preferable, as covered in this volume. I hope the series of books will satisfy both camps and enable practitioners at all levels to develop skills to practise esthetics, while respecting tooth tissue.

We intend this series to challenge your thinking and approach to the growing subject area of esthetic dentistry, particularly by showing different management of common clinical situations. We do not need to rely on a single formula to provide a smile make-over, promoting only one treatment modality where both the dentist and their patients are losing out; the patient losing valuable irreplaceable enamel as well as their future options.

For those seeking an MI approach the book will provide a suitable range of effective procedures in esthetic dentistry.

Professor Brian Millar BDS FDSRCS PhD FHEA

PREFACE

It has been a great pleasure and honour to edit and write Volume 3 of the new Elsevier series entitled *Essentials of Esthetic Dentistry*, which focuses on dental esthetics and caters for both dental undergraduates and qualified practitioners alike.

When I was asked originally to compile and edit the content for a new tome with the strap line *Minimally Invasive Esthetics*, I did feel a pang of concern about the direction and motive of the textbook and the series in relation to the appreciation of minimally invasive (MI) approaches by the dental profession as a whole. Surely, I thought, all operative dentistry should be esthetic and the preservation of natural, biological tissues must be all clinical operators' primary aim and objective? Or, in my naivety, is the more invasive one (or multiple) visit and 'smile make-over' the positive direction forward?

It was at that moment I appreciated the real value of this new volume and its important position in dental literature. There is a vital, and perhaps unmet, need to highlight the considerable and significant differences between dental cosmesis, which aims to deliver operative care solely for the improvement of the appearance of biologically healthy dental and oral tissues–and dental esthetics, which aims to repair and correct esthetically all oral and dental tissue defects created by underlying pathology or trauma. The former approach often relies traditionally on cutting away significant quantities of biologically sound tissues and replacing them with artificial restorative materials; whereas the latter focuses on the MI repair, refurbishment or replacement of minimal quantities of defective tissues, and often with directly placed, adhesive dental materials.

With these definitions in mind, I developed the contents for this important volume with a logical theme, starting with the discussion of possible patho-physiological aetiologies of biological tooth damage. Three of the more common MI tooth preserving operative solutions to treat such conditions have been dis-cussed and described in detail: dental bleaching, the judicious use of adhesive resin composite restorations to re-constitute teeth effectively in both the anterior and posterior dentition, and the use of MI techniques for replacing missing teeth, both directly and indirectly. The authoritative scientific and clinically evidence-based contributions from carefully selected world-class experts in these areas of MI operative dentistry have highlighted the way in which high-quality esthetics can be achieved with minimal biological cost and acceptable longevity, without long-term detriment to the patient. In all cases, communication among dentist, team and patient is of paramount importance in ensuring the patient's expectations are appreciated, managed and met. Some of the high-quality, contemporary operative techniques detailed in this volume may require further education/skill enhancement by restorative practitioners but should ultimately be within the remit of those dental professionals tasked with taking team care forwards into the future, where MI dentistry will surely underpin patient care, and so benefit the patient and the profession as a whole.

Professor Avijit Banerjee BDS, MSc, PhD (Lond), LDS,
FDS (Rest Dent), FDS, RCS (Eng), FHEA

CHAPTER 1

Common Clinical Conditions Requiring Minimally Invasive Esthetic Intervention

M. THOMAS

INTRODUCTION

Minimum intervention dentistry is the concept of a patient-centred, team-care holistic approach to maintaining life-long oral and dental health. The 'minimally invasive (MI)' concept is to preserve pulp vitality and as much natural tooth tissue for a lifetime. The main consideration underpinning the MI concept is achieving accurate identification and diagnosis of dental problems at the earliest stage. In providing a pro-active approach to the prevention of dental disease, MI dentistry aims to prevent the cycle of destructive restorative dentistry where existing dental treatment is replaced as a result of wear and deterioration, leading to further preparation and weakening of the remaining tooth structure and concomitant stress to the pulp. With an ageing population and an increase in the number of teeth retained throughout life, the need to preserve natural tooth tissue is of paramount importance.[1]

However, MI dentistry as a pro-active approach to modern dental care must not be interpreted as a 'do nothing' technique. A clinician adopting an MI approach to dental care is neither ignoring nor avoiding the (often raised) esthetic issues. The MI concept enables an esthetic intervention to be made with minimal harmful biological effect, which will therefore be of benefit in optimizing the natural appearance of tooth structure. Advances in dental materials and operative techniques encourage a less traditional and aggressive approach to be adopted, whilst achieving an improved outcome and prognosis.

In a society where appearance and esthetics are a driving factor, with high expectations for oral health and appearance, it is critical to identify dental characteristics that will impact on people's psychosocial well-being. Modern dentistry encompasses a variety of materials and techniques to enhance the esthetic outcome of managed dental care within the MI framework. These techniques are explored throughout this publication. In this chapter some clinical conditions will be discussed (Table 1.1) where MI options for esthetic intervention may be considered, including:

- Tooth discolouration, including trauma
- Hypoplastic conditions
- Dental caries
- Crowding
- Missing teeth
- Tooth wear.

TABLE 1.1   CAUSES OF DENTAL DISCOLOURATION

Cause of discolouration			Pathology	Visual changes	Possible management options
Developmental defects					
	Hereditary defects				
		Amelogenesis imperfecta	Fourteen different subtypes. Disturbance of mineralization or matrix of enamel formation	Yellow-brown to dark yellow appearance	Bleaching Micro-abrasion Composite bonding
		Dentinogenesis imperfecta	Type I – disorder of type I collagen	Bluish or brown in appearance, opalescence on trans-illumination	Bleaching Bonding Veneers
			Type II – hereditary opalescent dentine	Opalescent primary teeth. Enamel chips away to expose EDJ. Once dentine exposed, teeth show brown discolouration	Bonding Veneers Full coverage crowns
			Type III – brandywine isolate hereditary opalescent dentine	Outward similar appearance to Types I and II. Multiple pulpal exposures in primary dentition. Dentine production ceases after mantle dentine has formed	Bonding Veneers Full coverage crowns Replacement of teeth may be required if severe
	Metabolic disorders				
		Alkaptonuria	Incomplete metabolism of tyrosine and phenylalanine. Promotes build-up of homogentisic acid	Brown discolouration	Bleaching Bonding Veneers
		Congenital hyperbilirubinaemia	Deposition of bile pigments in the calcifying dental tissues	Purple or brown discolouration	Bleaching Bonding Veneers
		Congenital erythropoietic porphyria	Accumulation of porphyrins in teeth	Red-brown discolouration. Red fluorescence under ultra-violet light	Bleaching Bonding Veneers

TABLE 1.1 *Continued*

Cause of discolouration			Pathology	Visual changes	Possible management options
		Vitamin D dependent rickets	Defects in enamel matrix formation	Pitting and yellow-brown discolouration	Bleaching Micro-abrasion Bonding
		Epidermolysis bullosa	Pitting of enamel, possibly caused by vesiculation of the ameloblast layer	Pitting and yellow-brown discolouration	Bleaching Micro-abrasion Bonding
		Ehlers–Danlos syndrome	Areas of hypoplastic enamel and irregularities in region of EDJ	Pitting and brown or purple-brown discolouration	Bleaching Micro-abrasion Bonding
		Pseudo-hypoparathyroidism	Defects in enamel matrix formation	Pitting and yellow-brown discolouration	Bleaching Micro-abrasion Bonding
		Molar incisor hypomineralization (MIH)	Unknown aetiology. Hypomineralized enamel affecting incisors and permanent first molars	Asymmetrical appearance in arch. Enamel defects vary from white to yellow to brown areas	Bleaching Micro-abrasion Bonding
Intrinsic discolouration					
	Acquired defects				
		Trauma	Pulpal haemorrhage may lead to accumulation of haemoglobin or other iron-containing haematin molecules within the dentine tubules	Grey-brown to black	Bleaching
		Internal resorption	Increased volume of pulpal space and pulpal tissue	Pink	Extirpation and obturation of pulpal space
		Systemic infectious disease, e.g. rubella	Generalized hypoplasia due to disturbance of the developing tooth germ	Pitting or grooving leading to yellow-brown discolouration	Bleaching Micro-abrasion Bonding Veneers

TABLE 1.1 *Continued*

Cause of discolouration		Pathology	Visual changes	Possible management options
	Localized infection	Localized hypoplasia due to disturbance of the developing tooth germ	Pitting or grooving leading to yellow-brown discolouration	Bleaching Micro-abrasion Bonding
	Excessive fluoride intake	Enamel most often affected. Change in mineral matrix from hydroxyapatite to fluorapatite	Flecking to diffuse mottling. Colour changes range from chalky white to dark brown appearance	Bleaching Micro-abrasion Bonding
	Administration of tetracycline	Chelation to form complexes with calcium ions on the surface of hydroxyapatite crystals, mainly in dentine but also in enamel	Depends on type of tetracycline used, dosage and duration of administration. Yellow or brown-grey discolouration	Bleaching Bonding Veneers
	Amalgam	Migration of tin ions into the dentine tubules	Grey-black discolouration to dentine	Bleaching Bonding using opaque materials
	Eugenol and phenol containing endodontic materials	Staining of the dentine	Orange-yellow discolouration	Bleaching
Extrinsic discolouration				
	Direct stains	Food and drink, e.g. tea, coffee, red wine. Smoking	Usually multi-factorial. Chromogens incorporated into the plaque or acquired pellicle	Varies from mild yellow to more severe brown-black discolouration	Good oral hygiene May benefit from bleaching
		Chromogenic bacteria	Incorporated into plaque	Varies from yellow to green-black discolouration	Good oral hygiene May benefit from bleaching
	Indirect stains	Chlorhexidine and other metal salts in mouthrinses	Precipitation of chromogenic polyphenols onto tooth surface	Brown to black discolouration	Good oral hygiene May benefit from bleaching
Caries		Cariogenic bacteria, fermentable carbohydrate, susceptible tooth surface, time	Demineralization and eventual proteolytic destruction of organic matrix	White spot lesion to black arrested decay	Micro-abrasion Bonding Direct or indirect restoration

EDJ, enamel–dentine junction.

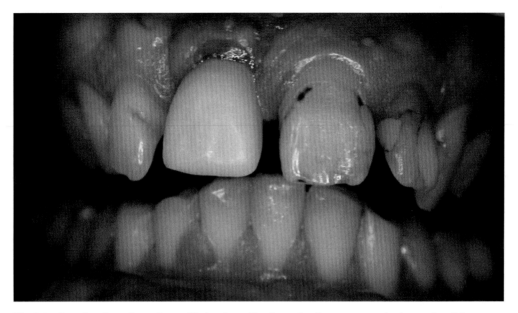

Fig. 1.1 Anterior view of a patient suffering from discolouration from wear, cavitation and staining around the margins of existing restorations, requiring esthetic modification.

DISCOLOURATION (Fig. 1.1)

Discolouration of the teeth may occur for a number of reasons, including:

- Developmental defects

- Intrinsic discolouration, including trauma

- Extrinsic discolouration.

In addition, teeth become darker with age due to the continuing deposition of secondary dentine and the gradual wear of enamel allowing the colour of the underlying dentine, and to some extent the pulp, to become more profound. Any change that affects the light transmitting and reflective properties of teeth may result in a patient's request for esthetic intervention. This may be achieved by the use of materials to replace or cover defective or missing tooth structures, but techniques to alter the appearance of the teeth, such as tooth whitening treatments, may be adopted which require minimal or no removal of sound enamel and dentine and rely on treating the cause of the discolouration rather than masking its effects.

DEVELOPMENTAL DEFECTS

Developmental defects can pose an esthetic problem,[2] as well as the teeth being more prone to wear and the damaging effects of the caries process. In addition,

COMMON CLINICAL CONDITIONS REQUIRING MINIMALLY INVASIVE ESTHETIC INTERVENTION

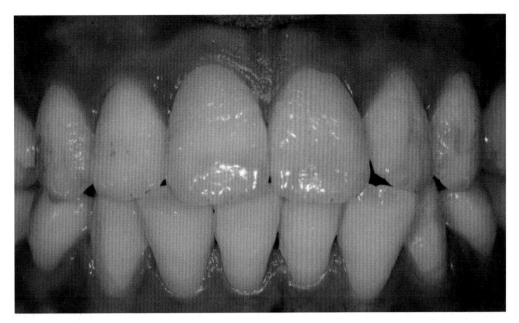

Fig. 1.2 Anterior clinical view showing developmental pitting and staining affecting the maxillary dentition, suitable for MI esthetic intervention with direct resin composite restorations.

developmental defects may result in symptoms of sensitivity and surface roughness, both combining to increase levels of plaque biofilm retention (Fig. 1.2). An early diagnosis is therefore important to enable careful planning and management.

Hereditary defects, such as hypodontia, amelogenesis imperfecta and dentinogenesis imperfecta, may affect the primary and secondary dentition equally. Management of defects in the primary dentition requires consideration of the child's self-perception and the parental expectation of treatment outcomes in addition to functional concerns and dental care inexperience, which will naturally be present at a young age. An esthetic intervention, using a biological MI approach, may provide the opportunity for a positive initial treatment experience and enable a good rapport and motivation to be established, making further management on development of the secondary dentition easier to accept later in life (Figs 1.3 and 1.4).

Metabolic disorders, such as alkaptonuria, congenital hyperbilirubinaemia or congenital erythropoietic porphyria, whilst rare, will result in discolouration of the dentition during development. Enamel defects may also be observed in cases of vitamin D-dependent rickets, epidermolysis bullosa, Ehlers–Danlos syndrome and pseudo-hypoparathyroidism.[3]

Acquired defects, resulting from trauma, systemic infectious disease, localized infection, excessive fluoride intake, or from administration of tetracycline

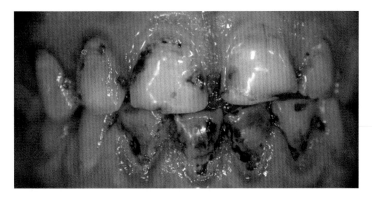

Fig. 1.3 Anterior view showing stained and pitted teeth with worn incisal edges. This was diagnosed as a mild case of amelogenesis imperfecta.

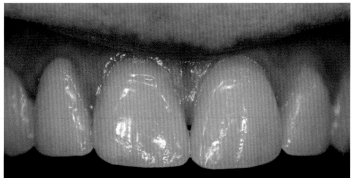

Fig. 1.4 The post-operative view of the case in Figure 1.3, following restoration with porcelain laminate veneers.

antibiotics during childhood or to the mother during pregnancy, may affect the dental tissues to a varying degree. Esthetic considerations, when a mild defect in the development of one or more teeth has occurred, may not be significant at a young age. However, as adulthood approaches, and social pressures affecting appearance become a more serious concern, demands for esthetic intervention may become increasingly prevalent.

INTRINSIC DISCOLOURATION

Intrinsic discolouration occurs when chromogens are deposited within tooth tissues. This is usually within the dentine and, once development of the tooth is complete, will be of pulpal origin (Fig. 1.5). However, staining agents may

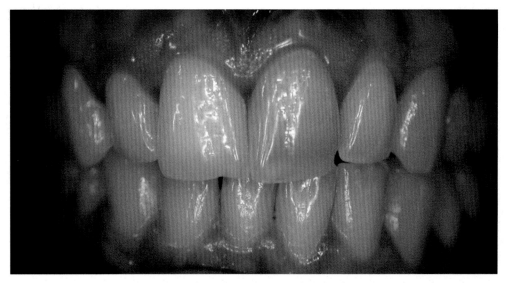

Fig. 1.5 Anterior view of a patient with a grey upper left central incisor with wear to the distal-incisal corner. The appearance of this tooth could be improved by bleaching and resin composite direct restoration.

enter the tooth through defects in the tooth structure. This will occur in the carious lesion and may also occur around the periphery of existing restorations. Cracking of the enamel, as a result of trauma, may also allow external staining agents to enter the tooth structure. Dentine may also become exposed as a result of toothwear or gingival recession, allowing external staining compounds to enter any patent tubules and intertubular dentine.

Pulpal haemorrhage may lead to discolouration of the tooth due to the accumulation of haemoglobin or other forms of iron-containing haematin molecules within the dentine tubules.[4] Bacterial invasion may result in further breakdown of these blood products leading to differing degrees of discolouration. If the tooth has been devitalized by trauma but the pulp chamber remains intact, bacterial invasion will not occur and re-vascularization may result in the tooth reverting to its normal colour.[5] A clear diagnosis of the cause of discolouration may therefore lead to the most minimal of interventions in order to achieve an acceptable esthetic outcome. If discolouration of the tooth was caused by blood pigments, agents can be developed specifically to remove or break down the haematin molecule within the dentine tubules in a tooth whitening procedure (see Chapter 3). The cause of the discolouration is therefore removed as opposed to the affected tooth structure.

Restorative dental materials may also affect the colour of the teeth. Eugenol and phenol-containing endodontic materials may stain dentine, causing a darkening effect. When an amalgam restoration is removed, a residual darkening/shadowing of the dentine may be noticed, due to the leaching of tin ions into the adjacent dentine.[6]

The deposition of tetracycline within teeth during development has been cited frequently as a cause of intrinsic discolouration, but new cases will become increasingly rare as a result of the improved awareness of the issues regarding the use of tetracycline during pregnancy and breastfeeding and in children up to 12 years of age. The effect of tetracycline on teeth is dependent on the medication used, the dosage and the period of administration. Affected teeth have a yellowish or brown-grey appearance, which is worse on eruption but can fade with time, although anterior teeth are affected by incident natural light changing the colour to brown as a result of photo-oxidative chemical processes. However, MI whitening treatment over an extended period can produce a pleasing esthetic result without the need for removal of sound tooth structure in many cases (see Chapter 2).

Excessive fluoride ion administration and intake will affect ameloblast function during enamel formation and maturation (Fig. 1.6). The effects are related to age and dose and both the primary and secondary dentition may be affected by

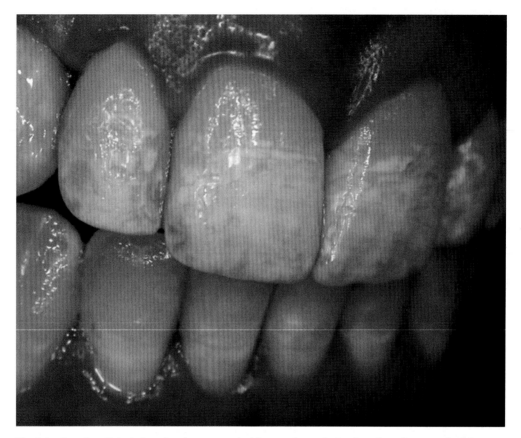

Fig. 1.6 Anterior clinical view showing a case of white spot hypoplasia, thought to have resulted from excessive fluoride intake by the patient as a youngster.

the resulting fluorosis. This may manifest as small areas of flecking through to opaque mottling of the enamel (Fig. 1.7). An increased porosity of the enamel may result in extrinsic stain deposition producing an internal effect[5] (Fig. 1.7). Similar hypoplastic effects to the enamel may occur locally following infection or trauma to the primary dentition affecting the underlying, developing secondary tooth germ. A large number of maternal or foetal conditions, such as infection or vitamin and mineral deficiency, may have a more generalized effect on the developing dentition. The outcome in terms of requiring an esthetic intervention will vary depending on severity of the condition and the individual patient's demands, but the principles of MI care can still be applied when considering the degree of operative intervention required. Again, care planning will centre around a true diagnosis of the cause of discolouration and an understanding of the histological location of the pigments/chromogens involved directly within the tooth structure. This will affect whether treatment will involve the removal of such molecules or masking their effects physically, but always using MI techniques.

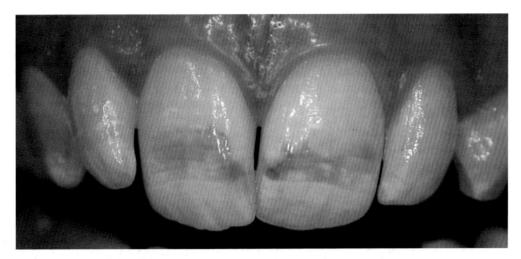

Fig. 1.7 Anterior clinical view showing a case of hypoplasia with associated brown discolouration affecting the labial surfaces of the two upper central incisors.

EXTRINSIC DISCOLOURATION

Chromogens affecting the tooth surface may be derived from a wide variety of sources. Examples include smoking tobacco products, tannins from tea, coffee, red wine and polyphenol compounds which provide the colouring to foods. External staining is usually multi-factorial and is transient, being removed with meticulous oral hygiene, the staining being a result of the chromogens being incorporated into surface plaque biofilm or acquired pellicle. Chromogenic bacteria within plaque may also produce a staining effect if allowed to stagnate long term. Exposure of dentine, as a result of tooth wear or gingival recession, may result in the externally sourced chromogens being incorporated into the dentine tubules and intertubular dentine structure.

The use of chlorhexidine in mouthrinses to reduce gingival inflammation has led to an increased incidence of surface staining, although this has been reported with mouthwashes containing other compounds. The staining mechanism is thought to be due to precipitation of chromogenic polyphenols within food and drink, and caused by chlorhexidine adsorbed onto the tooth surface.[7] Again, however, the staining can be removed straightforwardly and a good esthetic outcome can be achieved with the minimum of intervention.

DENTAL CARIES

The consequences of dental caries may result in an esthetic intervention being required to restore the appearance of the teeth as well as their function and strength. This may be as a result of cavitation resulting from the advanced caries process leading to the eventual undermining of the structural integrity of the tooth. However, the early carious lesion will produce a change in the appearance of the enamel surface as demineralization causes porosity within the prismatic structure of enamel. As the demineralization process continues, the characteristic frosty white appearance of the white spot lesion becomes visible due to a change in the relative local refractive index within the enamel lesion. The increased tooth surface porosity may permit dietary chromogens to become trapped, producing the darker appearance of the arrested brown spot lesion. When the lesion has spread into the dentine, this will undermine eventually the overlying enamel and, before cavitation occurs, a greyish shadowing may be visible on the tooth surface. Within the dentine lesion, colour changes may result from the Maillard reaction, where biochemical reactions occur between carbohydrates and proteins in the presence of an acid environment produced by the action of bacteria within the lesion. However, this effect is not uniform and dietary chromogens will also contribute to the changes in appearance of carious dentine if exposed for a sufficient time (Fig. 1.8).

As the carious lesion, in its early stages, is repairable, optimal management depends on accurate early detection, diagnosis and intervention before gross demineralization and proteolytic destruction require a more invasive operative approach. Risk assessment to identify high or low susceptibility to the disease allows appropriate standard or active preventive care and a non-operative preventive care approach to be adopted. Historically, caries has been classified based on a system of past experience of the disease as originally proposed by G.V. Black.[8] However, in the 2011 United Nations declaration on the control and prevention of non-communicable diseases, the importance of oral health was acknowledged and highlighted. This has led to the development of a global programme aimed at developing and implementing a new paradigm for caries management based on a preventive approach to healthcare.[9] Plaque control, dietary

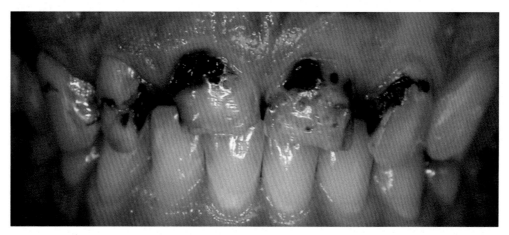

Fig. 1.8 Anterior clinical view of dental caries affecting the upper incisor and canine teeth. Excavation and esthetic MI reparative intervention is required.

modification and the use of fluoride should therefore be regarded as standard care for the control of dental caries to allow preventive, non-invasive remineralization treatments to be effective. This MI approach will aim to preserve the biological and structural integrity of the tooth in the long term.

An MI biological approach should also be adopted when operative intervention is required for treatment of a cavitated, progressing carious lesion.[10] This approach involves:

- Excavation of the biologically unrepairable, diseased enamel and dentine only, keeping cavities as small as possible.

- Physically and chemically modifying/optimizing the remaining cavity walls in order to restore cavities with suitable restorative adhesive materials, which will:

  · Support and strengthen the remaining tooth structure.

  · Promote remineralization and potentially have antibacterial activity.

  · Seal off any remaining bacteria from their nutrient supply, so arresting the caries process in the tooth.

  · Restore the appearance and function, enabling and enhancing the ability of the patient to remove the surface plaque biofilm, with suitable long-term success.

DENTAL CROWDING (IMBRICATION)

Crowding of teeth may lead to a patient request for an esthetic intervention. Carefully planned and judiciously used orthodontic alignment can provide a biologically sensitive, MI method of overcoming the adverse esthetic consequences of crowding. Although orthodontic treatment may not provide a quick improvement, the long-term consequences of a more rapidly executed, tissue-destructive restorative approach are the antithesis of an MI, biologically sound and ultimately long-term stable approach to dental care, in providing an acceptable esthetic outcome with teeth in stable final positions.[11]

MISSING TEETH

Missing teeth may require replacement to restore functional and/or esthetic harmony. When teeth are extracted, movement of adjacent and opposing teeth may occur, disrupting the established occlusal pattern and leading to alterations in comfort and function of the remaining dentition. The effects of an abnormal occlusion are subject to continuing debate throughout the dental profession, with a rapidly expanding literature: research based and empirical. Similarly, the care approach adopted in cases where an abnormal occlusion has been identified is subject to much discussion and varying opinions. This may range from minimum intervention to maximum preparation and re-alignment, adopting either a conformative or a re-organized approach.

When considering the replacement of missing teeth, it is the responsibility of the clinician to be convinced, along with the patient, that the replacement will produce significantly more benefit than harm. Consideration should be given to appearance, occlusal stability, ability to masticate, speech, retention of the position of the remaining teeth, restoration of the vertical dimension of occlusion and other particular circumstances, such as the ability of wind instrument players to create an embouchure. If the balance is strongly in favour of replacement, the clinician must decide on the most suitable technique for replacement. These interactive discussions between the dentist and the patient must be frank and honest, outlining all the potential benefits and pitfalls and must be comprehensively documented. Indeed, communication and documentation are the cornerstones to successful patient management.

The options available will include:

•   A removable partial denture, which may be made with a metal base, an acrylic base or from a flexible material.

•   A removable bridge retained using precision attachments, telescopic retainers, or a combination.

•   A fixed bridge retained with full or partial coverage extra-coronal restoration(s), inlay(s), or adhesive winged abutment(s). The design of the bridge may be cantilevered from a single adjacent tooth, or involve abutments on either side of the space to be filled. In addition, a variety of materials may be considered for construction of the restoration, all requiring different thicknesses for optimal mechanical and esthetic properties to provide sufficient strength and appearance. All of these factors, in turn, affect the degree of preparation required to the remaining teeth and therefore the degree of intervention required (see Chapters 8 and 9).

•   The placement and restoration of a dental implant or implants.

Today, in some parts of the world, implants are a relatively common dental procedure;[12] they have the advantage over alternative options for the fixed replacement of a missing tooth or teeth in that minimal/no biological or physical alteration to the adjacent hard tissues is necessary. Implants would therefore appear to be the ultimate MI approach to the replacement of a missing tooth or teeth. However, alteration to the underlying hard and soft tissues may be required in order to provide sufficient support for the fixture(s) and restoration. Therefore, although minimal intervention may be applied to the remaining dentition, surgical intervention may be a necessary part of the procedure in order to achieve a successful outcome. However, as has been demonstrated in one of the clinical cases in this chapter, an acceptable esthetic outcome, in appropriate circumstances, may still be achieved without the use of surgical intervention to replace missing hard and soft tissues.

TOOTH WEAR

Tooth wear, also known as tooth surface loss, is increasing in prevalence and severity. The incidence of moderate tooth wear is increasing in young adults although the overall incidence of severe tooth wear appears to be less common;[13] this indicates an increased requirement for dental care to manage this condition[14] (Fig. 1.9).

The MI concept for the esthetic management of the wear to teeth requires an accurate diagnosis of the aetiological factors of erosion, attrition, abrasion and/ or abfraction, which often occur in combination to varying degrees. This will then allow the cause(s) of tooth wear to be managed and an appropriate care strategy to be implemented, which aims to:

• Preserve remaining tooth tissue

• Achieve an esthetic improvement

• Restore and provide long-term stability to the dentition.

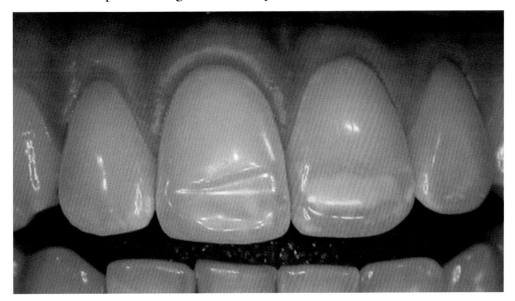

Fig. 1.9 An anterior view showing the result of erosive wear affecting the labial surface of the two upper central incisor teeth.

In order to meet these aims, the approach to restorative care should involve the use of suitable techniques and materials to protect and ensure the survival of remaining tooth tissue. This approach accepts that there should be the need for repair and renewal of restorations as required instead of the further loss of sound tooth tissue through further destructive tooth preparation.[15] The use of resin composite materials, with minimal long-term pulpal or structural complications to the tooth, is a more conservative and esthetically acceptable alternative to the use of porcelain restorations.[16] The long-term consequences to the dentition from extensive preparation to the tooth structure and pulpal damage as a result of using conventional indirect techniques can no longer be advocated routinely when advances in materials and cements now allow an MI, biologically based approach to the restoration of the worn dentition.

CONCLUSIONS

Clinicians have a responsibility to patients to meet their esthetic desires and aspirations by using techniques that are minimally tissue destructive, biologically sound and ethical in order to provide satisfactory short-term and long-term solutions to clinical conditions requiring intervention. The 'golden rule', which has been quoted many times throughout history, to 'do unto others what you would have them do to you'* should be kept very much in mind when making treatment decisions at all times.

CLINICAL CASE 1.1

There is a false perception that MI dentistry equates to always carrying out the least amount of operative dentistry and confining this to the simplest procedures. As this case demonstrates, an MI approach to dentistry does not preclude the use of involved and potentially complex procedures such as implant dentistry.

A female patient, aged 58, presented with a missing upper right central incisor tooth (Fig. C1.1.1). This had been lost several years previously as a result of trauma and she had worn an acrylic based removable partial denture since then. Her presenting concern was to consider an alternate method of replacement and have a tooth of improved appearance and characterization rather than the denture currently provided.

Examination revealed that the upper right central incisor tooth and the four third molar teeth were absent. The remaining teeth were sound with a number of small restorations present. No active caries was detected. An acrylic based

---

*   THE HOLY BIBLE, NEW INTERNATIONAL VERSION®, NIV® Copyright © 1973, 1978, 1984, 2011 by Biblica, Inc.® Used by permission. All rights reserved worldwide.

COMMON CLINICAL CONDITIONS REQUIRING MINIMALLY INVASIVE ESTHETIC INTERVENTION

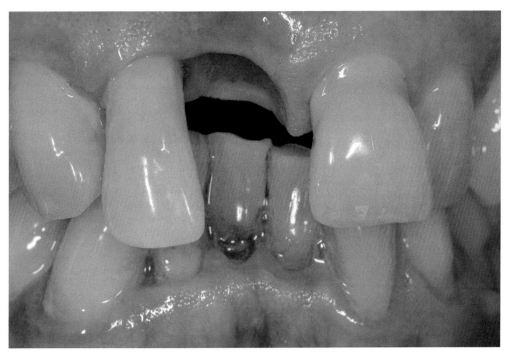

Fig. C1.1.1 Retracted anterior view without the denture in place, showing the missing UR1 tooth space.

removable partial denture replaced the missing incisor tooth. This had a reasonable fit with a scalloped margin to the adjacent upper right lateral incisor and upper left central incisor teeth. The retention was provided by clasping to the first molar teeth. The denture tooth was a stock tooth made of a single resin material and was a poor match in colour, shape and size to the adjacent teeth. The gingival tissue beneath the denture in the saddle area and around the adjacent teeth was inflamed. The scalloped design of the denture around the adjacent teeth was a plaque retentive factor and this lead to a localized loss of periodontal attachment to these teeth with probing depths of 5 mm and bleeding on probing. On smiling, the upper lip retracted to the gingival third of the maxillary dentition, without exposing the gingival margin. On closure, there was an increased overbite with an incisal overjet of 2 mm.

Radiographic examination (Fig. C1.1.2) showed that there was loss of bone support to the adjacent teeth as well as a reduced alveolar contour in the position of the missing tooth, resulting from the loss of this tooth several years ago. There was sufficient volume to enable consideration of the placement of a dental implant.

Options were discussed for the replacement of the missing upper right central incisor tooth. These were:

• Provision of a new removable partial denture, of improved design to remove the plaque stagnation features associated with the current denture, and

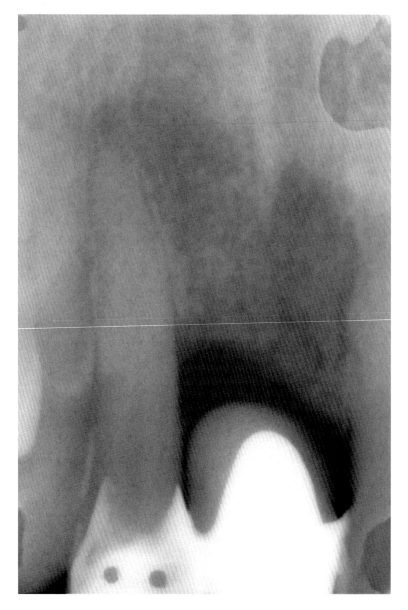

Fig. C1.1.2 Initial peri-apical radiograph showing bone levels/quality prior to implant placement.

using a customized resin tooth to improve the appearance over the current stock denture tooth. The patient, however, wished to avoid a denture if possible, although she recognized the improvement in appearance that could be gained using a customized tooth.

- Provision of fixed bridgework, of a resin bonded design to the adjacent incisor teeth. However, the reduced level of periodontal support to the adjacent teeth was a concern regarding the long-term effect to these teeth of the additional loading that would result from their use, either singly or in combination, as bridge abutment(s). In addition, the increased overbite did not provide space for an abutment wing to be fitted without the need for preparation of the

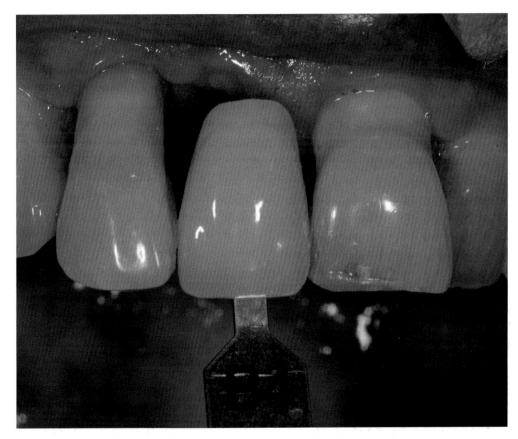

Fig. C1.1.3 Shade-taking photograph for the replacement tooth.

abutment tooth or teeth or reduction of the opposing incisors. Occlusal space could have been provided using orthodontic techniques involving appliances or the use of the Dahl technique for tooth intrusion.

• Placement and restoration of a dental implant. Assessment of the alveolus revealed that there was sufficient bone volume and density for the placement of a dental implant fixture. Although there was a reduced hard and soft tissue height compared to the rest of the maxillary arch, the position of the lip line on smiling meant that this area was not of an esthetic concern in considering the final outcome of the restoration.

After documented discussion with the patient, a decision was made to proceed with the placement and restoration of a dental implant (Fig. C1.1.3). Initial surgery for the placement of the implant involved raising a small muco-periosteal flap, preparation of the osteotomy site using a series of preparation drills, and placement of the implant fixture. The healing abutment was fitted at the time of fixture placement, removing the requirement for second surgical interven-tion. An adhesive bridge was provided to act as an interim replacement of the missing tooth during the primary phase of osseointegration. A course of

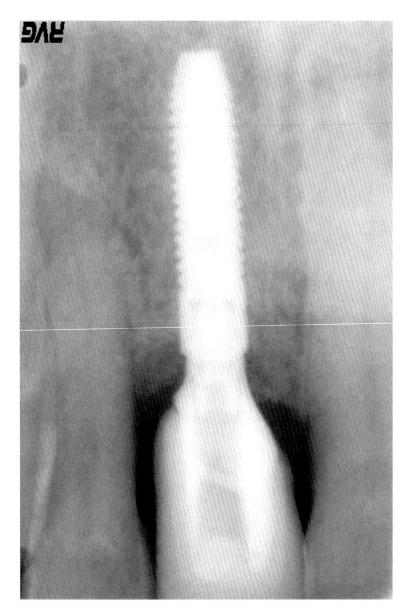

Fig. C1.1.4   Final peri-apical radiograph after implant placement and restoration showing good osseointegration.

treatment involving debridement of the existing pockets and introduction of a new oral hygiene regimen for the patient lead to healing of the inflammation of the soft tissues in the upper incisor region, and a reduction in probing depths to 2 mm was recorded after 3 months.

Following a 3-month period of osseointegration (Fig. C1.1.4), a customized abutment was milled to provide support for an all-ceramic crown. This was characterized to match the remaining dentition and contoured to allow no interferences on excursive movements of the mandible. The use of clinical photography enabled good characterization details to be reproduced in the final

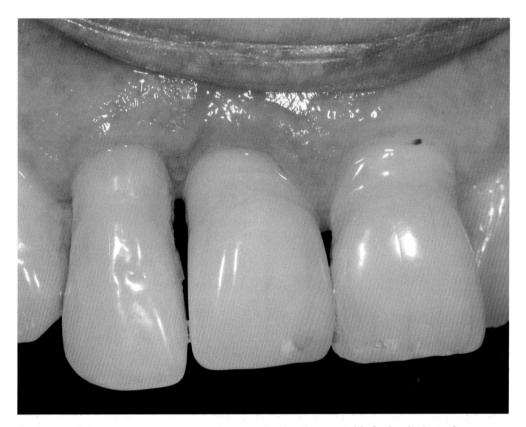

Fig. C1.1.5   Retracted post-operative anterior view showing the acceptable final esthetic result.

restoration (Fig. C1.1.5). The proximal contour allowed easy and effective inter-dental cleaning to be achieved.

This case demonstrates an MI approach to tooth replacement, respecting the biology of the oral tissues. In considering the patient requirements for comfort and appearance, a dental implant could be placed with a single surgical procedure without augmentation of the existing hard and soft tissues.

CLINICAL CASE 1.2

This clinical case study demonstrates the use of an MI resin composite technique to alter the shape of localized microdontia, affecting a lateral incisor tooth (Fig. C1.2.1).

A 19-year-old fit and well female patient presented requesting an improvement in the appearance of her teeth. She was concerned specifically with the appearance of a peg-shaped upper right lateral incisor tooth (Fig. C1.2.2). This had been of similar appearance since eruption, but she had not sought treatment as she had not been so conscious of its appearance. In researching the options for

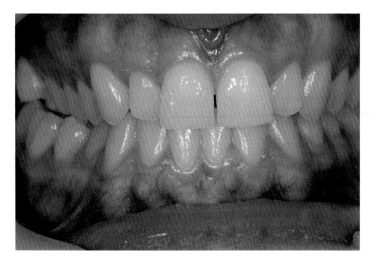

Fig. C1.2.1   Retracted anterior pre-operative clinical view in occlusion.

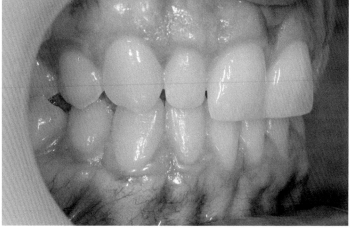

Fig. C1.2.2   Retracted right-hand side anterior clinical view showing the full extent of the diminutive lateral maxillary incisor.

her treatment prior to presentation, she enquired if she was a suitable candidate for veneers to her upper teeth.

An initial examination revealed the presence of 14 teeth in both maxillary and mandibular arches with the third molar teeth absent. There was no history of tooth restoration and no caries was detected. The periodontal health was good with an excellent standard of oral hygiene evident. There was a cross bite in the premolar and molar region on the right-hand side with a shift in the mandibular midline position to the right by half a unit. However, canine guidance was maintained on lateral excursive mandibular movements and there were no signs or symptoms of any further changes to the masticatory system.

The upper right lateral incisor tooth was smaller in size proportionately to the adjacent teeth (Fig. C1.2.2). There was a slight diastema between the maxillary central incisors, but the upper left lateral incisor was of proportionate size to the remaining teeth.

The patient had been an irregular dental attendee as she had not experienced problems with her teeth and therefore had not prioritized regular visits to a dentist as part of her lifestyle. She was an avid viewer of reality television shows, however, and had seen transformations being made to dentitions by 'smile make-overs'. This had influenced her decision to request the use of veneers to change the appearance of her teeth.

A detailed discussion revealed that her concern was limited to the appearance of only one tooth. Her perception of veneers was that these could be provided without the need for any preparation to the teeth and would last a lifetime. Although little hard tissue preparation would be required to provide

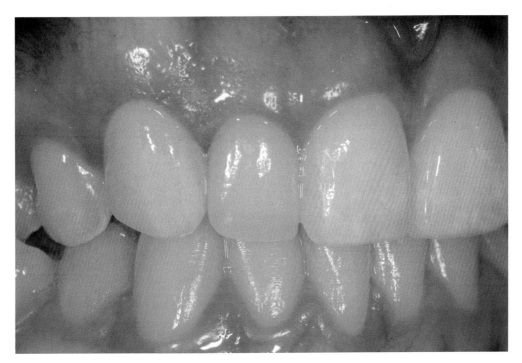

Fig. C1.2.3   Retracted right-hand side post-operative view after the UR2 has been built up with an esthetic direct resin composite.

thin porcelain laminate veneers to all the upper incisor teeth, so achieving a symmetrical relationship between these, the management of this case was limited to the reversible bonding of resin composite materials to the upper right lateral incisor tooth in order to reshape this tooth to match the adjacent teeth more closely.

The upper right canine and all four incisors were isolated using rubber dam, a split dam technique allowing unrestricted access to the upper right lateral incisor tooth. Gingival retraction cord was placed to retract the labial gingival margin and separation strips placed between the adjacent teeth. Acid etching was carried out to the dental enamel and direct bonding of resin composite materials was carried out to reshape the tooth. Finishing and polishing was carried out using ultra-fine diamond burs, polishing discs and mops (Fig. C1.2.3).

This case demonstrates the use of a simple, reversible clinical technique to achieve an improvement in the appearance of the dentition for a patient with the minimal amount of intervention and biological risk. This also demonstrates the importance of a full and detailed documented discussion with the patient when planning the appropriate management of a case in order to meet the request and requirement of the patient using the most appropriate clinical technique.

CLINICAL CASE 1.3

This clinical case demonstrates the use of an MI micro-abrasion technique to improve dental appearance.

An 18-year-old fit and well female presented complaining of a mottled appearance to her teeth (Fig. C1.3.1). She remarked that this appearance had been present since the teeth had erupted into position, but this had caused her no concerns regarding her appearance until now, as she was planning to leave home to commence university studies. However, on discussing the appearance of her teeth, her only concern was to improve the appearance of the two upper central incisor teeth. She also did not wish to make these two teeth appear perfect as she was aware that this would not match with her remaining teeth. She was also aware of the importance of an MI approach as she had a friend who had received treatment with porcelain laminate veneers who had experienced problems with sensitivity and the veneers debonding on repeated occasions.

Examination revealed a healthy dentition with no restorations present. Twenty-eight teeth were present, with early indication of all four third molar teeth due to erupt shortly. No caries was present, her oral hygiene was excellent, and all soft tissues were in good condition. There was a mottled appearance to the enamel of all teeth, producing a white striated appearance, with brown

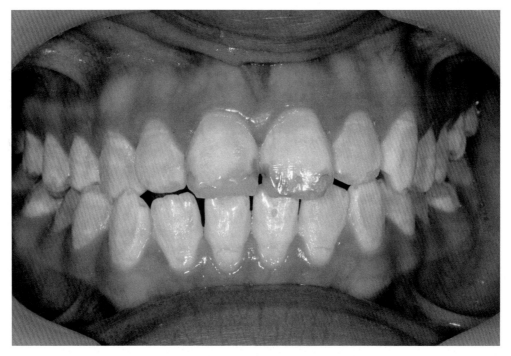

Fig. C1.3.1   Retracted anterior view showing the hypoplastic upper central incisors.

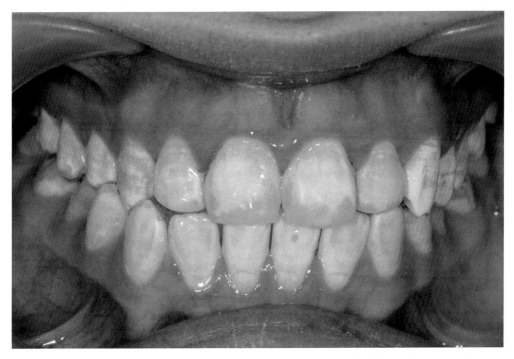

Fig. C1.3.2 Retracted anterior view, on completion of micro-abrasion and addition of nano-hybrid resin composite.

discolouration and chipping of the enamel on the incisal third aspect of both upper central incisor teeth. There was a small amount of brown discolouration and minor areas of chipping to the remaining maxillary teeth (Fig. C1.3.2).

From the history and examination, a diagnosis of enamel hypoplasia was concluded, of unknown origin. The patient had not been brought up in an area with a high level of fluoride in the water supply and had not received, to her knowledge, fluoride supplements during her development. Her siblings did not have the same characterization to their teeth.

Discussion with the patient helped to explain the options available for treatment of the upper central incisors as well as for the remaining dentition in order to improve the appearance. This included the options for tooth whitening, micro-abrasion and localized resin composite restorations. However, the treatment agreed and consented for was to provide micro-abrasion and localized resin composite restoration to the two maxillary central incisor teeth only. Micro-abrasion was carried out using Opalustre (Ultradent), consisting of 6.6% hydrochloric acid together with silicone carbide particles (particle size 20–160 μm) in a water soluble paste, followed by localized bonding of a nanohybrid resin composite of high translucency. Finishing was carried out using polishing discs, composite polishing paste, and a polishing mop.

The final esthetic result was pleasing to the patient and achieved her wishes of providing a localized improvement in the appearance of her dentition. This MI treatment technique permitted preservation of the existing tooth structure. The patient is also aware of further treatment being available to alter the appearance of her teeth further should she wish this in the future.

ESSENTIALS

- Minimum intervention oral care is the concept of a patient-centred, holistic, team-care approach to maintaining life-long oral and dental health.

- The biological concept of MI dentistry aims to preserve natural tooth tissue and pulp vitality for a lifetime.

- The main consideration for the MI concept is achieving the accurate identification and diagnosis of dental problems at the earliest stage.

- A clinician adopting an MI approach to dental care is not ignoring or avoiding the esthetic issues of dental treatment.

- The first rule of dentistry, 'do no harm', is an essential requirement of biological MI dentistry when applied to clinical conditions requiring esthetic intervention.

PATIENTS' FAQS

Q. What stains teeth?

A. Stained teeth can be caused by drinking tea, coffee, red wine, colas and consuming other stain-producing foods such as berries, soy sauce, mustards and ketchups. Smoking will also stain the teeth.

Q. How do I stop my teeth staining?

A. Avoid smoking. Limit the amount of coffee, tea and other stain producing foods you eat. Brush your teeth regularly with a good quality toothbrush and toothpaste, for 2 minutes at a time. Visit your dentist regularly for examination and professional cleaning.

Q. What is tooth whitening?

A. Tooth whitening is a technique used to treat mild to moderate staining to the teeth. A strong oxidizing agent is used to lighten/bleach the teeth and is a conservative and often highly effective way to brighten your smile.

Teeth with yellow stains are the easiest to lighten, but the process does not affect any crowns, veneers or other dental restorations that you have.

The average treatment time is 4–6 weeks, depending on the severity of the stain, but you may notice results after just a few days.

Q. What is bonding?

A. Bonding is the application of a composite-resin material to the tooth surface. This requires treatment of the tooth surface using a mild acid to enable bonding to be effective and long lasting, but does not require preparation of the tooth structure. This is an effective technique for treatment of stained teeth and can also be used to reshape teeth.

It may be advisable to wear a nightguard to protect the bonding if you are prone to clenching or grinding the teeth.

Further reading

Banerjee A, Watson TF. Pickard's Manual of Operative Dentistry. 9th ed. Oxford: Oxford University Press; 2011.

Kelleher M. Ethical issues, dilemmas and controversies in 'cosmetic' or esthetic dentistry. A personal opinion. Br Dent J 2012;212:365–7.

Kelleher MGD, Bomfim DI, Austin RS. Biologically based restorative management of tooth wear. Int J Dent 2012;2012:Article ID 742509.

Palmer RM, Smith BJ, Howe LC, Palmer PJ. Implants in Clinical Dentistry. London: Martin Dunitz; 2002.

Watts A, Addy M. Tooth discolouration and staining: a review of the literature. Br Dent J 2001;190:309–16.

REFERENCES

1. Kateb E-L, Heming M. 'Dentistry in a decade': Recent lessons from the Adult Dental Health Survey. Dent Update 2011;38:658–9.

2. Coffield KD, Phillips C, Brady M, et al. The psychosocial impact of developmental dental defects in people with hereditary amelogenesis imperfecta. J Am Dent Assoc 2005;136:620–30.

3. Watts A, Addy M. Tooth discolouration and staining: a review of the literature. Br Dent J 2001;190:309–16.

4. Marin PD, Bartold PM, Heithersay GS. Tooth discolouration by blood: an *in vitro* histochemical study. Endod Dent Traumatol 1997;13:132–8.

5. Weatherall JA, Robinson C, Hallsworth AS. Changes in the fluoride concentration of the labial surface enamel with age. Caries Res 1972;6:312–24.

6. Wei SH, Ingram MI. Analysis of the amalgam tooth interface using the electron microprobe. J Dent Res 1969;48:317.

7. Addy M, Moran J, Griffiths A, Wills-Wood NJ. Extrinsic tooth discolouration by metals and chlorhexidine. Surface protein denaturation or dietary precipitation? Br Dent J 1985;159:281–5.

8. Black GV. A Work on Operative Dentistry: The Technical Procedures in Filling Teeth. Chicago: Medical–Dental Publishing; 1917.

9. Fisher J, Johnston S, Hewson N, et al. FDI Global Caries Initiative; implementing a paradigm shift in dental practice and the global policy context. Int Dent J 2012;62(4):169–74.

10. Banerjee A, Watson TF. Pickard's Manual of Operative Dentistry. 9th ed. Oxford: Oxford University Press; 2011.

11. Kelleher M. Ethical issues, dilemmas and controversies in 'cosmetic' or aesthetic dentistry. A personal opinion. Br Dent J 2012;212:365–7.

12. Palmer RM, Smith BJ, Howe LC, Palmer PJ. Implants in Clinical Dentistry. London: Martin Dunitz; 2002.

13. The UK Health and Social Care Information Centre. Adult Dental Health Survey 2009: summary report and thematic series. <www.ic.nhs.uk/pubs/dentalsurvey-fullreport09>; 2011.

14. Van't Spijker A, Rodriguez JM, Kreulen CM, et al. Prevalence of tooth wear in adults. Int J Prosthodont 2009;22(1):35–42.

15. Kelleher MGD, Bomfim DI, Austin RS. Biologically based restorative management of tooth wear. Int J Dent 2012;2012:Article ID 742509.

16. Nalbandian S, Millar BJ. The effect of veneers on cosmetic improvement. Br Dent J 2009;207(2):Article E(3).

CHAPTER 2

Dental Bleaching: Materials

M. KELLEHER

INTRODUCTION

Dental bleaching (tooth whitening) solves the minimally invasive management dilemma regarding the treatment of discoloured teeth without damaging them structurally or biologically, in either the short or the long term. Bleaching is a chemical process involving the oxidation of organic material that is broken down to produce less complex molecules. Most of these smaller molecules are lighter in colour than the larger complex molecules from which they originated.

HOW TEETH BECOME DISCOLOURED (Fig. 2.1)

The minimal interprismatic proteinaceous matrix present in enamel acts like a wick drawing up ions and small molecules from extrinsic oral fluids. Complex molecules including pigments and dyes stain this interprismatic matrix. A pigment is a coloured substance composed of a colour-bearing group (a chromophore) and other molecules. Pigments may, or may not, attach to the organic matrix within the interprismatic spaces. A dye is a pigment with reactive (hydroxyl or amine) groups that can attach to organic matter. Common dyes within the human diet come from chocolate, coffee, tea, curry sauces, tomato sauces and red wine. Melanoidins are formed from the breakdown products of cooked vegetable oils and are also a common cause of dental discolouration (see Box 2.1).

Metal compounds can interact with dyes to form larger compounds that produce different colours of stain. Iron and copper-containing metallic compounds are often involved in causing darker intrinsic dental stains.

BOX 2.1 **CLINICAL RELEVANCE OF** **TYPES OF DISCOLOURATION**	• The type of initial discolouration affects bleaching effectiveness and shade retention • Discolouration due to ageing or fluorosis changes shade more quickly than teeth discoloured due to tetracycline drugs • Different tetracycline drugs produce different discolourations • Bleaching tetracycline-stained teeth in the yellow/brown range often requires 6–9 months and is easier than bleaching those tetracycline-stained teeth in the blue/grey discolouration range. Remember this by 'Yellow-brown WILL bleach, blue-grey MAY bleach'

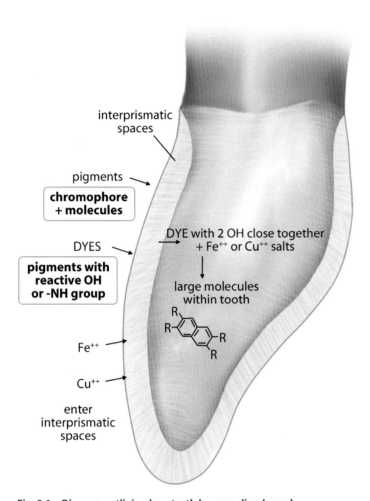

Fig. 2.1 Diagram outlining how teeth become discoloured.

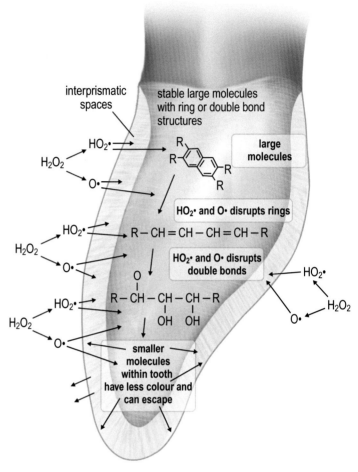

Fig. 2.2 Diagram outlining the mechanism of action of hydrogen peroxide, degrading larger molecules into smaller molecules that are lighter in colour. Some of these can then escape from the tooth, thereby producing a lighter looking tooth.

The oxidative bleaching process involves the breakdown of ring structures and other consecutive, conjugated double bonds in complex molecules. This results in a loss of colour caused by unwanted dark molecules in the non-cellular matrix. Hydrogen peroxide works by converting these large molecules into alcohols, ketones and terminal carboxylic acids. As these are smaller molecules they are then capable of being expelled through the tooth structure and from its surface. The net outcome is that the tooth is bleached and thereby appears lightened in colour (Figs 2.2 and 2.3).

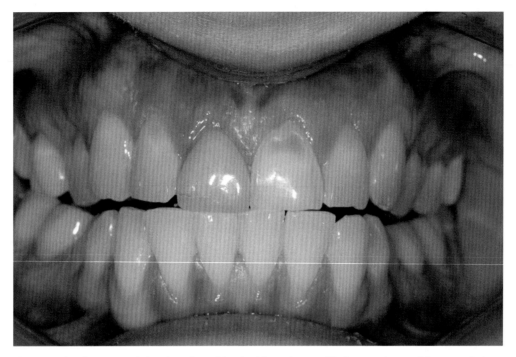

Fig. 2.3 The pigments and dyes have been bleached from the mandibular anterior teeth but remain in the labial surfaces of the maxillary anterior teeth.

CHEMISTRY OF BLEACHING

An oxidation/reduction (redox) reaction takes place during bleaching, where the hydrogen peroxide (Box 2.2) oxidizing agent releases free radicals with unpaired electrons, thereby becoming reduced in the process. The discoloured molecules within teeth accept the unpaired electrons and become oxidized, with a concomitant reduction in the overall discolouration. Hydrogen peroxide produces different free radicals, namely $HO_2\bullet$ and $O\bullet$, both of which are highly reactive. The perhydroxyl ion ($HO_2\bullet$) is the stronger and more reactive of the two free radicals. For $HO_2\bullet$ to be made readily available, the bleaching material needs to be alkaline. The optimal pH for $HO_2\bullet$ release is approximately pH 10.

BOX 2.2
CHEMICAL FORMULAE OF HYDROGEN PEROXIDE

The empirical formula for hydrogen peroxide is H_2O_2

The structural formula is HO–OH

The molecular weight of hydrogen peroxide is 34.0

It is a rapidly reacting and unstable material

From October 2012, the EU limit for use by dentists, or other dental professionals with suitable training, will be 6% hydrogen peroxide, which is equivalent to approximately 18% carbamide peroxide

CARBAMIDE PEROXIDE

The empirical formula for carbamide peroxide is $CO(NH_2)_2H_2O_2$. The structural formula is:

$$NH_2-C(=O)-NH_2 \qquad HO-OH$$

The molecular weight of carbamide peroxide is 94.1.

Carbamide peroxide is a stable compound that slowly releases about one third of its volume as hydrogen peroxide. In other words, a 10% carbamide peroxide gel will release about 3.5% hydrogen peroxide slowly over 3–4 hours while a 21% carbamide peroxide gel will release about 7% hydrogen peroxide.

HOW HYDROGEN PEROXIDE WORKS

The bleaching effect is caused by the degradation of high molecular weight, complex organic molecules that reflect a specific wavelength of light responsible for the colour of the stain in the dental substrate. The degradation products have relatively low molecular weights and result in a reduced colour reflectance. The bleaching process results in a reduction, or elimination, of those molecules causing the discolouration. Both enamel and dentine change colour as a result of the passage of the peroxide through the tooth tissues.

During dental bleaching the low molecular weight hydrogen peroxide readily penetrates through interprismatic enamel to enter dentine and, eventually, the pulp. The free radicals have unpaired electrons that react rapidly with, and attack, most organic molecules, generating further free radicals. These react with other unsaturated bonds, resulting in the disruption of the electron configuration of those molecules. Hydrogen peroxide is capable of undergoing numerous reactions, including molecular additions, substitutions, oxidations and reductions. It is a strong oxidant and can form other free radicals by homolytic cleavage. The various chemical reactions produce a change in the absorption energy of the large discoloured molecules within the enamel and dentine and these are broken down into smaller molecules with the concomitant loss of the unwanted discolouration.

In the process of bleaching, highly pigmented carbon ring compounds within the tooth can be broken down and turned into relatively simple chain molecules. Many of these chains have consecutive conjugated double bonds that are broken subsequently into single bonds. These chemical reactions result in hydrophilic

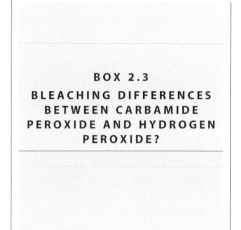

BOX 2.3

BLEACHING DIFFERENCES BETWEEN CARBAMIDE PEROXIDE AND HYDROGEN PEROXIDE?

- 10% carbamide peroxide solution is equivalent to 3.5% hydrogen peroxide and also contains 6.5% urea

- Bleaching with carbamide peroxide is slower, safer and longer lasting but it needs more time to be effective as the hydrogen peroxide is released slowly

- Hydrogen peroxide on its own is unstable and breaks down in minutes into a perhydroxyl free radical (HO$_2$•) and O• then into H$_2$O+O$_2$

- Urea breaks down into carbon dioxide and ammonia, elevating the pH, helping the bleaching by increasing the hydrogen peroxide release period, and allowing penetration well into the tooth structure

colourless, or lightly pigmented, structures. Complex molecules, in particular those forming metallic compounds, appear dark whereas simpler molecules appear lighter. By breaking the larger molecules into smaller ones, most of the stains are dissipated.

The terms 'whitening' or 'lightening', while in common usage, are confusing and do not describe 'bleaching' which is due to a chemical reaction. 'Lightening' or 'whitening', for instance, could refer to the removal of superficial or extrinsic stains whereas bleaching is a deeper and <u>not readily reversible</u> process.

Theoretically, if the bleaching process were to be continued indefinitely, damage could occur to the enamel matrix proteins. Optimal bleaching involves changing the teeth to an esthetically pleasing tooth shade, usually agreed in advance with the patient, while still preserving the hardness, health and strength of the teeth.

For differences between bleaching with carbamide peroxide and hydrogen peroxide, see Box 2.3 above.

SAFETY OF CARBAMIDE PEROXIDE

Carbamide peroxide is formed from hydrogen peroxide and urea. Urea is a normal body constituent and thus has no adverse biological consequences. Hydrogen peroxide is found in all cells as an endogenous metabolite. The human liver, the principal site of its metabolism, produces about 270 mg of H$_2$O$_2$ per hour. A standard 1.2 mL tube of 10% carbamide peroxide gel contains approximately 0.12 mg of carbamide peroxide so there is a very wide clinical safety margin relative to the liver's routine metabolism. Moreover, the carbamide peroxide is contained within a viscous gel and the released hydrogen peroxide that might escape from within the applicator tray is decomposed rapidly by the protective salivary catalase and peroxidases. This ensures the biological safety of the clinical bleaching process at the concentrations used for traditional dental bleaching (10% carbamide peroxide in a custom-made mouthguard is the current gold standard).

SYSTEMIC DEFENCE MECHANISMS AGAINST HYDROGEN PEROXIDE

All cells contain protective enzymes against hydrogen peroxide (catalase, peroxidases and selenium-dependent glutathione peroxidases). The highest levels are found in the liver, duodenum, spleen, blood, mucous membranes and kidney. Most of the catalase is found in red blood cells that can degrade hydrogen peroxide within a few minutes. The overall decomposition reaction of hydrogen peroxide in the presence of catalase is:

$$H_2O_2 + H_2O_2 \rightarrow 2H_2O + O_2 \text{ (water and oxygen)}$$

In the presence of peroxidases the reaction is:

$$H_2O_2 + 2RH \rightarrow 2H_2O + R-R$$

Hydrogen peroxide solutions below 35% are classified as a non-irritant to skin. There is no evidence in the available literature that hydrogen peroxide is a skin sensitizer in humans. However, occasional positive patch tests have been reported.

Biologic membranes are permeable to hydrogen peroxide. Hydrogen peroxide is taken up readily by cells of the oral mucosa, but it is metabolized rapidly. There is uncertainty as to the extent to which hydrogen peroxide enters the blood circulation from the bleaching process, given the variable quantities of existing endogenous hydrogen peroxide. In 1985 the toxicity of hydrogen peroxide was reviewed by the International Association for Research on Cancer (IARC), and in 1993 by Li and the European Centre for Ecotoxicology and Toxicology of Chemicals. These reviews concluded that there are no reasons for concern about the use of hydrogen peroxide in the concentrations employed in dentist-prescribed at-home bleaching.

DENTAL SENSITIVITY

Temporary dental hypersensitivity is a well-documented adverse effect of bleaching. Approximately 70% of patients experience some sensitivity during nightguard vital bleaching using 10% carbamide peroxide. This sensitivity is mild and transitory, usually persisting for about 24 hours following the completion of bleaching. Increased sensitivity is associated mainly with the use of heat and very much higher concentrations of hydrogen peroxide in attempts to accelerate the bleaching process. The predictors for patients developing dental sensitivity in vital teeth are:

• Existing dental sensitivity (a mild pre-existing reversible pulpitis).

• The use of higher concentrations of carbamide or hydrogen peroxide.

• Changing the bleaching gel more than once a day/night.

• Using heat as an adjunct to accelerate the bleaching reactions.

TOOTH RESORPTION

There are no reports of 10% carbamide peroxide (equivalent to 3.5% hydrogen peroxide) held within a mouthguard, causing hard tissue resorption. Resorption occurs frequently as a result of trauma to teeth (Fig. 2.4). The severity of damage to a tooth is related to the type of injury sustained, the force involved and whether the tooth was dislodged, intruded or laterally luxated. Severe damage or excessive drying of the periodontal ligament, the time out of the mouth or a failure to store the tooth properly, all significantly increase the risks of resorption of a traumatized tooth. The risks of late resorption are also related

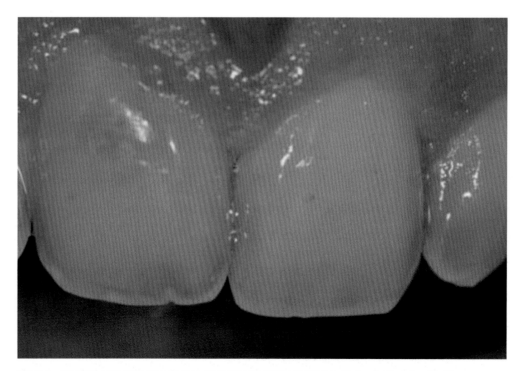

Fig. 2.4 Cervical resorption produces a pink discolouration ('pink spot') due to the blood in the resorbing vascular tissue below the thin enamel surface. The UR1 had a history of two episodes of trauma and one course of orthodontic treatment, but none of bleaching.

to damage to the cementum, contamination of the root, or a failure to endodontically treat or splint the already badly damaged tooth appropriately.

Cervical resorption is occasionally observed in bleached, root-filled teeth but only when a very high concentration of hydrogen peroxide (30–38%) is applied in conjunction with heat to the **already damaged** root or adjacent tooth surfaces.

EFFECTS ON THE HARDNESS OF TEETH

There are numerous laboratory studies to show that peroxide-containing tooth bleaching products do not affect the enamel microstructure. The abrasion resistance of enamel is not lowered by bleaching, nor is its microhardness or mineral content. The critical pH for enamel is 5.5, below which the hydroxyapatite mineral ions dissociate. The vast majority of carbamide peroxide products have a pH of 6.5 to 7. Even if a high concentration of hydrogen peroxide is used, there is no reduction in the hardness of enamel or dentine, let alone dissolution of tooth structure.

PULP CONSIDERATIONS

Hydrogen peroxide penetrates readily and quickly to reach the pulp. The higher the concentration, the more rapidly it appears in the pulp. Following exposure to hydrogen peroxide, histological studies have shown a mild inflammatory response that is limited to the superficial layers of the pulp immediately subjacent to the dentine–pulp interface.

These observations are consistent with the mild discomfort reported by patients as early as 15 minutes following their teeth being exposed to hydrogen peroxide for the purpose of bleaching them. Despite the uptake of hydrogen peroxide, the pulp appears to suffer no irreversible damage as a consequence of bleaching, even when using up to 40% hydrogen peroxide on intact teeth. There are no reports of teeth becoming non-vital even with very prolonged (6–9 months) use of 10% carbamide peroxide in studies where patients were followed up over 7 years later.

EFFECTS OF BLEACHING ON SOFT TISSUES

The American Dental Association *Guidelines for the acceptance of peroxide products* were published in 1994.

These guidelines required an evaluation of the effects of bleaching on the soft tissues of the mouth, including the tongue, lips, palate and gingivae. To date,

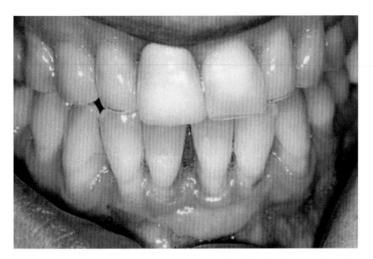

Fig. 2.5   Carbamide peroxide at 10% was used to bleach the natural teeth to match an existing old ceramic crown rather than replacing it with a darker one.

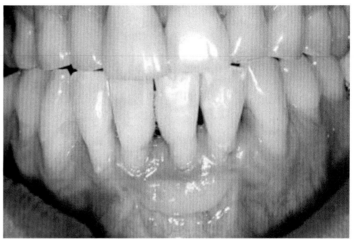

Fig. 2.6   After bleaching the maxillary and mandibular teeth, the lower incisors' 'black triangle disease' was reduced with direct resin composite at no biological cost. Note, the free gingival graft, present for 32 years, was not affected by the bleaching and the resin composite bonding (usually abbreviated to "B&B").

none of the published studies on the use of 10% carbamide peroxide have reported any adverse effects on the various soft tissues of the mouth. Where mild transient damage to gingival tissues has occurred, it appears to have been related to physical trauma caused by a poorly fitting mouthguard or gel tray.

In nightguard vital bleaching, during which the carbamide peroxide is contained within a customized mouthguard, the risks of adverse effects on soft tissues are limited (Figs 2.5 and 2.6).

AMALGAM RESTORATIONS

Some laboratory studies have demonstrated the release of small amounts of mercury from dental amalgam restorations when bleached. The levels are well within the limits of mercury exposure established by the World Health Organization (WHO) and do not pose a risk to patients. Notwithstanding these findings, it is prudent to replace any amalgam restorations in anterior teeth with temporary tooth-coloured restorations prior to bleaching. This will avoid the very limited risk of producing a green discolouration caused by the corrosion of copper, a common constituent of dental amalgam restorations (Figs 2.7 and 2.8).

TOOTH-COLOURED RESTORATIVE MATERIALS

Tooth-coloured restorative materials are not affected by the bleaching process and as a consequence they may appear darker following bleaching relative to their adjacent natural teeth. It is important for a dentist to discuss this with

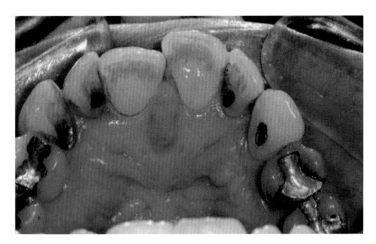

Fig. 2.7 Palatal amalgams should be removed and replaced prior to bleaching thin anterior teeth.

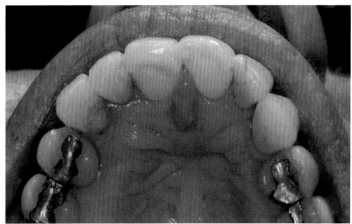

Fig. 2.8 Removal of the amalgam restorations and replacement with direct resin composite stops the theoretical risk of teeth turning green during bleaching. Some direct resin composite has been bonded to other teeth after the bleaching to minimise the Class 2 Div 2 appearance.

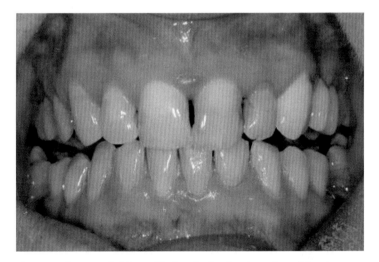

Fig. 2.9 The upper left lateral incisor had a discoloured mesial resin composite restoration and the tooth itself was darker than the adjacent canine crown, a light coloured, bonded metal/ceramic bridge abutment.

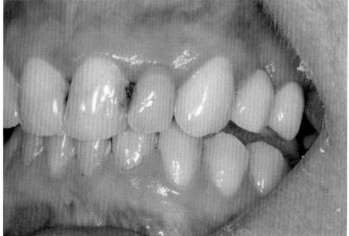

Fig. 2.10 The darker maxillary teeth will bleach but the existing restorations will not. Lighter natural teeth will match the bridge better, but the composite restorations within them will need to be changed in order to match the newly bleached teeth.

patients before they agree to bleach their teeth. Patients are frequently unaware of which of their teeth have restorations.

Expensive and potentially tissue destructive re-makes of previously well colour-matched crowns or other indirect restorations can become necessary at a significant biological and financial cost for patients who have used 'over-the-counter' or internet-sourced bleaching products, without previously consulting a dentist for advice on the risks of restoration colour mismatch caused by selective bleaching of the natural tooth tissues (Figs 2.9–2.11).

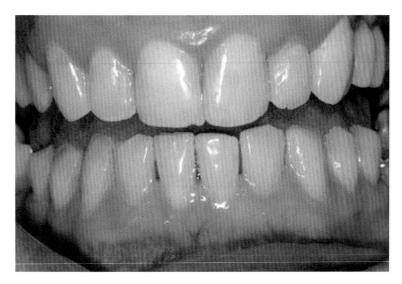

Fig. 2.11 New resin composite restorations were placed 1 week after cessation of nightguard vital bleaching with 10% carbamide peroxide. The natural teeth were now a better colour match for the pre-existing UL3 to UL5 bridge which therefore did not need to be changed because it was originally lighter in colour than the adjacent teeth. If it had been darker, then bleaching the natural teeth could have meant changing the bridge, possibly at very significant biological and financial costs to the patient. This bleaching approach and resin composite replacement treatment were minimally invasive, safe biologically and cost-effective for the patient.

MANAGING PATIENT EXPECTATIONS

Patients who have sourced and used such bleaching products or devices described above may present to the dentist subsequently requesting the replacement of their now apparently darker restorations. Some are surprised at the 'hidden' costs of the extensive and often invasive operative dentistry required in placing new restorations in order to match their newly bleached teeth.

In managing these esthetic bleaching cases, it is imperative that the dentist and their team evaluate the real concerns the patient has regarding their dental esthetics. Bleaching is a minimally invasive process but its limitations in the management of each individual case must be explained and discussed with the patient. Patients' expectations of available levels of esthetic correction must be managed by the oral healthcare team. These discussions must be clearly documented, with signed copies given to the patient. The use of digital photographic records, with suitable reference shade tabs included, should be encouraged, before, during and after treatment is complete, in order to help deal with any future concerns the patient may have. It must be made clear that the effects of dental bleaching are not permanent. The balance between this biologically favourable approach and the tissue-destructive operative option (crowns, veneers) should be explained fully. Relapse of colour changes achieved by bleaching is covered in Box 2.4.

ADHESIVE BONDING AND 'COLOUR REBOUND'

Bond strengths between enamel and resin-based restorations are reduced for the first 24 hours after bleaching. Thereafter, there is no difference in the bond strengths of composite resin to bleached or non-bleached enamel.

BOX 2.4 RELAPSE	Bleaching with carbamide peroxide is followed by a colour relapse in 1–2 weeks depending on the concentrations used. Higher concentrations demonstrate faster and greater colour change initially but also longer and greater colour rebound. The colour usually stabilizes by 1–2 weeks at a level still significantly different from baseline

'Colour rebound' is a term used in bleaching to describe changes in the colour of teeth after bleaching. These effects are linked to the loss of oxygen from teeth and any associated rehydration if the teeth have been isolated under a rubber dam. Rebound, whilst largely completed in the first 24 hours after bleaching, may take up to 7 days to stabilize. Therefore, it is prudent to delay post-bleaching restorative procedures for a week or so after completion of bleaching to allow stabilization of the colour before trying to colour match restorations, particularly if these are indirect restorations, to ensure optimal colour matching and bond strength.

Any residual oxygen still left within the teeth can produce inadvertent oxygen inhibition of a resin composite luting cement. As a precaution, therefore, it is sensible when planning any such restorations for completion after bleaching, to confiscate the mouthguard from the patient one week ahead of the preparation stage for any such indirect restorations. By doing this the patient will not be able to further bleach their teeth prior to taking the shade, or indeed between preparation and fitting of the supposedly 'definitive' restorations.

The patient should also be warned not to use any sort of over-the-counter bleaching product during this time, as this would affect the composite luting bond strengths and possibly also the colour match of the final restorations. If the patient is still unsure about having achieved their desired colour change, it is wise to postpone the supposedly 'definitive' restorative treatment until they confirm that they are happy to proceed with it. For information on colour regression after nightguard vital bleaching, see Box 2.5.

BOX 2.5 COLOUR REGRESSION AFTER NIGHTGUARD VITAL BLEACHING	The American Dental Association (ADA) 'seal of approval' requires that 85% of the original colour change is maintained at 3 months and that 75% is maintained at 6 months. To date, only nightguard vital bleaching with 10% carbamide peroxide bleaching products have gained this ADA seal of approval, which is based on multiple randomized, double blind, controlled clinical trials

CHAIRSIDE OR 'IN-OFFICE' BLEACHING

'Chairside' bleaching is carried out in the dental surgery chair using relatively high concentrations of unstable, rapidly reacting, hydrogen peroxide usually in the range of 15–38%. Hydrogen peroxide at a concentration of 25% is equivalent to 75% carbamide peroxide; 38% hydrogen peroxide is equivalent to 114% carbamide peroxide. For comparison purposes this is more than 11 times the concentration of the safer and more stable 10% carbamide peroxide material used normally for nightguard vital bleaching in a customized tray (see Box 2.6).

The higher the concentration of hydrogen peroxide, the greater the risk of harm to soft tissues or eyes from accidental contact, and suitable protection must be worn by both the patient and operating team to prevent injury/burns.

Chairside bleaching can and often does cause soft tissue damage. To avoid such damage, strenuous efforts need to be made to protect all the patient's soft tissues. The use of a rubber dam or another form of effective isolation is essential when using the highest concentrations (Fig. 2.12). Damage appears as a white burn of the epithelium and such burns are painful and distressing for the patient (Fig. 2.13).

In the event of an adverse soft tissue reaction, the area should be washed thoroughly and the patient reassured. The painful area normally takes a few days to a week to heal. Scarring is not usually a problem, as the ulceration is superficial. Burns to the fingers or cheek can happen if the material is touched accidentally (Fig. 2.14).

BOX 2.6
'IN OFFICE' (CHAIRSIDE) VS NIGHTGUARD VITAL BLEACHING

- The use of bleaching lights during in-office (chairside) techniques has, to date, not been shown in any randomized controlled, double blind, independent clinical trials to improve the longevity or effectiveness of bleaching

- Immediate change in the light-activated material seems more likely to be related to the chemical catalyst employed rather than to the bleaching light itself

- Dehydration effect of isolation and having the teeth full of oxygen at that stage accounts for much of the initial colour change

- Even multiple in-office (chairside) bleaching treatments are not nearly as good as nightguard vital bleaching with 10% carbamide peroxide at 3 or 6 months

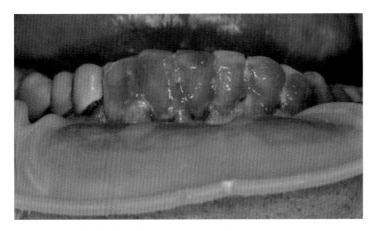

Fig. 2.12 Chairside bleaching using 38% hydrogen peroxide with paint-on dam and OptraGate retractor in position.

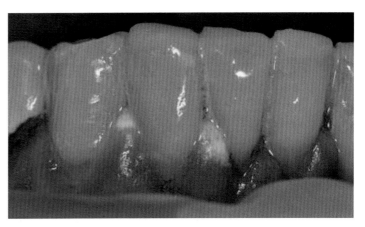

Fig. 2.13 White gingival epithelium burn following leaking of the high concentration hydrogen peroxide onto the thick periodontal tissues. This superficial epithelium sloughs off quickly leaving a red, painful ulcerated area that may affect temporarily adequate oral hygiene procedures in this area.

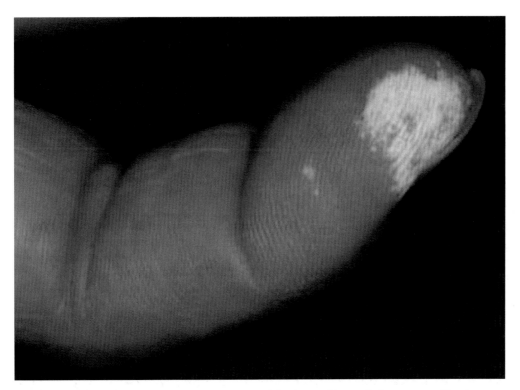

Fig. 2.14 Painful burn caused by accidental contact of the finger with 38% hydrogen peroxide when cleaning up after chairside bleaching.

CLAIMS MADE REGARDING DENTAL BLEACHING

Some manufacturers of bleaching products, or the dentists using these, advocate using the nightguard approach with 10% carbamide peroxide for a few weeks prior to undertaking chairside bleaching. As so-called 'evidence' for the supposed efficacy of this treatment protocol, the 'before' photographs are taken often before any bleaching has occurred or, indeed, sometimes before any pre-operative cleaning of the teeth has been carried out to remove any extrinsic stains, but certainly when the teeth are still hydrated and with no extra oxygen in them. The 'after' photographs are then taken immediately when the rubber dam comes off, i.e. before the teeth can rehydrate or 'colour rebound' has occurred, which usually takes a few days. This dubious photographic practice can easily mislead patients into thinking the treatment on offer produces dramatic beneficial results.

Ideally, the comparative shade change photograph should be taken at least 1 week after the bleaching is complete to have any credibility, and should be undertaken by a person who has no vested interest in the product being used and preferably using an objective colorimeter reference indicator.

Another approach marketed to patients for rapid results is to carry out 'power bleaching' in the surgery with 22–38% hydrogen peroxide first and then get the patient to complete the nightguard vital bleaching at home with 10% or 15% carbamide peroxide to 'maintain the bleaching effect'. There has been no difference found at the 3- or 6-month stage of the results with this approach as opposed to the more straightforward, cost effective and much safer nightguard vital bleaching with just 10% carbamide peroxide in a customized tray.

There is, however, an extra fee claimable by the dentist for the chairside bleaching and the possibility of extra pulp sensitivity for the patient, together with a risk of soft tissue damage due to the high concentrations of hydrogen peroxide used in the 'in-office'/chairside/'in-surgery' bleaching. Incidentally these terms all mean the same thing, i.e. bleaching with high concentrations of <u>chemically catalysed</u> hydrogen peroxide. The photographed shade changes, which are sometimes further enhanced by opening up a couple of the F stops on the camera between the 'before and after' photographs or using software to enhance the shade change, sadly do not last, as judged from independent, unbiased trials. At 3 or 6 months such results are no better than those achieved with the scientifically proven nightguard bleaching which can be obtained more safely and at a fraction of the cost or risks to the patient.

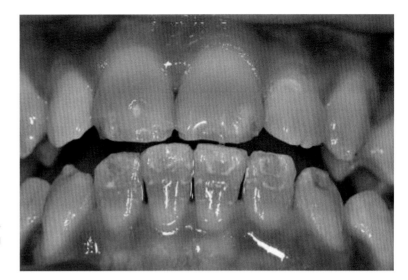

Fig. 2.15 Tetracycline-stained teeth cannot be bleached effectively with chairside or in-office bleaching. Prolonged nightguard vital bleaching with 10% carbamide peroxide will work eventually (6–8 months) on yellow/brown tetracycline stained teeth but will not work well on grey or blue tetracycline-stained teeth.

There is an interesting, subtle, but important issue of <u>responsibility</u> for the dental colour change. With chairside bleaching the dental professional is responsible solely for getting a satisfactory result as judged by the patient. In terms of the time required to achieve this change, it usually involves four separate appointments of approximately an hour each, with the time for isolation and protection or clean up time not included in that hour, to get a result similar to that achievable by a patient bleaching their teeth, in their own time and at their own pace, with nightguard vital bleaching. The subtlety in the transfer of responsibility is that with nightguard vital bleaching it is the **patient's responsibility** to obtain the colour change they want, regardless of how long it takes them to do so. That is particularly important when dealing with, for example, tetracycline staining, where the stable tetracycline orthophosphate is located deep within the dentine and takes many months of treatment to bleach it satisfactorily (Fig. 2.15).

PATIENT 'AT RISK' GROUPS

The only individuals known to be at any risk from bleaching with hydrogen peroxide are patients with very rare conditions such as acatalasaemia or glucose-6-phosphate dehydrogenase (G6PD) deficiency. This makes the individual more susceptible to the activity of peroxide as they are less capable of metabolizing it. Acatalasaemia is a rare condition with an incidence of 0.2%. G6PD is a disorder of erythrocytes in which the metabolic problems of the affected cells result in inadequate detoxification of hydrogen peroxide. The incidence of G6PD deficiency in Europe is about 0.1%.

ASSESSING EFFICACY AND EFFECTIVENESS OF DENTAL BLEACHING

American Dental Association (ADA) guidelines for endorsing bleaching systems or products are strict and require manufacturers to show both the safety-in-use of products and their efficacy. The data required for their 'seal of approval' includes:

- Findings from two randomized prospective double blind clinical trials, involving the comparison of the test material with a non-active control material.

- The assessment of the effects of treatment over a period of 2–6 weeks.

- The measurement of tooth colour at the start and at the end of treatment using two different systems of colour measurement.

- Colour duration measurements should take place at 3 and 6 months to assess whether the colour improvement is maintained. It is a requirement for the ADA seal of approval that 85% of any colour change is maintained at 3 months and 75% of colour change is maintained at 6 months.

MOUTHRINSES AND TOOTHPASTES

Over-the-counter mouthrinses such as Bocasan (Oral B, P&G) and Peroxyl (Colgate Palmolive) are available freely. Bocasan releases approximately 7% hydrogen peroxide and Peroxyl contains 1.5% hydrogen peroxide. The concentrations of hydrogen peroxide in mouthrinses do not bleach teeth. They may, however, have some minor, short-term, beneficial effect on oral hygiene and possibly in the management of certain extrinsic stains.

Toothpaste can remove superficial extrinsic stain only. No toothpaste can bleach teeth because the maximum hydrogen peroxide concentration allowed in toothpastes by EC law is 0.1% and at that level it is useless because it is immediately inactivated by salivary catalase and peroxidase.

Further reading

American Dental Association Council on Dental Therapeutics. Guidelines for the acceptance of peroxide containing oral hygiene products. J Am Dent Assoc 1994;125:1140–2.

Cooper JS, Bokmeyer TJ, Bowles WH. Penetration of the pulp chamber by carbamide peroxide bleaching agents. J Endod 1992;18:315–17.

ECETOC. Joint assessment of commodity chemicals No. 22: Hydrogen peroxide (Cas. No. 7722-84-1). Brussels: European Centre for Ecotoxicology and Toxicology of Chemicals; 1993.

Feinman RA, Madray G, Yarborough D. Chemical, optical and physiologic mechanisms of bleaching products: a review. Pract Periodontics Aesthet Dent 1995;3:32–6.

Frysh H. Chemistry of bleaching. In: Goldstein RE, Garber DA, editors. Complete Dental Bleaching. Chicago: Quintessence Books; 1995. p. 25–32.

Haywood VB. History, safety and effectiveness of current bleaching techniques and applications of the night guard vital bleaching technique. Quintessence Int 1992;23:471–88.

Heithersay GS, Dahlstrom SW, Marin PD. Incidence of invasive cervical resorption in bleached root-filled teeth. Aust Dent J 1994;39:82–7.

IARC. Hydrogen peroxide: evaluation of the carcinogenic risk of chemicals to humans. IARC Monographs 1985;36:285–314.

International Symposium on Non Restorative Treatment of Discolored Teeth. Chapel Hill, North Carolina, September 25–26, 1996. J Am Dent Assoc 1997;128(Suppl.):1S–64S.

Kelleher M. Ethical issues, dilemmas and controversies in cosmetic and aesthetic dentistry. A personal opinion. Brit Dent J 2012;212(8):365–7.

Kelleher MG, Roe FJ. The safety-in-use of 10% carbamide peroxide (Opalescence) for bleaching teeth under the supervision of a dentist. Br Dent J 1999;187:190–4.

Leonard RH Jr, Van Haywood B, Caplan DJ, Tart ND. Nightguard vital bleaching of tetracycline-stained teeth: 90 months post treatment. J Esthet Restor Dent 2003;15(3):142–52.

Li Y. The safety of peroxide-containing at-home tooth whiteners. Compend Contin Educ Dent 2003;24:384–9.

Patel V, Kelleher M, McGurk M. Clinical use of hydrogen peroxide in surgery and dentistry – why is there a safety issue? Brit Dent J 2010;208(2):61–4.

Schulte JR, Morrissette DB, Gasior EJ, et al. The effects of bleaching application time on the dental pulp. J Am Dent Assoc 1994;125:1330–5.

Sterrett J, Price RB, Bankey T. Effects of home bleaching on the tissues of the oral cavity. J Can Dent Assoc 1995;61:412–17, 420.

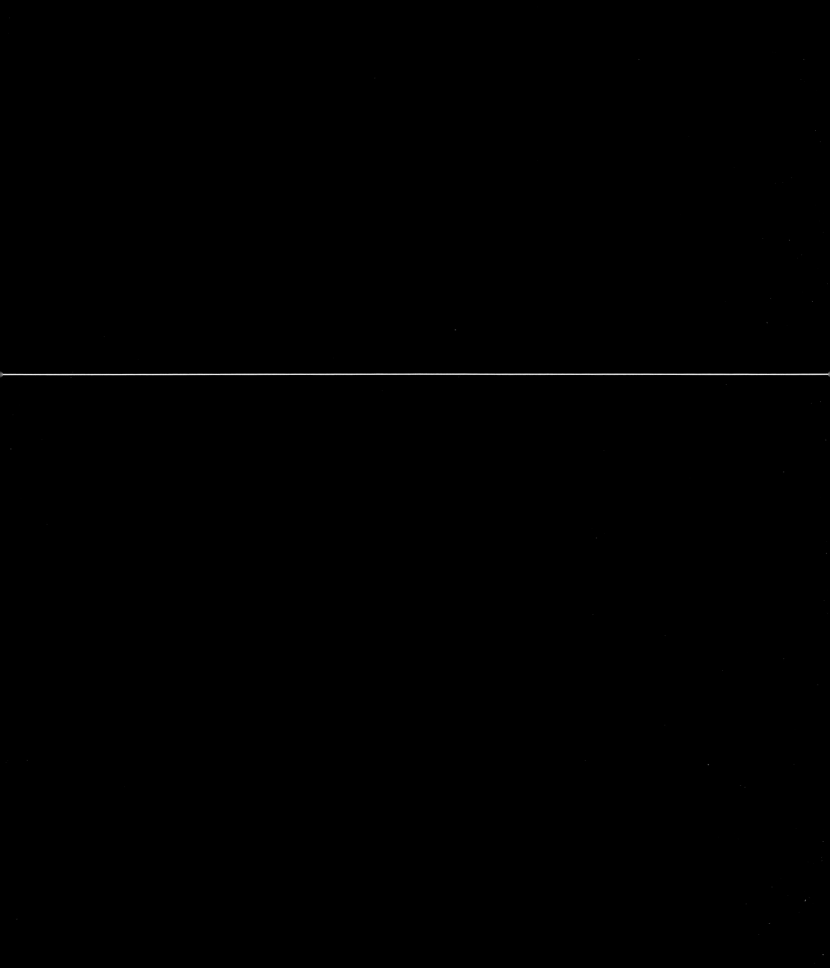

CHAPTER 3

Dental Bleaching: Methods

M. KELLEHER

INTRODUCTION

The aim of this chapter is to consider the indications for nightguard vital bleaching (NgVB) and to outline the clinical technique. Clinical assessment, tray designs and issues pertaining to existing restorations are discussed.

NgVB has revolutionized minimally invasive (MI) tooth preserving esthetic dentistry in that it produces a safe, effective and evidence-based method of improving the appearance of discoloured teeth. NgVB involves the patient placing a viscous 10% carbamide peroxide gel in a customized mouthguard that is worn by the patient while asleep, or for at least two hours at a time (Figs 3.1–3.3).

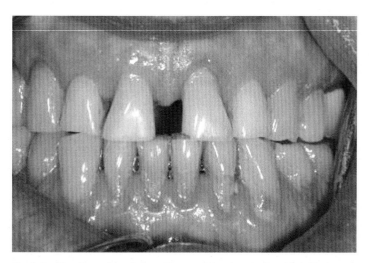

Fig. 3.1 Discoloured teeth in a 60-year-old patient before bleaching.

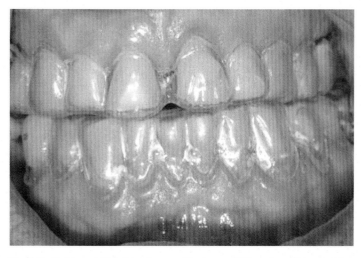

Fig. 3.2 Scalloped bleaching trays with viscous 10% carbamide peroxide gel within them in situ.

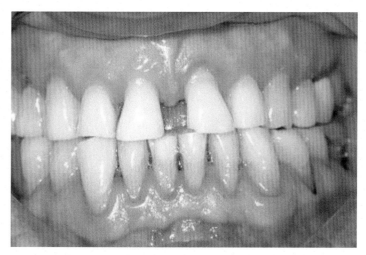

Fig. 3.3 Appearance of the teeth after 3 weeks of bleaching.

HISTORY AND DEVELOPMENT

Carbamide peroxide is an oxygen-releasing antiseptic and appears in various pharmacopoeia as such. It was the treatment of choice for 'trench mouth' in World War One (1914–1918), the name given at that time to acute necrotizing ulcerative gingivitis (ANUG/AUG/Vincent's infection). This destructive, rapidly progressive gum disease was common in soldiers in the trenches during the Great War due to the combination of smoking, stress and lack of effective oral hygiene.

The use of a viscous gel formulation within a customized mouthguard with reservoirs was described by Haywood and Heymann in 1989, based on the empirical post-orthodontic use of carbamide peroxide in 'finishers' (clear retainers) by Klusmier in 1962 to reduce periodontal inflammation after orthodontic treatment. Klusmier noted that a side effect of this treatment, undertaken primarily for gingival health reasons, was to lighten the colour of the teeth.

Haywood and Heymann from 1989 onwards were responsible largely for the further clinical development and the scientific evaluation of the technique. They based these developments on earlier separate works by Klusmier, Wagner, Austin and Munro, who noted independently the lightening of teeth as a side effect of using carbamide peroxide in the management of gingival tissue conditions.

The most acceptable evidence for good clinical practice is based on the results of prospective randomized, double-blind, controlled clinical trials. Such trials are relatively rare in dentistry, but a number of such trials have confirmed the safety and efficacy of NgVB. Colour changes have been reported as lasting for up to 4 years. Teeth can be re-bleached safely or 'touched up' easily using this technique, usually taking just 1 night per week of the time required to get the original colour changes. In other words, if it took 4 weeks to get a satisfactory colour change initially, it will take just 4 nights of bleaching to 'touch up' to the initial bleached colour.

PATIENT MANAGEMENT AND EXPECTATIONS

Assessment of patient expectations of the outcomes of bleaching is important and should be carried out at the earliest opportunity. With NgVB, the main issue is patient compliance in wearing the mouthguard containing the bleaching gel for the required periods of time. Patients who gag at the impression stage are unlikely to be particularly compliant with this bleaching technique.

If patients indicate an interest in dental bleaching (or 'tooth whitening'), it is good practice to have information packs available for them. This general information can be placed on the practice (or hospital) website, or emailed/posted to patients prior to consultation in order to give them basic, regulated and reliable

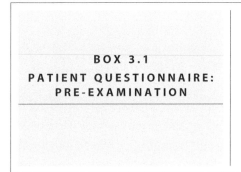

BOX 3.1
PATIENT QUESTIONNAIRE: PRE-EXAMINATION

- What outcome do you wish to achieve?

- Have you tried any other treatment to whiten or bleach your teeth? If so, how did you find the results?

- What do you think has caused your problem?

- What would you consider a satisfactory solution?

- How long do you think treatment might take to achieve your desired result?

information on dental bleaching and time also to reflect on the advantages and disadvantages ahead of their dental consultation appointment. This can reduce misunderstandings caused by the injudicious reliance on the Internet as a source of reliable or allegedly accurate patient information.

There is no reason to avoid the use of occlusal coverage trays in patients with a history of temporomandibular dysfunction (TMD). It is prudent, however, to warn patients with a history of TMD that they may experience some mild discomfort. There are no reports of patients undergoing NgVB complaining of TMD during or after the bleaching process. In contrast, some TMD patients may experience some relief of their symptoms, given that the soft bleaching tray may double as a soft 'TMD device' or a so-called 'occlusal biteguard'.

A pre-examination questionnaire may be a useful adjunct prior to the consultation (see Box 3.1). Please note, if somebody answers 'very white' teeth, be aware that their expectations may be too high and these will need managing. 'Somewhat lighter teeth' is a much more realistic treatment objective.

NIGHTGUARD VITAL BLEACHING CLINICAL PROTOCOL

The protocol for NgVB is based on that developed by Haywood and Heymann (1989) and is as follows:

- A thorough history is taken, a detailed clinical examination is carried out and a differential diagnosis is made in respect of the cause(s) of the dental discolouration.

- Restorations in the target area and in the adjacent and opposing teeth are recorded. Veneers or crowns are charted, as these, together with other existing restorations, will not change colour with bleaching and may need costly replacement if they no longer shade match after bleaching.

Fig. 3.4 Recession and erosion are already obvious on the upper teeth. An air blast onto these teeth detects individual sensitivity pre-bleaching and this information needs to be recorded. These teeth are likely to become more sensitive when bleaching and this will probably therefore affect patient compliance. The patient has a thin periodontal biotype in both upper and lower jaws that could recede further if the bleaching tray edges were left rough and damaged them physically.

- A note is made as to the biotype of the periodontal tissues (Fig. 3.4).

- A 3-in-1 syringe is used to blow air around the teeth to be bleached and any sensitivity is recorded. Patients should be warned that if any teeth are sensitive at the time of this initial examination that these teeth are likely to get much more sensitive with bleaching. Patients presenting with sensitivity may need to bleach for 1–2 hours only at a time, rather than for the typical overnight period. In such cases, satisfactory bleaching results will take a proportionately longer time to be achieved.

- Tooth wear (tooth surface loss) caused by chemical erosion is noted as the affected teeth may be sensitive and become hypersensitive temporarily with bleaching. Attritional tooth wear rarely causes an issue when bleaching.

- The shade is agreed with the patient by reference to a value-orientated (light to dark) dental shade guide (Box 3.2). This shade is recorded in the notes and a written record of this agreed shade should be given to the

**BOX 3.2
EFFECT OF THE INITIAL SHADE**

- The yellower the teeth are at baseline, the greater the magnitude of the bleaching response in most cases. Only moderately dark yellow/brown teeth will bleach predictably

- Blue/grey teeth due to some of the tetracyclines are very difficult to bleach

- Younger subjects experience greater lightening of their teeth but often suffer more relapse. Nevertheless, most of the initial shade improvement remains at 6 months post-treatment using NgVB of moderately dark yellow/brown teeth

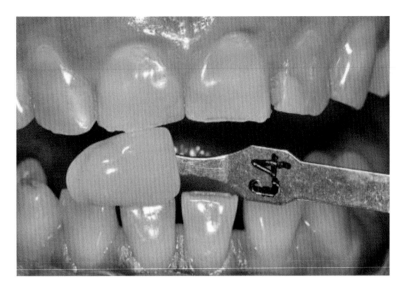

Fig. 3.5   The shade tab should be photographed beside the teeth. The letter and the number should be clearly visible for the patient's photographic records in case of any dispute as to the tooth colour prior to bleaching or relating to efficacy of bleaching. The brown-yellow discolouration is due to a combination of oxytetracycline and demethylchlortetracycline, both of which are stable compounds deep within the dentine and usually take 6–9 months to bleach. Chairside bleaching is of no use in such cases.

patient with a diagram or clinical photograph of any restorations present and visible (Fig. 3.5).

- Patient expectations must be assessed carefully. If a patient whose teeth are already white, with reference to a shade guide tab, insists that they are still too dark, it is probably unwise to proceed with bleaching as the outcome from the patient's perspective is unlikely to be satisfactory. A diagnosis of possible dysmorphophobia (body dysmorphic disorder or distortion of body image) might need to be considered in these cases.

- Radiographs, if appropriate, justifiable and indicated clinically, are taken and a note is made of any relevant findings, including the periapical status, the presence of sclerosis, atypical pulp morphology or pulp size (Fig. 3.6 and see Fig. 3.11).

- The option of bleaching one arch rather than both or bleaching a single, darkened tooth preferentially (Figs 3.7 and 3.8) should be discussed with the patient. It sounds counter-intuitive to many dentists, but a surprising number of patients wish only to have one arch bleached, usually the arch with the most visible teeth when they smile and this is only sometimes for financial reasons.

For advantages and disadvantages of tray-applied NgVB bleaching, see Box 3.3. In the case depicted in Figures 3.6–3.8, only when the upper right central incisor is as light as the others should a full tray be used to bleach the remaining arch. Note, it is inadvisable to accomplish this the other way around, i.e. bleaching all teeth to start with and then trying to bleach further the darker one, preferentially, at the end. This is because if, for any reason, bleaching fails to get the darkest tooth as light as the others at the end of bleaching, then the

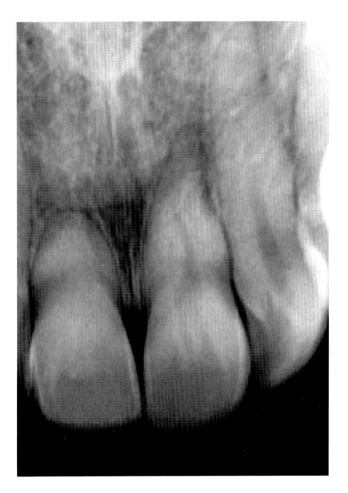

Fig. 3.6   The radiograph shows shortening and sclerosis of the clinically darker coloured upper right central incisor by comparison with the upper left one.

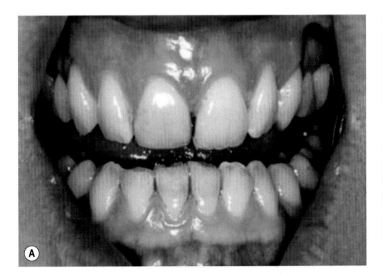

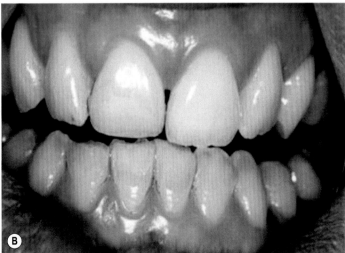

Fig. 3.7A,B   The short, sclerosed upper right central incisor should be bleached preferentially for a few weeks first because the increased amount of tertiary dentine, which is clear on the radiograph, causes it to appear darker. On the positive side, it should not be sensitive when bleaching because of the obliteration of dentine tubules and a reduction in the pulp space observed on the diagnostic radiograph.

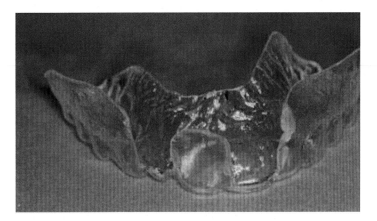

Fig. 3.8   A single-tooth bleaching tray is used to bleach one tooth preferentially. Cutting windows in the bleaching tray over the adjacent teeth allows the salivary peroxidase and catalase to inactivate the carbamide peroxide immediately on contact with the saliva, and thereby avoiding bleaching the adjacent teeth unintentionally.

treatment will have appeared to make the problem of the darker tooth worse by comparison. If there has been any previous attempt to conceal the darker tooth with direct resin composite, for example, then all the resin tags created in the previous adhesive bonding process need to be cut back to at least 50 μm below the enamel surface and the whole of the labial and palatal surfaces 'check etched' by applying standard phosphoric acid gel to the surfaces for 15 seconds, washing it off, drying it carefully with a 3-in-1 syringe and checking that the surfaces appear 'frosty' white. Any unaltered areas probably still have retained resin composite tags within the enamel that will prevent effective bleaching in that area. These will need to be removed to allow more predictable bleaching. However, if a porcelain veneer is in place, it is possible to place the reservoir for the 10% carbamide peroxide on the <u>palatal aspect</u> of the tooth and this will allow slow bleaching with the hydrogen peroxide passing though the palatal enamel, palatal dentine, pulp, labial dentine and finally through to the residual labial enamel, where it will be stopped by the resin holding the porcelain veneer in position (Fig. 3.9).

BOX 3.3 TRAY-APPLIED NGVB BLEACHING: ADVANTAGES/ DISADVANTAGES	<ul><li>Advantages of at-home NgVB include it being known to be the gold standard with the most long-term evidence for its efficacy and safety</li><li>It causes less post-operative discomfort</li><li>Lower cost of the initial treatment and easy top up treatments for the patient</li><li>Less chair time for the dentist</li><li>The main disadvantage with home bleaching is that it takes time and relies on good compliance by the patient</li><li>Trays have to be designed and fit properly to stop salivary enzymes destroying the hydrogen peroxide that is released gradually from the viscous carbamide peroxide</li></ul>

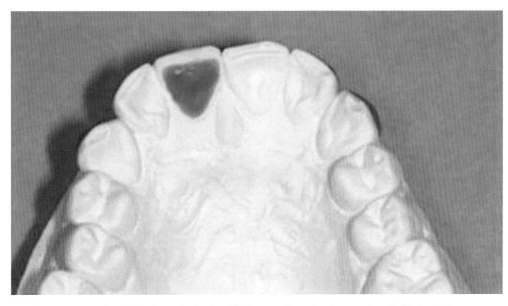

Fig. 3.9 It is possible to bleach teeth slowly with the use of a palatal reservoir to hold the 10% carbamide peroxide gel.

- Any structural or histological abnormalities of enamel and dentine, the extent and sufficiency of any restorations and the presence or absence of pulpal or periodontal conditions should be noted (Figs 3.10–3.12).

- Check the patient's gag reflex by running a finger along the expected extension of the bleaching tray.

- If patients retch, or are unable to tolerate impressions/having an appliance in their mouth for prolonged periods while awake or asleep, then NgVB is unlikely to be successful.

- Patients who retch frequently can have a history of having had an invasive procedure such as tonsillectomy or extraction of teeth under general

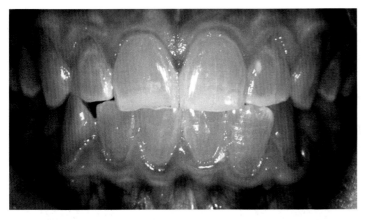

Fig. 3.10 Dentinogenesis imperfecta (hereditary opalescent dentine) due to brown opalescence colour.

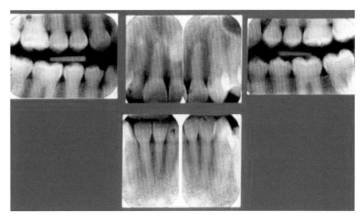

Fig. 3.11 Radiographs of the patient in Figure 3.10 showing complete obliteration of the pulp canals at age 17 years.

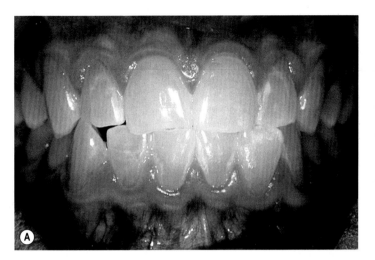
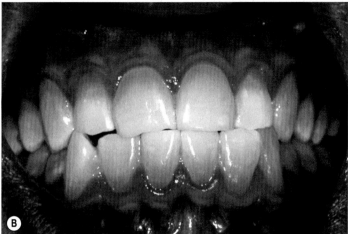

Fig. 3.12 (A) Dentinogenesis imperfecta appearance after 3 months of NGVB with 10% carbamide peroxide. (B) Appearance after seven months of NGVB. Note the more dark dentine there is in each part of the tooth the darker it remains.

anaesthesia. Patients who have experienced a difficult general anaesthetic frequently show great reluctance to have an appliance in their mouth. It is prudent to discuss such details as part of the patient's history, prior to incurring the costs of making them customized bleaching trays. Retching when an impression is being taken may be a warning of future difficulties with wearing a mouthguard.

• The alternative options to bleaching must be discussed. Patients should be informed that any existing restorations will not change colour and that their presence on one surface of the tooth can inhibit complete bleaching. Ensure that all orthodontic resin adhesive cement is removed down to sound enamel after any fixed appliance orthodontic treatment phase has been completed. In this case the teeth need to be 'check etched' briefly with phosphoric acid and the enamel washed and dried to make sure it has gone "frosty" in order to ensure the complete removal of any adhesive resin cement, as described previously.

• If existing restorations are currently lighter, the patient should be advised that bleaching can lighten the natural teeth to help improve the colour match.

• If the natural teeth are lighter than adjacent restorations within the bleaching target area, then further bleaching will make the situation look worse. Patients with existing restorations need to be warned to control the rate of bleaching and not to over-bleach the natural teeth. It is prudent to limit the amount of bleaching gel given to such patients and to review them at 1-week intervals. Patients need to be told that if the natural teeth start to go lighter than their restorations, they must stop bleaching immediately and return to the surgery for reassessment.

- Once the care plan is agreed, and consent gained, an alginate impression of the teeth is then taken. It is advisable to dry the teeth and use a finger to wipe or sweep some alginate around all the occlusal and labial aspects of the dried teeth prior to insertion of the loaded tray. This minimizes the formation of air bubbles and helps produce an accurate cast. This, in turn, will allow a well-fitting bleaching mouthguard (also called a bleaching tray) to be constructed. The teeth to be bleached are identified on the laboratory instruction card, together with an indication of the outline and extension of the tray. The teeth to be bleached are blocked out with plaster or resin (see tray design). This is usually done for each tooth on the cast from one first molar around to the other.

- The thickness of the material to be used in the construction of the tray needs to be specified as this is a customized medical device and covered by the EC Medical Devices Directive (MDD). The tray material should be strong in the thin section. A 1 mm clear preheated blank is usually suitable. If the patient is a bruxist, a thicker material (2 mm) is indicated. The material should be adapted easily and capable of being finished to a smooth edge to prevent trauma to the gingival tissues and tongue. It should be non-allergenic, stable, and easy to clean.

TRAY DESIGN

The purpose of the tray is to hold the gel in contact with the teeth to be bleached. Different designs of tray are indicated depending on the viscosity of the bleaching gel. Poorly designed or badly made trays will not produce the desired outcome. For the effects of tray design, see Box 3.4. If there are specific teeth that need localized bleaching, a useful clinical tip is to first dry the teeth concerned prior

BOX 3.4
EFFECT OF TRAY DESIGN

- An evaluation of the effect of tray design on the degree of colour change using 15% carbamide peroxide suggested that trays with reservoirs had significantly greater amounts of colour change initially than trays without reservoirs, but had more sensitivity than such trays with 10% carbamide peroxide

- Reservoirs are sensible if the carbamide peroxide gel is viscous to allow the tray to sit near the necks of the teeth and thereby prevent inactivation of the gel by salivary enzymes at the cervical areas of the teeth

- Failure to bleach the necks of the teeth is often due to poor fit of the trays thereby leaving the gel short of the gingival areas or open to inactivation by the ever present salivary peroxidase or catalase enzymes

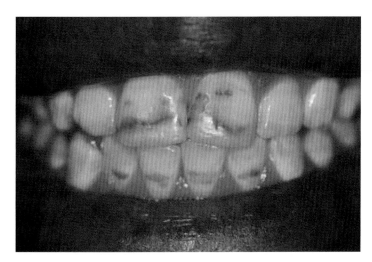

Fig. 3.13 Localized brown fluorosis with banding and white fluorosis. In this case removing the brown fluorosis is the patient's priority. Patients should be warned that the white fluorosis ('secondary flecking') will not be removed but will probably be less obvious when viewed against the bleached teeth.

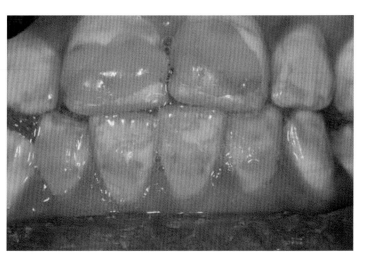

Fig. 3.14 The teeth are dried with a 3-in-1 syringe and some hybrid resin composite shade C4 is applied over the darkest brown part of the un-etched enamel and photocured in position.

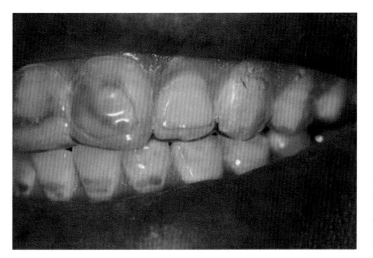

Fig. 3.15 Bleaching tray in position with reservoirs to hold the 10% carbamide peroxide gel just over the brownest areas of the two central incisors.

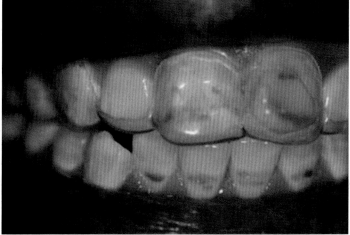

Fig. 3.16 A window has been cut in the bleaching tray over the lateral incisors to allow the protective salivary enzymes access to destroy any perhydroxyl ions that spread onto these teeth and thereby prevent any inadvertent bleaching.

to sculpting temporarily some resin composite of a contrasting shade, which is then limited to the target areas only. This is then light cured in position without the use of etching or adhesive (Figs 3.13–3.20).

An alginate impression is taken, with the cured resin composite masking the darkest areas. The composite is then removed and the patient given another appointment to fit the customized tray. When the alginate is cast, the resin composite additions will appear as positive excesses on the model that will match exactly where the gel reservoirs are required. No further block out of the models

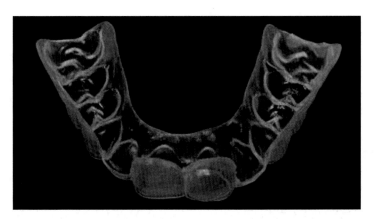

Fig. 3.17 The tray extends from the upper first molar to first molar to aid retention and stability of the tray in situ with the reservoirs over the labial of the central incisors and the windows cut out over both laterals.

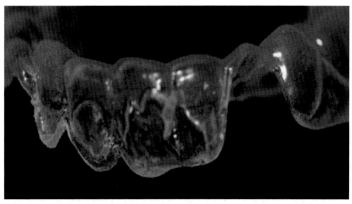

Fig. 3.18 The lower tray has the reservoirs just over the brownest surfaces of the lower incisors. The areas over the mandibular canines have been cut back to allow the salivary peroxidase and catalase access to these teeth, and thereby prevent undesirable bleaching of the lower canines.

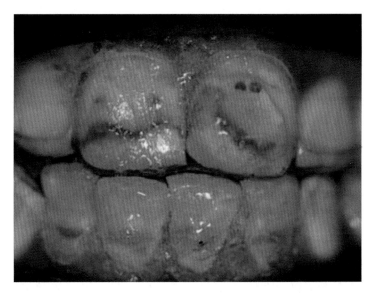

Fig. 3.19 The bleaching trays with the 10% carbamide peroxide gel in position.

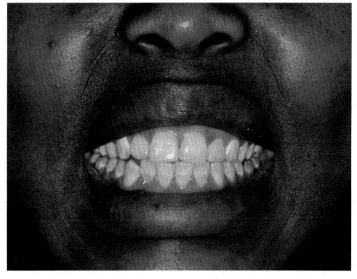

Fig. 3.20 Clinical appearance after 8 weeks of bleaching with 10% carbamide peroxide.

is required because, when the heated thermoplastic material is sucked down onto the model to make the bleaching tray, the reservoirs will be in the correct positions.

A window is cut over those teeth that are not to be bleached so that the protective salivary peroxidase and catalase can inactivate the gel and stop any unwanted bleaching of the adjacent teeth.

Trays with or without reservoirs?

The need for a reservoir is dependent largely on the viscosity of the bleaching material. Carboxypolymethyl cellulose (carbopol) is a thickening agent that is added to carbamide peroxide. The increased viscosity limits movement of the gel and prevents salivary ingress beneath the mouthguard. It is important to be able to seat the tray and still keep the carbamide peroxide bleaching gel in the correct position. It is impossible to compress a gel: it can only be displaced.

It is important to design the tray so as to avoid gel coming into unnecessary contact with soft tissues. The bleaching effect cannot be limited to an area of the teeth covered by the reservoir areas. However, reservoirs help to ensure that most of the effective bleaching gel is held over the target areas.

The presence of reservoirs also helps the loaded tray to seat fully on the teeth. If the tray does not seat properly, it will usually be short at the gingival margins, which may result in a failure to bleach adequately the cervical aspects of the target teeth. If the necks of the teeth are not covered by the tray then the protective salivary enzymes can react readily with the unprotected bleaching gel and rapidly inactivate the hydrogen peroxide, thereby stopping any effective bleaching in those areas.

Some commentators have suggested that reservoirs are unnecessary and that trays without reservoirs 'are more economical'. Trays with reservoirs can indeed be bulkier and require increased volumes of bleaching material. The counter argument is that if there is an inadequate amount of bleaching gel in the target areas then trays without reservoirs are a false economy. Keeping saliva away from the gel helps keep it active for longer periods. Reservoirs hold the viscous bleaching gel in the tray for several hours and this allows the gel to continue releasing low levels of perhydroxyl ions, thereby sustaining the bleaching process.

If there is a veneer of any type on the labial aspect of the tooth, then the reservoir should be placed on the palatal aspect of the tooth so that the 10% carbamide gel will accumulate preferentially on that side (Fig. 3.9). No perhydroxyl ion will penetrate any restorative material. The bleaching peroxide ions will, however, penetrate through the palatal enamel, palatal dentine and dental pulp to reach, albeit slowly, the dentine and enamel of the labial aspect of the tooth. In this way, existing porcelain veneered teeth can be lightened to a degree, but it can be a slow process and the patient needs to be informed and evidence of the warnings needs to be documented, to provide verification that the patient understood about the issues in advance and agreed to continue with treatment.

The viscous nature of the bleaching gel also has the advantage of improving the tray's retentiveness. Viscous 10% carbamide peroxide materials are designed for use with a reservoir and a list of those materials with the American Dental Association (ADA) seal of approval is available from their website.

The block-out material used to create the reservoirs is usually placed on the labial aspects of the teeth on the cast. Blocking out should stop about 1 mm

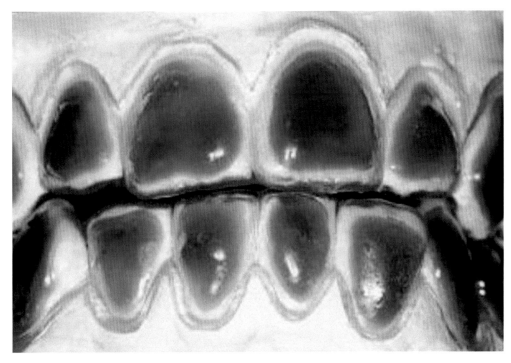

Fig. 3.21 Scalloped trays with reservoirs on the labial aspect. The material used for blocking out stops short of the incisal tips.

short of the incisal tip. The incisal area is mainly enamel and this area bleaches readily without the need for an overlying reservoir (Fig. 3.21).

The reservoirs can be of different sizes, depending on specific circumstances. The more bulbous or darker the tooth, the greater is the need for a reservoir. If the necks of the teeth are to be bleached, the reservoirs should extend over the gingival margin but in such a way that the tray does not pinch the soft tissues and is still capable of holding the gel in the cervical regions. In such cases, it is prudent to check that the patient does not have thin, friable periodontal tissues that may be traumatized by the extended tray (see Fig. 3.4).

Contraindications for this method of bleaching are limited but caution needs to be exercised when the clinical examination reveals a reduced width of thin attached gingiva and marked pre-operative cervical sensitivity. These conditions also restrict alternative treatments, such as ceramic veneers or direct resin composite bonding, thereby limiting the opportunity to satisfy these patients' esthetic demands (Fig. 3.4).

Scalloped trays (Fig. 3.22)

Scalloped trays follow the gingival margins. When the tray material has been adapted to the model, a permanent ink pen can be used to draw the outline of the underlying gingival margin on the labial aspect of the clear tray material. The tray is then removed from the cast and cut along this outline with sharp

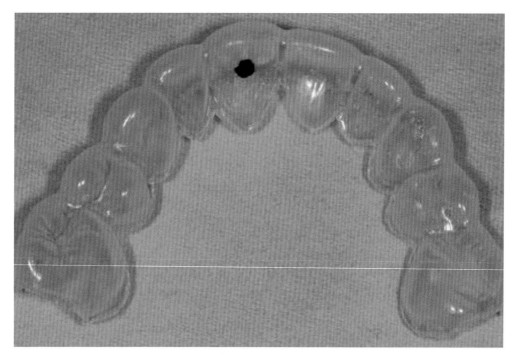

Fig. 3.22 A scalloped tray with a mark made with black permanent ink on the palatal aspect to remind the patient which tooth to bleach. One disadvantage of scalloped trays is that some patients find the margins on the lingual/palatal aspects irritating to the tongue, even when finished and smoothed.

scissors. Scissors have been designed specifically for this purpose and can produce a tray with a smooth edge that is well tolerated by the tongue. If the scalloping is positioned short of the gingival margin, some gel will extrude over the gingival tissues. This gel will be quickly inactivated by salivary catalase and peroxidase and consequently the necks of the teeth may fail to bleach.

Straight-line trays (Fig. 3.23)

Straight-line trays have been advocated on the grounds that they are easy to construct and hold an appropriate volume of bleaching material over the cervical margins of the teeth. These trays extend approximately 2 mm beyond the gingival margins and tend not to irritate the tongue. A disadvantage is that by having bleaching material held over the gingival tissues, there may be a mild, transient soft tissue reaction to the gel. Some dentists use this style of tray with 6% hydrogen peroxide (the EC 2012 legal limit) for an hour at a time. If that is to be done on an empirical basis, the material should be used sparingly and the patient should be instructed to swallow, breath in hard to try to dry the teeth and immediately insert the tray with the 6% hydrogen peroxide gel. This is in order to try to exclude the salivary peroxidase from inactivating rapidly the unstable hydrogen peroxide gel.

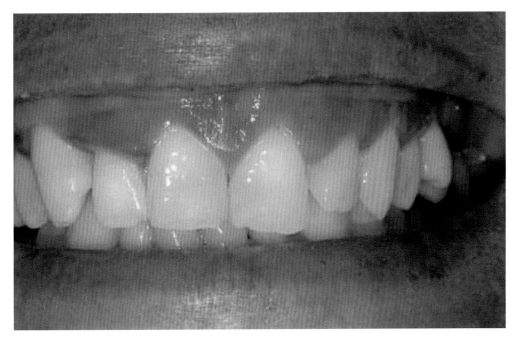

Fig. 3.23 Soft tissue redness caused by a tight fitting straight-line tray (i.e. cut straight across and not scalloped to follow the gingival margins) used with hydrogen peroxide gel. Reservoirs are indicated with this type of tray. They can be placed on the palatal as well as the labial aspects of the teeth, although this can make the tray somewhat bulky.

Single-tooth trays (Figs 3.24–3.26)

Single tooth trays are designed to bleach individual teeth. In such cases, a standard tray is adjusted by trimming it away from the labial aspect of the adjacent teeth. By cutting away the tray, the salivary enzymes inactivate any hydrogen peroxide coming in contact with the adjacent teeth that therefore will not bleach.

Combination trays

Combination trays are used in situations where, for example, it is planned to bleach the canines and one central incisor only. Combination trays are produced by modifying standard trays to hold the gel over the target teeth only. Cutting windows makes a tray less retentive and relatively flimsy. It is important to incorporate retention in such trays by extending them into normal undercuts in the premolar and molar regions.

LABORATORY TECHNICAL PROCEDURES

- An accurate plaster cast of the arch to be bleached is produced. The cast should be horseshoe shaped and have sufficient bulk to ensure adequate strength and rigidity. The base of the cast is trimmed to be parallel to the occlusal plane.

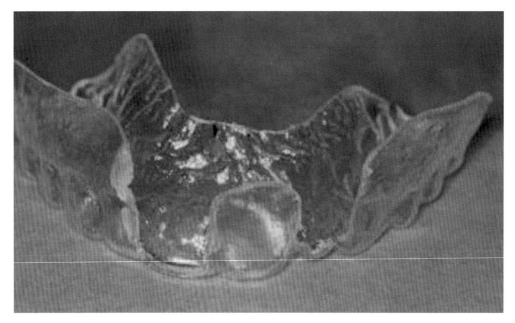

Fig. 3.24   Close-up of the labial aspect of a single tooth tray with the windows cut over the adjacent teeth to avoid bleaching them inadvertently.

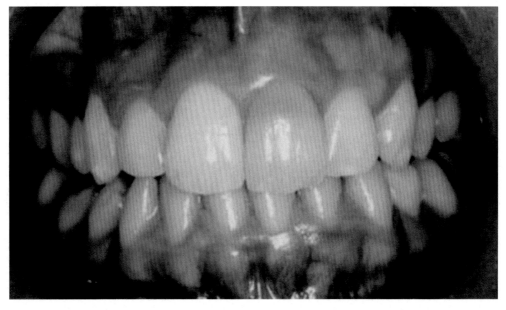

Fig. 3.25   It is only the discoloured upper left central incisor that requires bleaching.

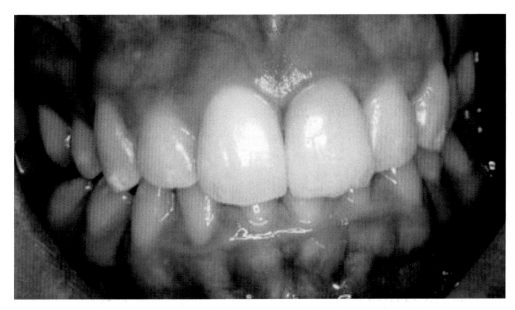

Fig. 3.26 The appearance after use of a single tooth tray and 10% carbamide peroxide for 2 months.

- Block-out resin is placed over the target teeth and light cured in position (Fig. 3.27).

- Cold mould seal is applied to the cast to help with the removal of the vacuum-formed thermoplastic material.

- The thermoplastic ethyl vinyl acetate comes in various thicknesses. If there is clinical evidence of tooth wear, or parafunctional activity, a thicker sheet of material should be used (2 mm).

- The modified cast is placed on the platform with the occlusal aspect facing the plastic sheet. The thermoplastic material is heated until it goes clear and is then adapted to the cast in a vacuum-forming machine (Figs 3.28 and 3.29).

- Following adaptation, the tray material is allowed to cool (Fig. 3.30).

- Excess material is removed with sharp scissors and a scalpel blade. If the necks of the teeth are dark, the material is trimmed back so that it just covers the gingival tissues on the cast. Check for any sharp edges using your finger.

- Finish the tray with burs, a scalpel and appropriate polishing systems (Fig. 3.31).

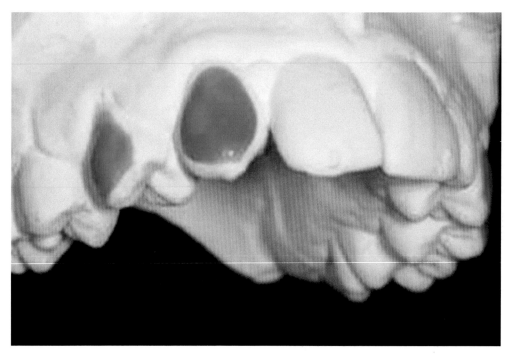

Fig. 3.27   Target teeth blocked out with a contrasting colour resin on the cast.

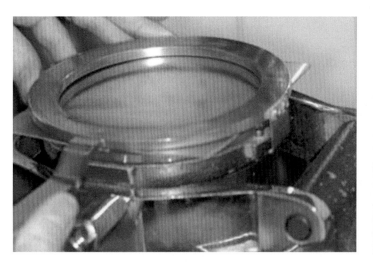

Fig. 3.28   The thermoplastic material is heated.

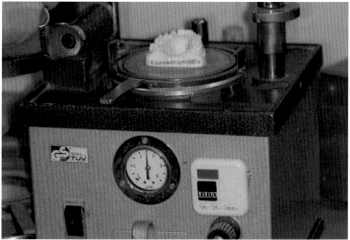

Fig. 3.29   The cast on the table of the vacuum-forming machine with the occlusal aspects facing upwards.

CLINICAL PROCEDURES

Fitting the tray

- The fit of the tray is checked. There should be no blanching of the soft tissues. This is especially important to check if the gingival tissues are thin and may be damaged by ill-fitting or sharp margins. The patient should be

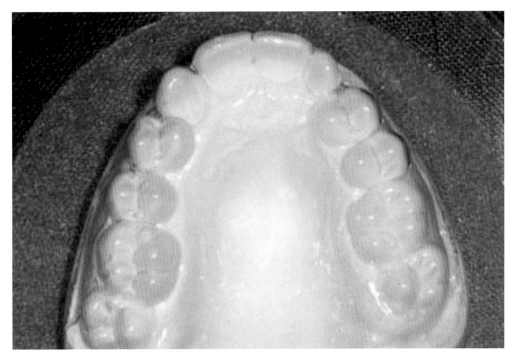

Fig. 3.30   Bleaching tray material adapted to the cast.

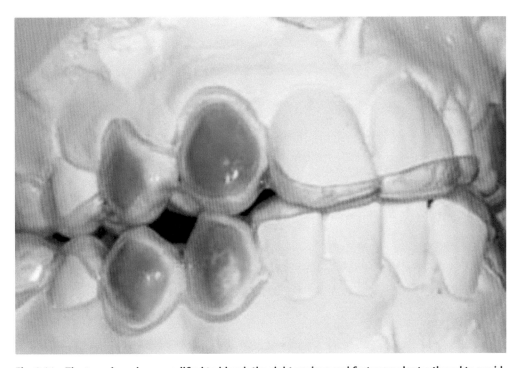

Fig. 3.31   The trays have been modified to bleach the right canines and first premolar teeth and to avoid bleaching the upper and lower incisors, and the second premolars.

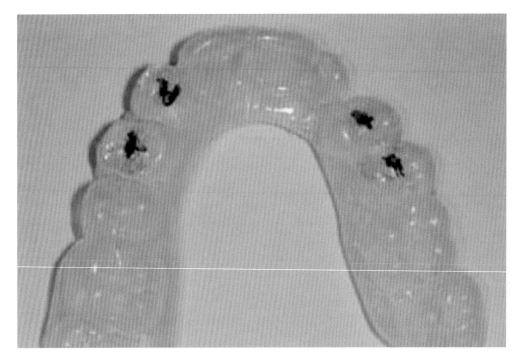

Fig. 3.32   The target teeth marked with a permanent ink felt tip pen on the outer aspect of the tray, to help the patient identify which teeth are to be bleached.

asked to identify any uncomfortable areas with their tongue. These areas should be adjusted as necessary.

- The teeth to be bleached can be marked on the outer surface of the tray with a permanent ink felt tip pen. This helps the patient identify where to place the bleaching gel (Fig. 3.32).

- The accuracy of the clinical photographs obtained at the consultation appointment is checked with the patient and then replaced in the notes. The agreed shade is confirmed with reference to the value orientated shade guide (arranged from lightest to darkest) and confirmed in the clinical records. The patient is given a note of the agreed existing shade.

- The appropriate amount of 10% carbamide peroxide is given to the patient along with written instructions (Box 3.5). Higher concentrations of carbamide peroxide bleaching gel may be prescribed but there is little scientific evidence of any real benefits in doing so. Higher concentrations can produce a more rapid response in some patients, but there is also an increased risk of sensitivity in others.

- The patient is given a protective (orthodontic retainer style) box for safe storage of the bleaching tray when not in use and instructions on tray maintenance.

BOX 3.5

INSTRUCTIONS FOR PATIENTS ON THE USE OF 10% CARBAMIDE PEROXIDE

1. Brush your teeth thoroughly in the normal fashion

2. Remove the tip from the syringe containing the 10% carbamide peroxide gel and push out a little of the contents into the appropriate parts of the tray towards the deeper and front parts of the mould of each tooth to be bleached

3. Place gel in the tray on the cheek and the tongue side of the back teeth. About half to three quarters of the syringe will usually be necessary if doing a whole arch of teeth

4. Seat the tray over the teeth and slowly press down firmly

5. A finger, a tissue, or a soft toothbrush should be used to remove excess gel that will flow beyond the edge of the tray

6. Rinse gently and do not swallow. The tray is usually worn overnight whilst sleeping but as long as it is worn for at least 2 hours, this will be effective

7. In the morning remove the tray and brush the residual gel from the teeth. Rinse out the tray in <u>cold</u> water only and brush it to remove the residual gel. Store it in a safe container

8. One or both trays can be worn overnight

9. If bleaching upper and lower teeth, it is best to bleach one arch at night and the other one for at least 2 hours during the day

10. Do not eat, drink or smoke while wearing the bleaching tray

11. Carbamide peroxide should not be exposed to heat, sunlight or extreme cold

Notes

1. It is counterproductive to change the bleaching gel more than once a day, as this has been shown to increase sensitivity, which in turn tends to delay completion of bleaching

2. It will probably take about 3–6 weeks to achieve a satisfactory result. Your dentist will advise you about your individual problems but the general rule is to keep bleaching until the teeth are an acceptable colour

	• Diagnosis	Y/N
	• Radiographs	Y/N
	• Photographs	Y/N
BOX 3.6	• Discuss options with patient	Y/N
A CLINICAL RECORD CHECK-LIST FOR BLEACHING SHOULD INCLUDE THE FOLLOWING INFORMATION WITH DATES	• Shade of teeth recorded and agreed with patient	Y/N
	• Discuss option of single arch bleaching	Y/N
	• Consent	Y/N
	• Impressions	Y/N
	• Mouthguard inserted Date:	
	• Material used and quantity:	
	• Time of recall:	
	• Shade after bleaching:	

- A log form should be given to the patient to record the use of the bleaching trays and the amount of material used.

- Patients who experience sensitivity of their teeth can be advised to use toothpaste containing 5% potassium nitrate but preferably without any *n*-lauryl sulphate, which is a surfactant that can cause gingival soreness in rare cases.

Evaluation of colour change

Sequential photographs should be taken to record changes in colour at review appointments, preferably with the same ambient light and camera settings. All changes in colour should be recorded in the patient's clinical records (Box 3.6).

Sensitivity

About 70% of patients experience significant sensitivity while bleaching. If this happens, bleaching should be stopped for a day or two and then recommenced on an every second or third night basis. Fluoride gel or toothpaste can be used to treat sensitive teeth. This can be placed in the tray and worn at night. Toothpaste with 5% potassium nitrate and without *n*-lauryl sulphate is also recommended for 30 minutes before starting the bleaching itself. It needs to be washed out with cold water before replacing it with the 10% carbamide peroxide gel.

Acidic drinks and fruit should be avoided as these are known to cause sensitivity. Very rarely, temporary discomfort of the gums, lips and tongue can occur. This usually reduces when bleaching stops.

Re-bleaching

Re-bleaching normally takes 1 night for each week of the original course. If it took 4 weeks to bleach initially, it will take 4 nights to 'top up' the bleaching.

ESSENTIALS: BLEACHING DO'S AND DON'TS FOR THE DENTIST

Do

- Take a history. Record the shade in the notes
- Make a diagnosis of the cause(s) of the discolouration
- Discuss options/costs
- Discuss the lack of guarantees if there is poor compliance plus 'the time to touch up'
- Check for secondary 'white flecking' in fluorosis
- Check if the patient has a gag reflex/retches
- Block out casts as appropriate
- Control the amount of bleach issued
- Have advice sheets on alternative treatments, e.g. bonding with resin composite or veneers
- Check for the presence of resin composite restorations
- Check on the radiographs for resin composites
- Warn that resin composites will not bleach and will have to be replaced
- Check for the presence of veneers, crowns, bridges in both arches
- Warn that these will not bleach and may need to be redone if the natural teeth change colour
- Keep high concentration hydrogen peroxide products separate from standard carbamide peroxide products and do not delegate this to anyone inexperienced in case they give patients the wrong concentration material. EU law is specific as to who can dispense extra gel

Do not

- Promise unrealistic results (e.g. "a dazzling Hollywood smile")
- Encourage patients to use stronger concentrations of carbamide peroxide or change the gel more than once a day
- Believe unsubstantiated claims from manufacturers of 'special' new materials
- Use higher concentrations than are legally allowed, i.e. 6% hydrogen peroxide = 18% carbamide peroxide
- Use non-ADA approved bleaching products
- Believe all products are the same
- Delegate the distribution of extra bleaching material to staff without checking

MANAGEMENT OF DISCOLOURED, NON-VITAL ANTERIOR TEETH

AIMS

To consider:

- Terminology and methods of dealing with dead ('non-vital') discoloured teeth.

- Describing the inside/outside bleaching technique.

OUTCOMES

The dental professional will be made more aware of predictable MI approaches to managing discoloured, dead, root-filled anterior teeth.

ASSESSMENT

The successful management of discoloured non-vital teeth is based on an accurate diagnosis followed by detailed care planning. A comprehensive history should be taken, including details of events that may have contributed to the discolouration. A detailed clinical examination, including special investigations as indicated clinically, should then follow.

A focused approach will reduce the chances of overlooking critical information to avoid failure of treatment. Patient input is critical. A full and frank discussion of individual patients' perceptions of their problem is especially important in assessing whether or not they have realistic expectations of the possible outcomes of treatment. Whatever care plan is agreed, it should provide the most realistic prospects of a durable, predictable, esthetically pleasing and cost effective result for the patient. This should also be achieved with the least possible biological damage, using an MI approach.

Patients with a low lip line may accept a mildly discoloured, dead, root-filled anterior tooth while those with a high lip line may find any significant discolouration unacceptable. Such discolouration is often the reason for seeking treatment (Fig. 3.33). Improving the appearance of a discoloured, non-vital anterior tooth can have a profound effect on the patient's self-confidence and oral health (Fig. 3.34). Marked discolouration of teeth can be a serious handicap that impacts on a person's self-image, self-confidence, physical attractiveness and, possibly, employability.

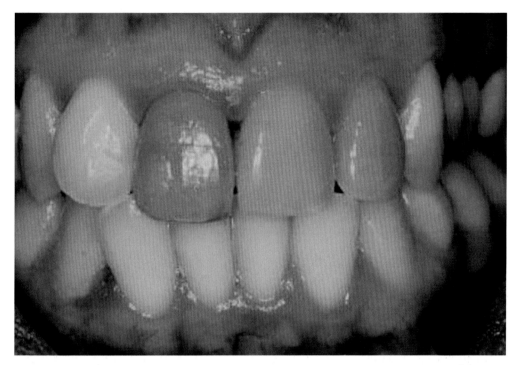

Fig. 3.33 The discoloured appearance of the non-vital upper right central incisor and the sclerosed upper left central and lateral incisors.

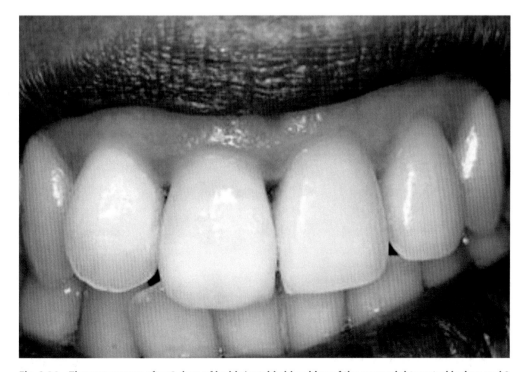

Fig. 3.34 The appearance after 3 days of inside/outside bleaching of the upper right central incisor and 2 months of conventional tray bleaching with 10% carbamide peroxide of the discoloured left central and lateral incisors.

AETIOLOGY (SEE CHAPTER 1)

The most common cause of discolouration in dead 'non-vital' teeth is the presence of residual pulpal haemorrhagic products. These are most likely to be retained in the pulp horn spaces and in the cervical region. The discolouration is caused usually by breakdown products of haemoglobin and other haematin molecules, which may permeate into the dentine of the tooth from the pulpal aspect.

Dental trauma can be a cause of discolouration of dead 'non-vital' anterior teeth. Patients may not give a clear history of the relevant trauma. The discolouration, whose onset may be gradual, is often painless and may only become apparent when others comment on it. Discolouration of a non-vital tooth may also be an incidental finding in a routine dental examination.

Incorporating blood or other stains into the tooth/restoration interface may cause, or substantially contribute to, discolouration. Materials used in endodontic procedures, including root canal sealants containing silver, eugenol, polyantibiotic pastes, and compounds containing phenol may cause darkening of the root dentine over time. Endodontic metal points, pins and posts inserted into root-filled anterior teeth are a possible cause of discolouration. In addition, leakage of restorations may be a causative/contributing factor (Figs 3.35–3.38).

MECHANISMS OF DISCOLOURATION

When teeth suffer significant trauma there is disruption of the pulp contents and its blood supply. This can result in haemorrhage into the dentine and subsequent tooth discolouration. The extent to which the products of pulp degradation contribute to tooth discolouration remains unclear. It is considered that pulpal ischaemia and subsequent pulp death, in the absence of bacterial contamination, does not produce dental discolouration to the same extent as catastrophic haemorrhage into the pulp chamber and the pulp–dentine complex. Following haemorrhage, the haemoglobin molecules may be found in the coronal dentine close to the pulp. They do not tend to penetrate far into the dentine tubules. This largely explains why inside/outside bleaching produces such satisfactory results as it addresses the source and location of the discolouration.

Any methods attempting to remove discolouration following trauma and haemorrhage into the pulp chamber should focus initially on the physical and then, later, the chemical removal of these breakdown products. The pulp chamber is surrounded by dentine and isolated from any inflammatory or healing response in the adjacent soft tissues. Therefore, normal healing, which occurs, for example, with a soft tissue bruise, and the eventual resolution of discolouration in the tissues, cannot occur. If the pulp does not survive following trauma and

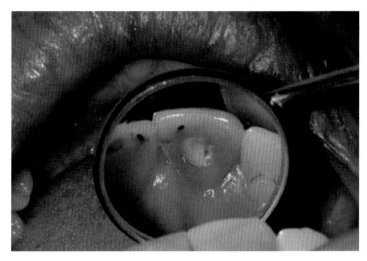

Fig. 3.35   Leaking and poorly sealed access cavity in discoloured root-filled teeth with metal pins in the incisal tips causes discolouration.

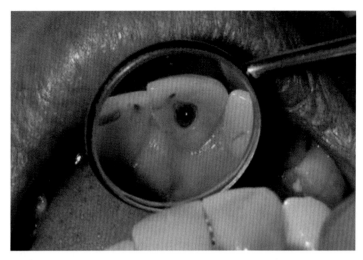

Fig. 3.36   Thorough ultrasonic removal of the debris is essential to eliminate old blood breakdown products.

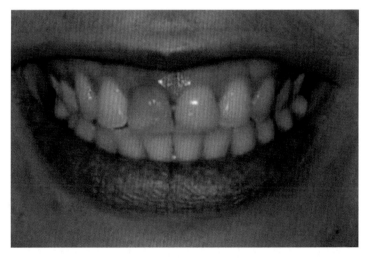

Fig. 3.37   Discoloured, dead root-filled upper right central incisor before inside/outside bleaching and rebuilding with direct resin composite without pins or a post.

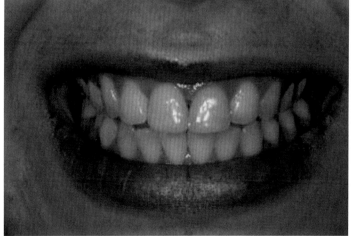

Fig. 3.38   Result following inside/outside bleaching for 2 days and followed 1 week later by direct free-hand resin composite repair without retentive pins or a post. No sound tissue was removed during this minimally invasive (MI), biologically respectful treatment.

haemorrhage, then haematin molecules remain within the pulp chamber and consequently the tooth appears discoloured. On the other hand, if re-vascularization occurs and the pulp survives, the tooth can revert to its normal colour within 2–3 months.

REVIEW

The colour of teeth can be monitored by using a shade guide or by taking clinical photographs with a shade tab beside the tooth. A record should be kept. Follow-up reviews of root canal treatment should include a check for discolouration using the shade guide or a photograph as a reference. If discolouration is observed, it is better to intervene sooner rather than later. Later discolouration may indicate, amongst other possibilities, leakage or degradation of the endodontic sealer or the material sealing the access cavity. Delaying treatment may well result in the discolouration becoming more difficult to manage successfully.

INSIDE/OUTSIDE BLEACHING (Figs 3.39–3.55)

Prior to undertaking inside/outside bleaching the dead tooth should be root-filled in a standard fashion under rubber dam isolation, using copious amounts of sodium hypochlorite irrigation. Hypochlorite is a bleaching agent mainly used as an antiseptic in endodontics, which also removes a degree of discolouration.

Inside/outside bleaching involves placing 10% carbamide peroxide gel simultaneously onto and inside a discoloured root-filled tooth, usually with the aid of a 'single tooth customized bleaching tray'. This allows penetration of hydrogen peroxide both internally and externally with the bleaching gel being protected from salivary deactivation by the tray itself.

Prior to bleaching, the contents of the pulp chamber should be cleaned thoroughly for 5 minutes with a very fine ultrasonic or airsonic tip. The root filling should be cut back with the ultrasonic or airsonic device to a level of approximately 3 mm below the enamel–cementum junction. Popular advice is to seal off the root canal filling with radiopaque glass ionomer or zinc polycarboxylate cement. However, in the real clinical situation, it can be difficult technically to

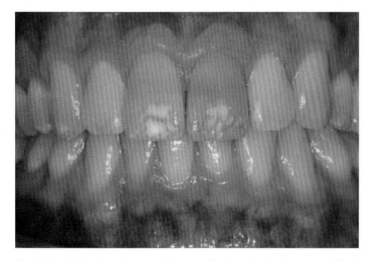

Fig. 3.39   A discoloured upper left central incisor that has been root-filled twice previously. The upper right central was sclerosed. Note the white fluorosis on both teeth.

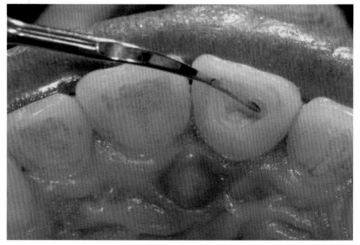

Fig 3.40   An ultrasonic tip is used for 5–10 minutes within the canal to vibrate blood products out physically and also any residual resin composite tags in the dentine. This is more of an MI approach than the use of burs.

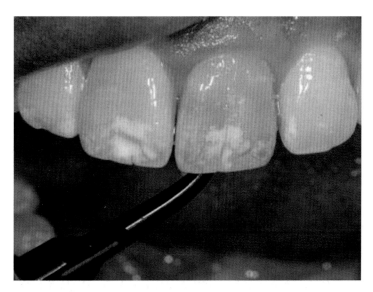

Fig. 3.41   The right angled needle attached to the syringe containing 10% carbamide peroxide gel is inserted into the deepest part of the chamber and used to fill up the whole chamber down to the gutta percha root filling, usually approximately 3 mm below the enamel–cementum junction. Note the mid-labial vertical crack in this tooth.

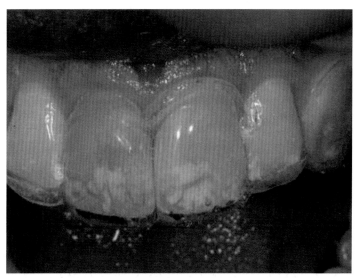

Fig. 3.42   The patient is told to wear the mouthguard all the time, with fresh 10% carbamide peroxide gel in it, including whilst asleep, but not when eating or drinking. During the day, the gel is changed every two hours and last thing at night. The patient does not need to wake up to change the material.

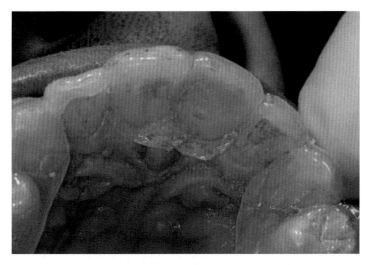

Fig. 3.43   The bleaching tray in the regions of both central incisors is filled with 10% carbamide peroxide gel and inserted immediately to cover both central incisors. The tray is cut back to provide windows over the lateral incisors in order to avoid bleaching them inadvertently.

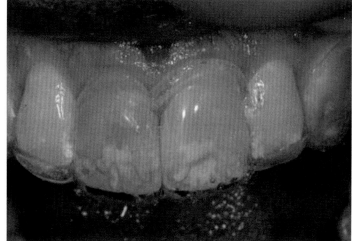

Fig. 3.44   The tray has been extended over the left central incisor that is having inside/outside bleaching, but is short in the cervical region of the upper right central that is not to be bleached at this stage. Two windows have been cut over the upper lateral incisors to allow the salivary peroxidase and catalase to stop unintentional bleaching of the lateral incisors.

place such a material to seal the gutta percha root filling accurately enough without the fluid restorative material being drawn down the internal dentine walls by capillary action. This unwanted situation will compromise effective bleaching of the neck of the discoloured tooth thereafter because the carbamide peroxide gel cannot penetrate through any restorative cements. Flowable

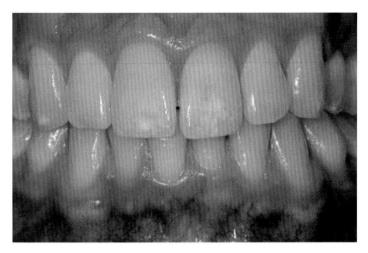

Fig. 3.45 The upper left central incisor took 3 days and nights to bleach. Only when it was lighter than the upper right central incisor was the upper right central incisor bleached with a conventional tray with 10% carbamide peroxide, but with windows cut back over both lateral incisors. Note that both the crack and the white fluorosis appear less obvious against a lighter background.

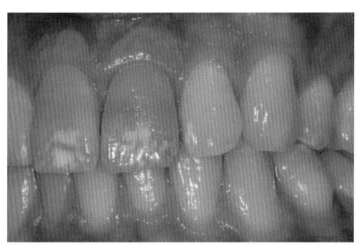

Fig. 3.46 Pre-operative clinical photograph. Always bleach the darkest tooth first until it is lighter than the others before considering any other adjacent bleaching. Differently designed trays are required for different situations.

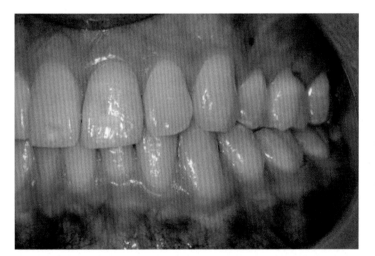

Fig. 3.47 The post-operative result was acceptable to the patient as it preserved tooth tissue.

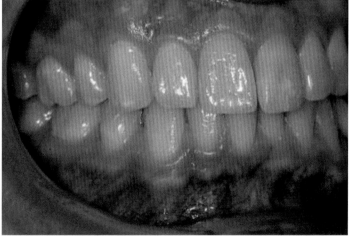

Fig. 3.48 The post-operative result was acceptable to the patient and he did not want other teeth bleached.

composite or compomer should be avoided because these are especially liable to flow into the neck of the chamber. If that happens, it is impossible to bleach the necks of the discoloured teeth. Conversely, a restorative cement of higher viscosity is unlikely to flow adequately to seal the gutta percha root filling effectively in the depths of the pulp chamber.

In cases of marked cervical discolouration, it is both possible and sensible to undertake bleaching <u>without sealing</u> over the root filling, <u>provided</u> patient co-operation is optimal and the access cavity can be kept bathed constantly in 10%

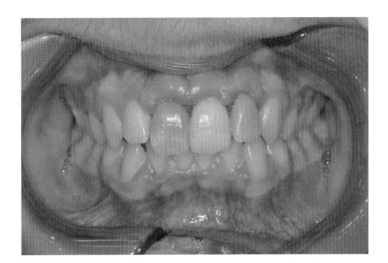

Fig. 3.49 Three discoloured and dead teeth following a sports injury. The upper right central incisor was grossly discoloured and there was significant soft tissue damage.

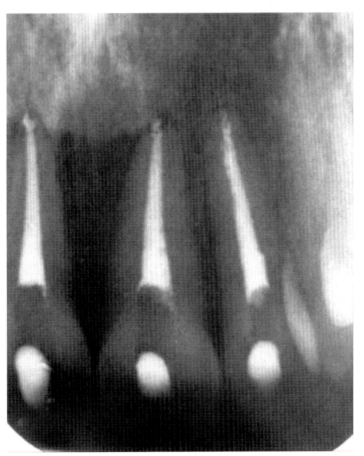

Fig. 3.50 A periapical radiograph showing the root-filled teeth with the gutta percha cut back to well below the enamel–cementum junction. (Endodontics by Mr Gavin Seal).

carbamide peroxide within the protective bleaching tray for the few days involved. This is because carbamide peroxide is a well proven oxidizing antiseptic that, if changed every 2 hours by the patient and protected within the bleaching tray being worn constantly, will readily and effectively inhibit Gram-negative anaerobic bacteria. Any tooth-coloured restorative material on the external <u>or internal</u>

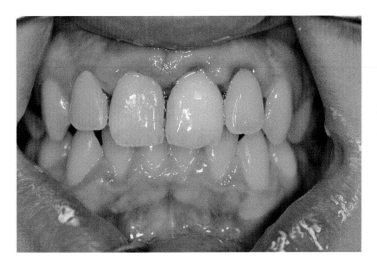

Fig. 3.51 The results of inside/outside bleaching after 2 days.

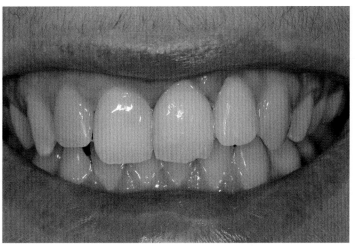

Fig. 3.52 The teeth were deliberately over-bleached to allow for 'rebound' in colour.

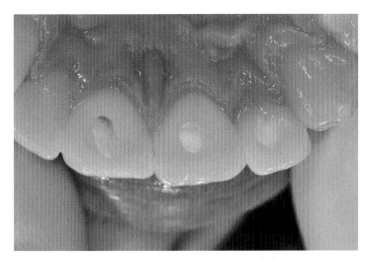

Fig. 3.53 The access cavities allowed for direct line access to apices but have not destroyed the structural strength/integrity of the teeth, most of which is manifest in the still intact marginal ridges.

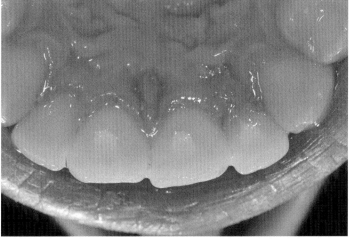

Fig. 3.54 The access cavities sealed with radiopaque and opaque white glass ionomer cement that is injected into the chambers with a fine needle. If these teeth ever need re-bleaching, white glass ionomer cement is much easier to see and remove than resin composite. Note how little of the palatal structure of the teeth has been lost and this has minimized further damage to the traumatized teeth.

surfaces of the tooth must be removed before bleaching, as the hydrogen peroxide cannot penetrate through these.

The endodontic access cavity is left open, but constantly covered both inside and outside with the bleaching gel in the protective tray except very briefly when eating and drinking, for the 2–4 day duration of the inside/outside bleaching procedure.

During the bleaching procedure, patients need to be advised to avoid tannin-containing foods such as curries, tomato-containing sauces and dark coloured fluids (red wine, coffee or strong tea) until the access cavity is restored. The

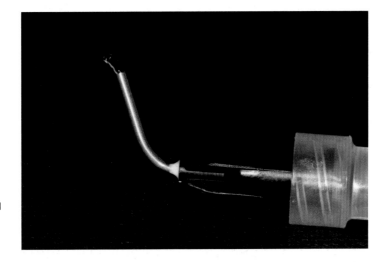

Fig. 3.55 The needle is made of soft bendable material to allow the viscous 10% carbamide peroxide gel to be injected directly inside the root well below the cemento-enamel junction.

worry about disruption of the root filling and the, largely theoretical, bacterial contamination of the root filling interface needs to be considered against the requirement for an acceptable esthetic result in the cervical region where the enamel is only 0.7 mm thick. It should be remembered that failure to bleach the neck of the tooth adequately could necessitate a destructive procedure, including the possible provision of a post and core restoration that will lead to hugely predictable radicular bacterial contamination. The 10% carbamide peroxide gel, both within the tooth and in the tray, is changed every 2 hours and last thing at night. The more often the gel is changed, the more rapid the bleaching will be. When changing the gel, in particular after eating, the access cavity is flushed out using a blunt, fine needle that is attached to a syringe of the gel in order to gain access to the neck of the discoloured tooth (Fig. 3.55). Due to its viscous nature, this syringing effect removes any trapped food debris and ensures that the cavity is filled with fresh, active, 10% carbamide peroxide gel.

The patient is instructed to stop bleaching when they are satisfied with the degree of lightening of the tooth. It is acceptable for the tooth to be bleached a little lighter to allow for 'rebound' of the colour. The patient is reviewed after 2–3 days to assess colour changes and to limit the time the access cavity is left open.

Following successful completion of bleaching, usually after 2–3 days, the pulp chamber is once again cleaned out thoroughly with the aid of an ultrasonic tip and dried with large paper points. The tooth is then restored provisionally with contrasting white-coloured glass ionomer cement. Following bleaching, the tooth frequently appears to be lighter than the adjacent tooth. This is understandable given the reduction in the volume of dentine within the root-filled tooth.

A resin composite restoration should <u>not</u> be placed immediately following completion of the bleaching process, because oxygen will be released from the tooth for up to a week. This could compromise the resin composite adhesive bond and thereby result in micro-leakage. Conventional, radiopaque, white glass ionomer cement is preferred because it is easier to see and remove if required at any stage.

As resin composites are difficult to remove from within the tooth without inadvertently removing residual sound tooth structure, there are benefits to selecting a white shade and radiopaque glass ionomer cement to replace lost dentine. It is possible to check that the appearance of the restored tooth will be acceptable by leaving some water inside the access cavity and placing the selected material, on a trial basis, to check that it will achieve the desired outcome. A trial assessment of the colour is preferable to having to remove a definitive restoration that fails to achieve the desired outcome.

Obviously, if there is any concern about the endodontic status, the tooth should be re-root treated prior to commencing any inside/outside bleaching using copious amounts of sodium hypochlorite as the irrigant.

'WALKING' BLEACH TECHNIQUE

It is important to minimize structural damage to initially avulsed, intruded, laterally luxated or otherwise traumatised discoloured teeth. Endodontic treatment with pulp extirpation and preliminary chemo-mechanical debridement should be commenced after 2 weeks of flexible splinting following the accident, and before the risks of inflammatory root resorption start to increase.

Endodontic access should be in a straight line to the apex, and the minimum amount of sound tooth tissue should be removed during the process in order to maintain the residual structural strength of the traumatized crowns. Once endodontic obturation has been completed, the teeth can benefit from inside/outside bleaching, which is more effective than the traditional 'walking bleach' technique using sodium perborate, which when mixed with water produces approximately 7% hydrogen peroxide.

When 6% hydrogen peroxide is mixed into a slurry/paste with sodium perborate and sealed in the tooth, as a version of the walking bleach technique, this combination releases a total of 17.6% hydrogen peroxide (i.e. above EU limits). If 12% hydrogen peroxide is mixed into a paste with sodium perborate, this produces a total of 25.6% hydrogen peroxide (which is over four times the EU limit), which has to be sealed effectively into the discoloured tooth (Table 3.1). These concentrations are 5–8 times the concentration of 10% carbamide peroxide and so increase dramatically the biological damage risk, as discussed previously. Once the wet slurry/paste is placed in the access chamber, it starts effervescing quickly and the pressure can blow the temporary sealing material out of the access cavity within the first hour. This results in an open access cavity with the effect of the

TABLE 3.1	THE CONCENTRATIONS OF RELEASED HYDROGEN PEROXIDE FROM DIFFERENT BLEACHING AGENT FORMULATIONS	
		Released hydrogen peroxide concentration
10% carbamide peroxide		3.5%
Sodium perborate and water		7.0%
Sodium perborate with 6% hydrogen peroxide		17.6%
Sodium perborate with 12% hydrogen peroxide		25%
'Power' or 'chairside' or 'in-office' bleaching		15–38%

hydrogen peroxide being nullified by salivary peroxidase and catalase gaining access to the pulp chamber. In this situation there is no protective mouthguard which is different to the case with inside/outside bleaching.

PROTOCOL FOR INSIDE/OUTSIDE BLEACHING

First appointment

1. Make and record the diagnosis.

2. Take clinical reference photographs.

3. Check the periapical status of the tooth with a long cone periapical radiograph. Be satisfied that the root space is obturated satisfactorily (Fig. 3.50).

4. Undertake any necessary endodontic revision prior to starting inside/outside bleaching using copious amounts of sodium hypochlorite.

5. Check that the tooth is asymptomatic and has a favourable prognosis.

6. Use a shade guide to estimate the shade before treatment. Agree the shade with the patient. Record this in the clinical records and give the patient a copy.

7. Warn the patient that any existing matching restorations within the target and adjacent teeth will not bleach. After bleaching, such restorations may well appear to be a darker colour than the bleached natural tooth. Such restorations may need to be replaced. In all such cases the patient should be warned of this esthetic and financial consequence of bleaching and replacement of restorations.

8. A diagram of the existing restorations is made and given to the patient, with a copy being kept in the clinical records.

9. Discuss other treatment options, highlighting the MI nature of bleaching.

10. Check the patient is not allergic to peroxide or plastic and that female patients of childbearing age are not pregnant or breastfeeding.

11. Provide the patient with a written care plan and estimates and obtain consent.

12. Provide the patient with written instructions and demonstrate what the treatment involves.

13. Make contemporaneous notes that this protocol has been completed.

Making the tray

An alginate impression is taken and cast in the laboratory. Proprietary resin or, failing that, plaster is used to block out the cast on the labial and palatal aspects of the target tooth, providing the desired extent and depth of the intended reservoirs.

Cold mould seal is applied to the cast. Softened bleaching tray material is then vacuum formed to the cast and once cooled is removed. Labial windows are cut out over the adjacent teeth with sharp scissors so that only the target tooth (or teeth) is covered. Any gel that strays onto the adjacent teeth will be inactivated by the patient's salivary peroxidase or catalase.

Second appointment

1. Check the bleaching tray for fit and comfort, and that the patient is able to place and remove it. Check that they can use the angled tip on the syringe of bleaching gel (Figs. 3.41 and 3.55).

2. Remove the access cavity restoration and reduce the root filling as necessary to a level at least 3 mm below the enamel–cementum junction. A fine ultrasonic or airsonic tip is the simplest way to do this. The pulp chamber is checked for any residual debris. The pulp cornuae and cervical region are cleaned ultrasonically or airsonically for at least 5 minutes (Fig. 3.40). The root filling can then be sealed off, if desired, but take care not to allow any restorative material to cover the discoloured labial dentine walls. Radiopaque, white glass ionomer cement is suitable for this purpose. It should be allowed time to set fully (3–4 minutes).

3. It is prudent to 'check etch' the inside of the tooth to see if all the exposed dentine takes on a cleaned appearance, indicating that the surfaces have been properly prepared and are free of any residual tooth-coloured filling material, in particular resin composite. Any resin composite on the labial aspect of the tooth should be removed. The outside of the tooth should

also be etched with phosphoric acid. A frosty appearance will confirm that the enamel is free of any residual resin composite tags.

4. The 10% carbamide peroxide gel is injected by the patient directly into the chamber of the tooth using a medium bore needle attached directly to a syringe of the material (Fig. 3.55). The tray with gel in the reservoirs only is inserted into the mouth. Excess gel is wiped away with gauze.

5. Provide the patient with enough gel and written instructions. Demonstrate again and check that the patient knows what to do. Check that the patient can insert the gel effectively into the tooth using the syringe and angled needle tip.

6. If the patient is unable to place the gel effectively, an immediate fall back situation is for the dentist to seal some 10% carbamide peroxide in the pulp space and have the patient use the tray to carry out external bleaching. However, this is not as effective as inside/outside bleaching.

Instructions for patients

1. Remove the top from the syringe containing the 10% carbamide peroxide gel. Screw the supplied blunt right-angled needle tip onto the syringe. Insert the tip of the needle into the cavity on the inside of the tooth to be bleached and fill with the gel.

2. Load the appropriate part of the bleaching tray with the 10% carbamide peroxide gel. A mark made on the outside of the tray with a permanent ink pen will help identify that part of the tray to be loaded.

3. Insert the tray and remove any excessive gel with a finger or a soft toothbrush.

4. Rinse the mouth gently with water and spit out.

5. Wear the tray at all times, except when eating or cleaning.

6. Every 2 hours and last thing at night, change the gel inside the tooth and also in the tray. Clean the inside of the tooth by flushing it out with the needle on the bleaching gel after eating and before re-inserting the new gel into the mouthguard and replacing it fill the inside of the tooth with the gel.

7. The tray can be cleaned with cold water only and a toothbrush.

8. Avoid highly coloured foods such as curries, tomato-containing sauces, and dark coloured fruits or vegetables, e.g. beetroot. Red wine, coffee and strong tea must be avoided until bleaching has been completed and the tooth is sealed with a filling.

9. If there are any problems, contact the practice immediately.

10. Stop bleaching when the tooth is the desired colour.

PROBLEMS AND TROUBLESHOOTING

POOR PATIENT COMPLIANCE

Appropriate patient selection and clear instructions should minimize this problem. Inability or unwillingness to follow the instructions will lead to failure or prolonged treatment time. The patient must understand their responsibilities and role in their treatment. Inside/outside bleaching should not be undertaken when a patient is not well known to the practitioner or there are problems of poor manual dexterity or of limited understanding of what is involved.

The patient must have reasonable manual dexterity and must be able to place the gel within the tooth. This can be checked before making the tray and opening the access cavity by testing whether the patient is able to hold the syringe effectively against the inside of the tooth. If the patient is unable or unwilling to do this, then alternative treatment options should be considered.

Patients complain rarely about food getting into the access cavity. This should not create any great difficulty, assuming the patient is properly briefed and capable of placing and using the bleaching gel syringe to flush out any food debris after eating (Fig. 3.55).

THE NECK OF THE TOOTH DOES NOT BLEACH

The neck of the tooth does not bleach when some restorative material residue, usually resin composite, is bonded to the internal dentine walls. Magnification should be used to ensure complete and safe removal of all materials covering the dentine, thereby allowing it to be bleached. It is prudent to 'check etch' the inside of the tooth where a clean dentine appearance indicates that its surface is free of residual tooth-coloured materials.

Failure to reduce the root filling to a level well below the enamel–cementum junction will hinder the penetration of the bleaching agent into the dentine at the neck of the tooth. Furthermore, the tray needs to be extended cervically to cover the gingival margin to hold the bleaching gel in and around the cervical region. Enamel is only approximately 0.7 mm thick in the cervical region and therefore it is important that the underlying discoloured dentine is adequately bleached. The soft metal needle on the syringe needs to be bent appropriately in order to ensure that the gel is deposited into the deepest part of the cavity below the cemento–enamel junction (see Fig. 3.55).

FAILURE TO BLEACH

If the tooth fails to bleach despite appropriate clinical technique and good patient compliance, the source of the discolouration is probably not pulpal blood in origin. A history of an amalgam restoration in the palatal access cavity may be the cause. Metal ions, which migrate from the amalgam into the adjacent tooth structure, are much more resistant to bleaching than the molecules originating from the pulp. If any amalgam is left in the tooth during bleaching, the tooth may take on a green tinge if copper was a constituent of the amalgam. It is essential to remove all amalgam debris by ultrasonics from within the tooth before undertaking inside/outside bleaching.

The presence of a labial porcelain veneer means the reservoir must be placed on the palatal aspect as the porcelain is impervious to the hydrogen peroxide. With this approach the tooth can be bleached successfully, but slowly, without removing the porcelain veneer.

COMBINED AETIOLOGY OF DISCOLOURATION

Where a tooth has been discoloured, for example, by tetracycline therapy and trauma, then the combination of discolouration may be very difficult to manage effectively.

'WALKING BLEACH'

This traditional technique involves the use of a mixture of water and sodium perborate that is sealed temporarily into the pulp chamber of the discoloured, root-filled tooth. The difficulty with this traditional approach is that the continual oxygen effervescence from the hydrogen peroxide frequently 'blows' the temporary dressing out of the back of the tooth and the wet environment makes it difficult to reseal the cavity. As a result, the hydrogen peroxide may not be contained adequately in the tooth for long enough to bleach the tooth. While 10% carbamide peroxide gel can be sealed within the tooth, this technique is not as effective as inside/outside bleaching.

'CHAIRSIDE'/'IN-SURGERY' BLEACHING

Chairside bleaching involves the use of high concentration (30–38%) hydrogen peroxide, sometimes together with heat applied both inside and outside the tooth. This technique involves the use of a material that is about 10 times the concentration of hydrogen peroxide released from 10% carbamide peroxide and is well above EU limits.

Rubber dam or light-cured dam must be used, given the caustic nature of the bleaching agent. If this aggressive clinical technique is used inside the tooth, the root filling must be carefully sealed off and care taken to avoid penetration of the bleaching gel through to the periodontal ligament. The high concentration hydrogen peroxide used may damage the periodontal ligament and compromise the clinical outcome. About 2% of teeth have a defect at the enamel–cementum junction and very high concentration material may damage the periodontal ligament cells if it leaches out in that area. External resorption has been reported with this approach, which, in effect, burns the periodontal ligament due to the very high concentration of hydrogen peroxide and heat. Inside/outside bleaching uses a material that is one-tenth of the concentration that is involved in chairside bleaching (Table 3.1) and is biologically benign as well as legal under EU law.

'RESTORATIVE' ALTERNATIVES TO BLEACHING NON-VITAL, DISCOLOURED TEETH (see also Table 3.2)

VENEERS

The placement of a veneer on a deeply discoloured anterior tooth will not provide a satisfactory result. The underlying discolouration is often most

---

TABLE 3.2 SUMMARY OF THE MANAGEMENT OF DISCOLOURED NON-VITAL ANTERIOR TEETH: FROM LEAST TO MOST INVASIVE

Review

Inside/outside bleaching with 10% carbamide peroxide

Walking bleach technique

10% carbamide peroxide releases 3.5% hydrogen peroxide

Sodium perborate and water releases 7% hydrogen peroxide

Sodium perborate and 18% hydrogen peroxide mixed together as a paste releases approximately 25% hydrogen peroxide

External bleaching

Chairside bleaching or home bleaching or a combination of both

Chairside bleaching using heat and a high concentration (30–38%) of hydrogen peroxide (highest risk of resorption)

Restorative techniques

Veneers – direct composite

Veneers – indirect composite

Porcelain veneers

Crown, with or without a post

Extraction and prosthetic replacement

(Least destructive → Most destructive)

noticeable in the cervical region where, after preparation, there is very little, if any, enamel to conceal the underlying dentine and the veneer has to be at its thinnest in that area. To mask the discolouration, it may be necessary to produce a thick over-contoured veneer, including an opaque layer, which compromises the appearance of the veneer and will not match the other incisors. Conversely, preparation for a veneer involving greater tooth reduction in the cervical area exposes a significant amount of discoloured dentine. It is common to find that discolouration gets worse the deeper the preparation, as dark dentine, in the cervical region, is no longer masked by the translucent enamel and the darkest dentine is nearest the pulp space.

A thick opaque veneer placed on a discoloured tooth will not match the adjacent more translucent teeth. The life expectancy of a thick veneer bonded to deep, discoloured dentine is uncertain. What is clear is that once the patient has had a veneer, the tooth will have been weakened further by up to 30% and the veneer will require a lifetime of maintenance, with the possibility of the further loss of tooth tissue, as and when, the veneer needs to be replaced.

CROWNS AND POST CROWNS

Preparations for crowns are destructive of the remaining tooth tissue. Preparation of a root-filled tooth for a conventional crown often results in a post being necessary to support a replacement core. Such an approach does not address the discolouration within the remaining root dentine. Gingival recession frequently exposes the margin of the crown and the discoloured root dentine. This is likely especially in a young patient when full maturation of the gingival tissues is likely to result in an unsightly gingival appearance. The esthetic issues associated with the provision of a single anterior crown, in particular a post crown, are well documented.

An aggressive, indirect restorative approach to the management of discoloured dead teeth weakens greatly the remaining tooth tissues, is biologically and financially costly, and may result in catastrophic root failure sooner rather than later. Recent developments in tooth-coloured resin bonded post systems have not overcome all the inherent structural or strength disadvantages of the post crown approach to dealing with these esthetic problems.

Inside/outside bleaching has reduced dramatically the incidence of unacceptable appearance of dead discoloured teeth. It removes the discolouration while maintaining the structure of the tooth. This is particularly important when a high lip line exposes the gingival margins.

PATIENTS' FAQS

Q. What causes tooth discolouration?

A. Tooth discolouration is caused by external (extrinsic) or internal (intrinsic) colourants or a combination of both (Table 3.3).

Q. What happens during bleaching?

A. Hydrogen peroxide penetrates through the enamel and dentine reacting with the discolouration within the tooth. Discolourations, including those on external tooth surfaces, are oxidized. Discolourations in enamel usually bleach relatively quickly while those in dentine usually take much longer to bleach.

Q. Are there any contraindications to bleaching teeth?

A. Yes. Existing fillings, veneers and crowns in the same or opposing jaw will not change colour. If tooth-coloured restorations match the existing teeth before bleaching, they will appear darker after the natural teeth have been bleached. This may mean that existing restorations, veneers or crowns may need to be replaced following bleaching. This may add greatly to the cost of treatment. Please ask your dentist to check for these before any bleaching is done.

Q. How much will it cost?

A. This varies according to the system being used, the severity of the problem, the condition of the discoloured teeth and the amount of time and material needed to achieve a satisfactory result. Please ask your dentist for a quotation.

Q. Will I have to sleep with the mouthguard in position?

A. Sleeping with the mouthguard in position is the most effective way of keeping the bleaching gel in contact with the teeth for prolonged periods of time. If this is a problem, and provided the loaded tray can be worn for at least 2 hours each day, bleaching will be effective but will take longer than would otherwise be the case.

Q. Are there any side effects?

A. The majority of patients suffer some tooth sensitivity during treatment. This resolves usually within a few days once bleaching has stopped. If the teeth are sensitive before bleaching, they will probably become more sensitive during bleaching. There have been no reports of long-term side effects of using tray or mouthguard bleaching with 10% carbamide peroxide. Even prolonged (6–9 months) use of this nightguard type of bleaching has been shown to be safe with no teeth needing root fillings or being damaged in any other way.

Q. Can sensitivity be reduced?

A. There are a number of ways of controlling sensitivity. Desensitizing toothpastes (usually those containing 5% potassium nitrate) can be used for 2 weeks prior to bleaching. Alternatively, desensitizing toothpaste can be placed in the mouthguard and applied for about 30 minutes before each period of bleaching. The toothpaste is then replaced with the bleaching gel. To limit the risk of sensitivity, the mouthguard with the bleaching gel may be worn for 1–2 hours only, rather than overnight. If the teeth are sensitive prior to bleaching, the gel should not be applied more than once a day and the mouthguard should be worn only for a few hours. Higher concentration hydrogen peroxide bleaching agents or those composed of 16% or 22%, carbamide peroxide, should not be used.

Q. Which toothpaste should be used when bleaching?

A. There is some evidence that brushing with toothpaste containing 5% potassium nitrate for 2 weeks prior to bleaching helps reduce the risk of sensitivity. Normal toothpaste is usually used during bleaching. NO toothpaste can bleach teeth but brushing with a good quality toothpaste can help reduce future stain formation.

Q. How long will bleaching take?

A. This depends on the cause of the discolouration and on patient compliance. It usually takes between 2 and 6 weeks of nightguard ('at home') bleaching for normal teeth to become lighter. Tobacco discolouration takes 3–6 months to bleach provided the patient stops smoking. Yellow/brown tetracycline discolouration may take up to 9 months to bleach. Deeply coloured blue/grey tetracycline discolouration is very difficult to bleach satisfactorily but there is usually some improvement with very prolonged bleaching (more than 9 months).

Q. Is chairside (also known as 'power' or 'in-surgery') bleaching better than nightguard vital ('home') bleaching?

A. The short answer is no. There is very limited scientific evidence supporting the long-term efficacy of light assisted chairside bleaching. The gold standard is nightguard vital bleaching using 10% carbamide peroxide. This method has the American Dental Association (ADA) seal of approval. Light assisted chairside bleaching may be useful for patients who are unable to tolerate wearing a mouthguard and in rare situations in which a 'kick-start' to bleaching might be advantageous.

Q. How long does bleaching last?

A. The effects of NgVB last on average 2–3 years before there is any noticeable deterioration. The colour change can remain stable for up to 7 years, but bleached teeth may need some 'touching up' or 'top-up bleaching' at 2–3 yearly intervals. If additional bleaching is required, the time taken is normally much less than that required for the initial bleaching. As a general rule, 'top up' bleaching takes 1 night for each week taken to complete the initial bleaching.

Q. What is the best material to use?

A. The most extensively researched material is 10% carbamide peroxide, releasing 3.5% hydrogen peroxide. The typical presentation is a thick gel for use in a customized mouthguard made from an accurate impression of the teeth.

Q. Why not use over-the-counter products as advertised on TV and in magazines?

A. Bleaching is managed best by a dentist who can diagnose the cause of the discolouration, assess the risks of any possible adverse effects and supervise bleaching (which may be part of more extensive treatment). This helps avoid colour mismatching of teeth and restorations. Many of the over-the-counter products have no proof of their safety or efficacy. Some products contain acids that may etch and damage the teeth and others contain titanium dioxide, as used in white paints. The titanium dioxide may appear to 'whiten' teeth, but the effect is almost always very short-lived. Many of the claims made in respect of over-the-counter products are misleading. 'Boil and bite' mouthguards for use with over-the-counter bleaching gels do not fit well. As a consequence they can be uncomfortable and may fail to protect the gel from deactivation by the saliva, thereby producing disappointing results.

Q. Are whitening toothpastes effective?

A. Whitening toothpastes primarily only remove superficial stains. Most supposedly whitening toothpastes contain only 0.1% hydrogen peroxide. None of these toothpastes have been shown to be effective at bleaching intrinsic discolouration. Regular toothpaste used together with a proper brushing technique is equally as effective as more expensive 'whitening toothpastes' at removing superficial tooth stains.

Q. How much peroxide gel is swallowed during bleaching with a mouthguard?

A. About 25% of the carbamide peroxide in the tray is swallowed. Most of the hydrogen peroxide that escapes from the tray is immediately inactivated by saliva before it is swallowed. Exposure to hydrogen peroxide is at its highest when the nightguard is inserted initially. The exposure reduces rapidly over time.

Q. Is swallowing hydrogen peroxide harmful?

A. Not at all. Most of the hydrogen peroxide released into the mouth during bleaching is inactivated immediately by normal saliva before being swallowed. Any gel that is swallowed is inactivated in the stomach. Any hydrogen peroxide that is absorbed and enters the circulation is very quickly and effectively inactivated by the red blood cells.

TABLE 3.3   CAUSES OF TOOTH DISCOLOURATION

Colour	Cause
Extrinsic colourants	
Brown or black	Tea/coffee/iron
Yellow or brown	Poor oral hygiene/tea
Yellow/brown/black	Tobacco/marijuana
Green/orange/black/brown	Bacteria
Red/purple/brown	Red wine
Intrinsic colourants	
Grey/brown/black	Pulp death with haemorrhage
Yellow/grey/brown	Pulp necrosis without haemorrhage
Brown/grey/black	Endodontic or other (e.g. amalgam) materials within the tooth
Yellow/brown	Pulpal obliteration/sclerosis
Brown/white lines/spots	Fluorosis. Excessive fluoride swallowed during tooth development
Black	Sulphur
Brown or grey	Minocycline taken after tooth formation (adult teeth)
Yellow/brown/grey/blue	Tetracycline taken during tooth development
	Doxycycline after tooth formation
	(Remember: 'yellow/brown will bleach; blue/grey may bleach')
Pink	Internal resorption
Grey/brown/black	Dental caries
Yellow/brown	Ageing
Other causes of discolouration	
Yellow/brown	Amelogenesis imperfecta
Brown/violet/yellow brown	Dentinogenesis imperfecta
Brown	Inborn errors of metabolism, e.g. phenylketonuria
Black	Porphyria

Further reading

Baldwin DC. Appearance and aesthetics in oral health. Community Dent Oral Epidemiol 1980;8:244–56.

Barbosa CM, Sasaki RT, Flório FM, Basting RT. Influence of in situ post-bleaching times on resin composite shear bond strength to enamel and dentin. Am J Dent 2009;22(6):387–92.

Dawson PF, Sharif MO, Smith AB, Brunton PA. A clinical study comparing the efficacy and sensitivity of home vs combined whitening. Oper Dent 2011;36(5):460–6.

Friedman S, Rotstein I, Libfield H, et al. Incidence of external root resorption and aesthetic results in 58 bleached pulpless teeth. Endod Dent Traumatol 1988;4:23–6.

Hasson H, Ismail AI, Neiva G. Home-based chemically-induced whitening of teeth in adults. Cochrane Database Syst Rev 2006;(4):CD006202.

Haywood VB. Frequently asked questions about bleaching. Compend Contin Educ Dent 2003;24:324–38.

Haywood VB, Heymann HO. Nightguard vital bleaching. Quintessence Int 1989;20:173–6.

Haywood VB, Leonard RH, Neilson CF, Brunson WD. Effectiveness, side effects and long-term status of nightguard vital bleaching. J Am Dent Assoc 1994;125:1219–26.

Heithersay GS. Invasive cervical resorption: an analysis of potential predisposing factors. Quintessence Int 1999;30:83–95.

Heithersay GS, Dahlstrom SW, Marrin PD. Incidence of invasive cervical resorption in bleached root filled teeth. Aus Dent J 1994;39:82–7.

Heymann HO. Tooth whitening: facts and fallacies. Br Dent J 2005;198(8):514.

Kelleher MG. The 'Daughter Test' in aesthetic ('esthetic') or cosmetic dentistry. Dent Update 2010;37(1):5–11.

Kelleher MG, Djemal S, Al-Khayatt AS, et al. Bleaching and bonding for the older patient. Dent Update 2011;38(5):294–6, 298–300, 302–3.

Kelleher M. The law is an ass: ethical and legal issues surrounding the bleaching of young patients' discoloured teeth. Fac Dental J 2014;5(2):56–67.

Kugel G, Gerlach RW, Aboushala A, et al. Long-term use of 6.5% hydrogen peroxide bleaching strips on tetracycline stain: a clinical study. Compend Contin Educ Dent 2011;32(8):50–6.

Leonard RH Jr, Bentley C, Eagle JC, et al. Nightguard vital bleaching: a long term study on efficacy, shade retention, side effects, and patient perceptions. J Esthet Restor Dent 2001;13:357–69.

Leonard RH, Van Haywood B, Caplan DJ, Tart ND. Nightguard vital bleaching of tetracycline-stained teeth: 90 months post treatment. J Esthet Restor Dent 2003;15:142–52.

Matis BA, Hamdan YS, Cochran MA, Eckert GJ. A clinical evaluation of a bleaching agent used with and without reservoirs. Oper Dent 2002;27:5–11.

Matis BA, Wang Y, Jiang T, Eckert GJ. Extended at-home bleaching of tetracycline-stained teeth with different combinations of carbamide peroxide. Quintessence Int 2002;33:645–55.

Meireles SS, Heckmann SS, Leida FL, et al. Efficacy and safety of 10% and 16% carbamide peroxide tooth-whitening gels: a randomized clinical trial. Oper Dent 2008;33(6):606–12.

Nathwani NS, Kelleher M. Minimally destructive management of amelogenesis imperfecta and hypodontia with bleaching and bonding. Dent Update 2010;37(3):170–2, 175–6, 179.

Nutting EB, Poe GS. Chemical bleaching of discoloured endodontically treated teeth. Dent Clin North Am 1967;655–62.

Patel V, Kelleher M, McGurk M. Clinical use of hydrogen peroxide in surgery and dentistry – why is there a safety issue? Br Dent J 2010;208(2):61–6.

Poyser NJ, Kelleher MG, Briggs PF. Managing discoloured non-vital teeth: The inside/outside bleaching technique. Dent Update 2004;31(4):204–10, 213–14.

Ritter AV, Leonard RH, St George AJ, et al. Safety and stability of nightguard vital bleaching 9–12 years post treatment. J Esthet Restor Dent 2002;14:275–85.

Rosenstiel SF, Gegauff AG, Johnson WM. Randomised clinical trial of the efficacy and safety of a home bleaching procedure. Quintessence Int 1996;27:413–24.

Russell CM, Dickinson GL, Johnson MH, et al. Dentist-supervised home bleaching with ten per cent carbamide peroxide gel: a six month study. J Esthet Dent 1996;8:177–82.

Settembrini L, Gultz J, Kaim J, Scherer W. A technique for bleaching non-vital teeth: inside/outside bleaching. J Am Dent Assoc 1997;128:1283–4.

Spasser HF. A simple bleaching technique using sodium perborate. New York State Dent J 1961;27:332–4.

Sulieman M, MacDonald E, Rees JS, et al. Tooth bleaching by different concentrations of carbamide peroxide and hydrogen peroxide whitening strips: an in vitro study. J Esthet Restor Dent 2006;18(2):93–100, discussion 101.

World Health Organization. Oral Health for the 21st Century. Geneva: WHO; 1994.

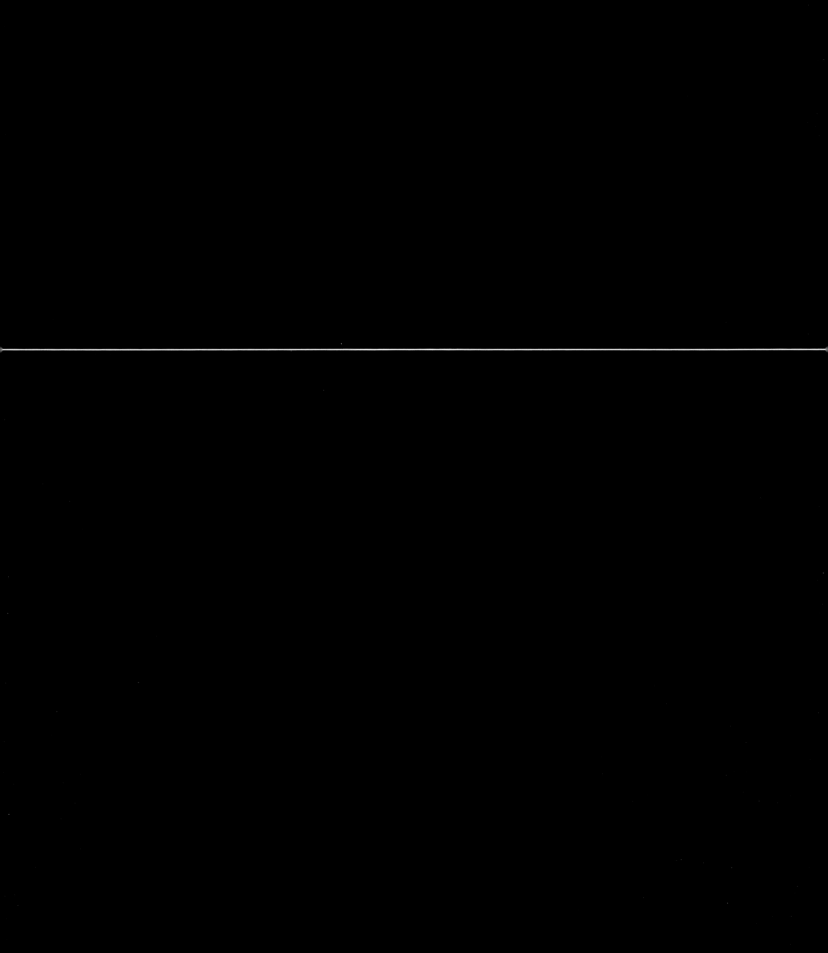

CHAPTER 4

Direct Anterior Esthetic Dentistry With Resin Composites

A. DOZIC, H. DE KLOET

INTRODUCTION

Due to the excellent adhesion to enamel and dentine, and the esthetics and adaptability of resin composite dental restorative materials, it is possible to place resin composite restorations directly in the oral cavity, preserving a maximum quantity of healthy tooth tissue as compared to many alternative indirect methods. The goal of this chapter is to show the care planning required and detailed operative procedures involved with handling resin composites, focusing on techniques used to achieve an optimal esthetic outcome with minimally invasive procedures. The underpinning minimally invasive care philosophy is based upon the remit that the ultimate esthetic benefits of the outcome must be superior to the operative and biological risks taken. In other words, the benefits must outweigh the risks.

The cases presented in this chapter have been selected from many patients complaining of compromised esthetics. These patients decided to be treated with direct resin techniques after careful care planning and extensive explanations/discussions of advantages, disadvantages and eventual risks of all different treatment options. Several cases are described in detail in order to share the pragmatic restorative approach and to encourage dentists to consider direct resin composite as a material of choice in many cases of compromised anterior appearance.

Many clinical situations could be managed with a direct resin composite minimally invasive approach instead of depending on orthodontic or fixed prosthodontic methods. Examples include widening of a narrow upper jaw (Fig. 4.1), closing diastemata (Fig. 4.2), replacing lost tooth substance in cases of severe erosion and wear (Fig. 4.3), reshaping teeth to camouflage crowding (Fig. 4.4), masking gingival recession and interdental 'black triangles' after the periodontal treatment (Fig. 4.5), refurbishing technically acceptable but unesthetic fixed prosthodontic restorations (Fig. 4.6), remodelling dislocated incisors, canines and premolars (Fig. 4.7), replacement of missing teeth (Fig. 4.8), masking discolourations (Fig. 4.9) and reshaping teeth with developmental disorders (Fig. 4.10).

DECISION MAKING

Appropriate treatment decisions can be achieved between the patient and the dentist/dental team through verbal and visual communication.

VERBAL COMMUNICATION

Before any esthetic treatment takes place, the dentist must be sure that the hopes and expectations of the patient have been understood fully and that they are aware of the possible outcome and risks of any potential rectifying treatment.[1-3]

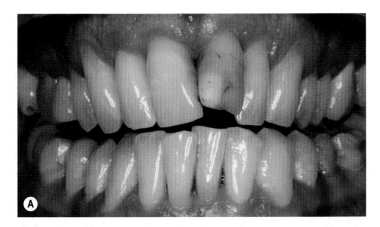

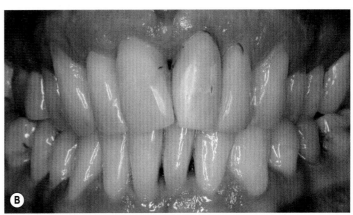

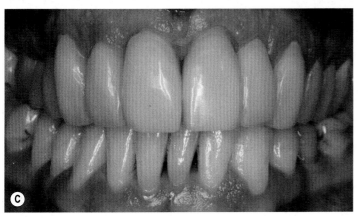

Fig. 4.1 A 38-year-old male patient with tapered maxillary arch form, moderate overbite, midline displacement and restored anterior teeth (#21 endodontically treated) has expressed a wish for an esthetic improvement to his smile. (A) Unesthetic appearance of the maxillary anterior teeth. (B) The first phase of treatment was to enhance colour of #21 and to correct the shape and position of the two central incisors. (C) One-and-a-half years later, the patient asked for further esthetic correction. This was accomplished by placing direct resin composite facings/veneers from #14 to #25.

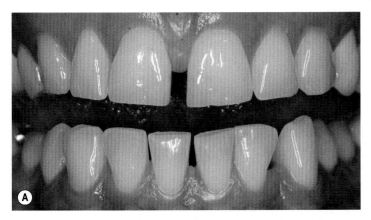

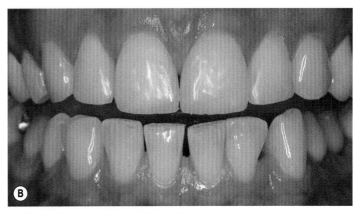

Fig. 4.2 A central diastema can be an unacceptable feature to many patients. To achieve optimal esthetics, it is sometimes advisable to reshape minimally all four incisors to prevent the excessive widening of the central incisors leading to a loss of proportion for these teeth. (A) The diastema is caused by a mild hypoplasia of the upper incisors. For that reason orthodontics was not the first choice solution for this 54-year-old female. (B) By removing 0.5 mm of the distal surface of the central incisors, enough space was created to widen all four incisors and a harmonic distribution of the maxillary anterior teeth was achieved.

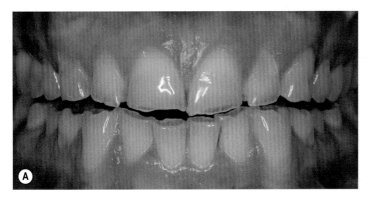
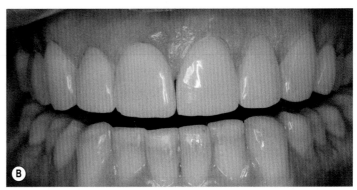

Fig. 4.3 Wear and erosion can cause not only functional problems, but also an unesthetic appearance. Once the cause has been dealt with, minimally invasive operative dental treatment may be necessary to prevent further loss of tooth substance. (A) The main complaint by this 24-year-old male was sensitivity of almost all his teeth, anterior and posterior, together with the sharp incisal edges. (B) In this case, direct resin composite was used to restore the original form and function. In the future it will be possible to treat posterior teeth individually with more definitive and invasive restorations if necessary.

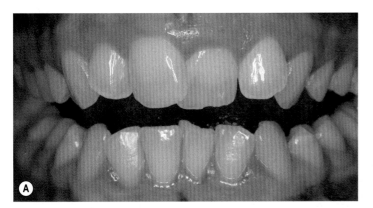
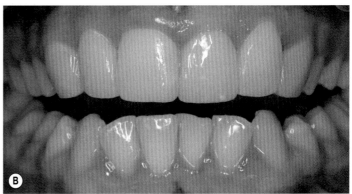

Fig. 4.4 The main reason for dental crowding causing an esthetic concern is the uneven light distribution among the upper incisors. If there is a stable occlusion and a disinterest in pursuing orthodontic correction, a pragmatic, minimally invasive solution using direct resin composite build-ups can satisfy many patients. (A) A 3 mm arch length discrepancy resulted in protrusion of #11 and #22, rotation of #12 and retrusion of #13, #21 and #23 in this 35-year-old female. (B) By thinning minimally the buccal enamel of the protruded and rotated teeth, shortening the incisal edges of the retruded teeth and reducing the central incisors mesially slightly, it was possible to create aligned upper teeth.

Communication ladder

- Patient's verbal evaluation of their esthetic concerns and the impact of this problem on their daily life.
- Patient's evaluation of their esthetic wishes, expectations and requirements.
- Dentist's recognition of the clinical problem.
- Evaluation of the technical possibilities and risks of different treatment options.

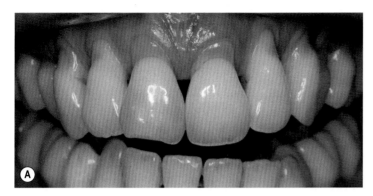
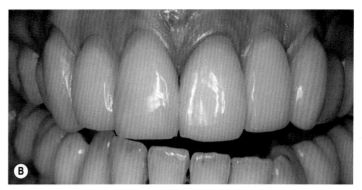

Fig. 4.5 Periodontal surgery aims to improve the periodontal health but can jeopardize the esthetics of a smile. (A) Recession in this case not only resulted in compromised esthetics but also in wear, discolouration and sensitivity of the exposed root surfaces. The black interproximal triangles were the most important reason to seek further restorative treatment for this 42-year-old female. (B) Without removing any tooth substance the natural anatomical crowns were lengthened towards the new gingival level. The original shape of the tooth crowns was restored in resin composite to the current gingival margin. Gingival shade indirect and direct composites now exist to enable a gingival effect.

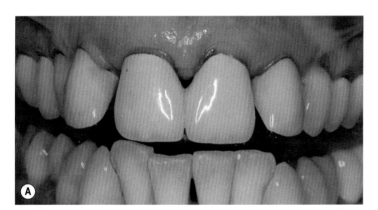
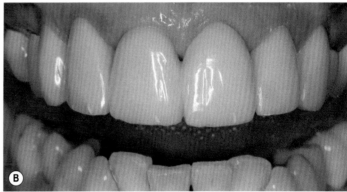

Fig. 4.6 In many cases, so-called 'permanent' restorations become unesthetic after several years in situ. (A) Five-year-old crowns made from porcelain fused to metal were a social problem for this 57-year-old woman, who was reluctant to smile in public. (B) After removing the cervical porcelain and metal, an opaque colour modifier (Kolor + Plus, Kerr) and opaque resin composite were used to reach a satisfactory cervical result.

- Estimation of the biological costs, i.e. the amount of tooth substance to be removed, long-term prognosis of the teeth (pulp vitality) and of the restoration, failure rates and future consequences.

- Dentist's graded judgment of the current appearance and that of the expected esthetic outcome. For example, the current appearance may be judged as 5 and the esthetic outcome judged between 7 and 8, out of 10. Using this subjective judgment method the dentist can set up the patient's expectations on a par with what is achievable realistically, to overcome future disappointment or disagreement.[3]

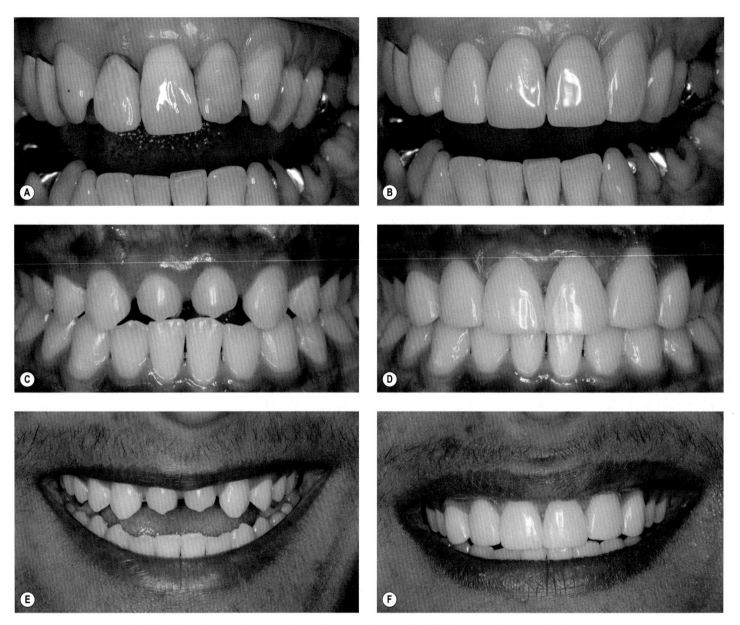

Fig. 4.7 Missing incisors (agenesis, trauma) can create severe esthetic issues, even when a diastema is closed by orthodontic treatment. (A) Tooth #21 was lost in an accident 40 years before the photograph was taken. It resulted in an asymmetrical, unesthetic look at the age of 56. (B) The left lateral is changed into a central, #23 in tooth #22 position and the first premolar is altered visually to appear like a canine. To make the esthetic outcome more pleasing, #11 and #12 (porcelain crown) have been treated with direct resin composite facings. (C) When two or more front teeth are lost by trauma, orthodontic treatment alone may not be sufficient to create an acceptable final result. In children, auto-transplantation may be a treatment option to help compensate for the loss of upper front teeth. (D) Two lower premolars were used to create central incisors, the canines changed into laterals and the first premolars into canines. (E) The smile of the patient, prior to this minimally invasive adhesive dentistry, was atypical and unesthetic. (F) After the treatment this 14-year-old boy was pleased with the final result.

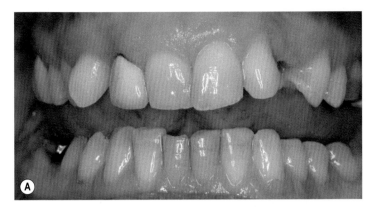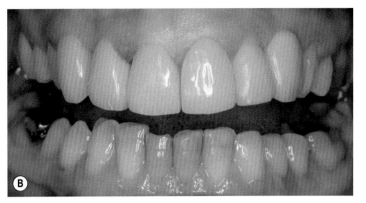

Fig. 4.8   Sometimes orthodontics may not be the first treatment choice, especially when a tooth is lost at an older age. (A) Tooth #23 was lost 10 years earlier due to trauma (root fracture) and the fixed adhesive partial prosthesis made subsequently debonded many times in this 47-year-old female. (B) To enhance the esthetics, not only was a direct resin composite adhesive bridge constructed, but also the remaining anterior teeth were treated with direct resin composite facings.

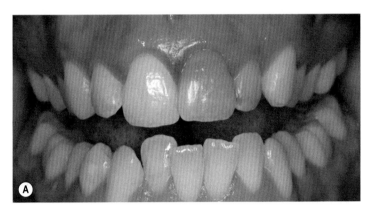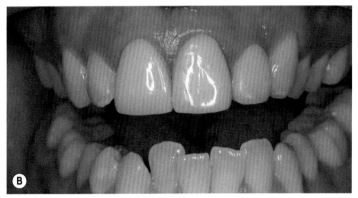

Fig 4.9   Discolouration of teeth has, in many cases, an endodontic cause (see **Chapter 1**). Non-vital bleaching is the first treatment option (see **Chapters 2 and 3**). When this is not successful, a direct facing/ veneer can be used to mask the discoloured tooth surface. (A) The discoloured central incisor #21 was protruded thus permitting the placement of direct labial veneers on the adjacent incisors in a 32-year-old male. (B) Following this care plan, there is less need to cut back the tooth to mask the discolouration. In other words, the more #11 is built up, the less invasively #21 has to be cut back.

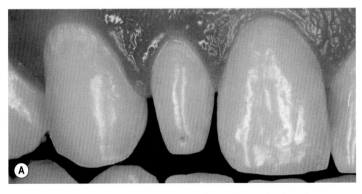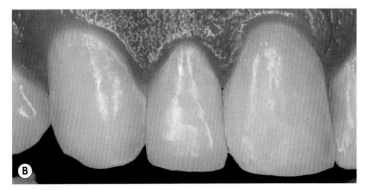

Fig. 4.10   Hypoplasia of lateral incisors is a common phenomenon and can compromise anterior esthetics. (A) Sometimes it can be necessary to build up the neighbouring teeth, but in the case of this 22-year-old male, there was an ideal space to create a natural, well-proportioned lateral incisor. (B) In most cases with hypoplastic incisors, it is wise not only to build up the mesial and distal surfaces, but also to make a labial facing because the hypoplasia includes the buccal surface too.

VISUAL COMMUNICATION

A relatively simple, non-invasive method to improve communication with patients is to show them, before any operative intervention is carried out, the esthetic result that could be achieved with the suggested treatment.

Digital imaging

Using digital imaging and image processing, a range of esthetic adjustments and outcomes can be illustrated outside the oral cavity (Fig. 4.11). However, it is important to acquire clinical photographs, after gaining full written consent, with controlled lighting conditions (e.g. ring flash or ambient lighting)[4-6] in order to have a faithful and standardized representation of any esthetic changes in the natural environment.

The standardized photograph of the original clinical situation can be adjusted digitally to present a multitude of esthetic results, using image processing software (e.g. Corel PaintShop Pro X4), a graphic pen tablet (Wacom Bamboo One), and the methodology developed by the authors.[7,8]

Direct resin composite mock-up

This refers to pre-treatment resin composite build-up without etching/bonding. One of the greatest advantages of the direct, intra-oral mock-up is the possibility

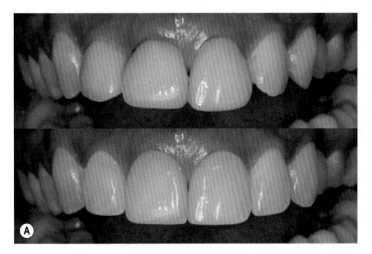
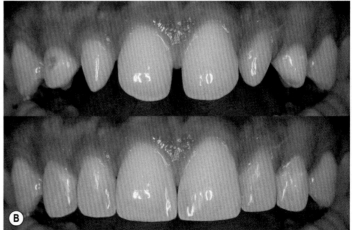

Fig. 4.11 Dental imaging is an ideal way to present the 'post-treatment' results to the patient for comment and analysis. The patient can judge the outcome and communicate their wishes precisely before the actual treatment is carried out, and can also get acquainted with the new situation. (A) Recently made porcelain veneers did not fulfil the esthetic desires of this 18-year-old woman. Dental imaging was used to understand more fully what her expectations were. (B) In this separate hypoplasia case, dental imaging was used to see if the planned build-ups could offer a natural looking distribution of tooth width across the front teeth.

of having a real-life esthetic dry run, prior to the actual start of any invasive treatment, of the restoration outcome in terms of size, shape and colour.[9,10] Moreover, a patient can visualize and experience the changes in their mouth and offer a judgment before any physical treatment commences. This close patient–dentist interaction will help increase trust and the acceptance of the final post-treatment esthetic alterations.[3] Finally, the dentist can use this opportunity to discover possible technical operative challenges that will have to be overcome during the treatment.

This procedure is an excellent way to assess the effect of ambient light conditions on treatment outcomes (the objective daily conditions under which humans perceive each other's teeth and surrounding tissues). Moreover, photographs of the mock-up can help the dentist and patient judge how tooth/restoration position may influence the surface light reflection and its perception in the original and finally adjusted clinical situations (Fig. 4.12).

Resin composite mock-ups can also be observed under ultra-violet incident lighting to help judge the optical fluorescence matching between the teeth and the selected resin composite shade (Fig. 4.13).

Colour determination

The fundamental colour destination for resin composite restorations can be determined using a VITA shade guide or an electronic device, which measures the full colour spectrum[11,12] (e.g SpectroShade, MHT, Italy) (Fig. 4.14A). The

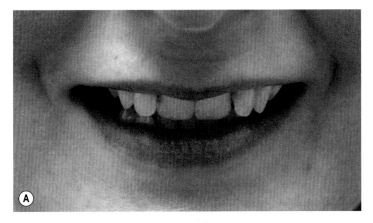
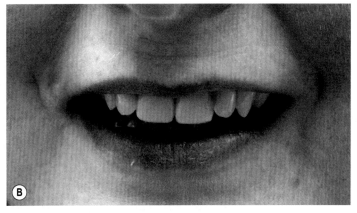

Fig. 4.12 Retroclined and retruded anterior teeth do not catch enough light compared to the other teeth in daylight. (A) In this mild Angle Class II/2 case the centrals appeared discoloured. Photographs are taken with tube luminescent (TL) lighting from the ceiling. (B) With a mock-up (temporary resin composite facings placed without etching) the dentist and patient can judge the effect of the alterations. This procedure is also suitable for the determination of colour.

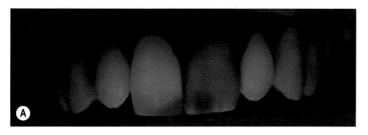
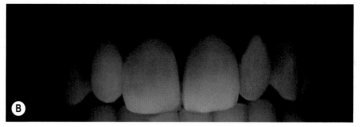

Fig. 4.13 Ultra-violet light makes the internal natural dental fluorescence visible (emission of blue light by radiation with ultra-violet light). There are large differences in fluorescence between teeth and restorative materials. (A) Ultra-violet light revealed two edge-repairs on teeth #11 and #21 and a thin resin composite veneer on #21 that lacked natural fluorescence. (B) When using a resin composite with moderate fluorescence, the new restorations are almost invisible, even under ultra-violet light.

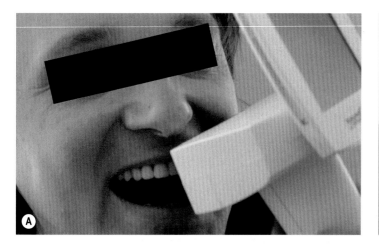
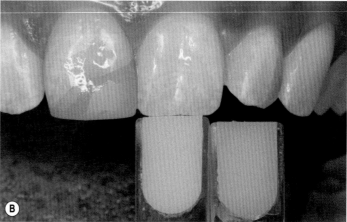

Fig. 4.14 Colour perception and selection is critical, especially when only one tooth is to be treated. (A) Digital means for colour determination (e.g. SpectroShade) can help a dentist judge colours more objectively. (B) In contrast to the standard, commercially produced VITA shade guide made from porcelain, a self-made 'in-house' resin composite shade guide is more versatile.

colour of most contemporary resin composites developed for layering techniques can be selected using layering keys, where the colour and translucency parameters are separated (Fig. 4.14B).[13–15] The finest colour tuning can be accomplished using the polymerized resin composite material itself placed directly on the surface of the teeth to be restored. When resin composite itself is used to determine colour, it is important to respect all optical characteristics of teeth including the relative thickness of the enamel/dentine, hue, chroma, value, translucency and fluorescence (Fig. 4.15).[11–17]

Resin composite build-up

In order to determine the amount of tooth tissue which may have to be removed to create a harmonious and esthetic result (e.g. in a severe crowding case), it can be useful to make a resin composite build-up on a plaster model of the

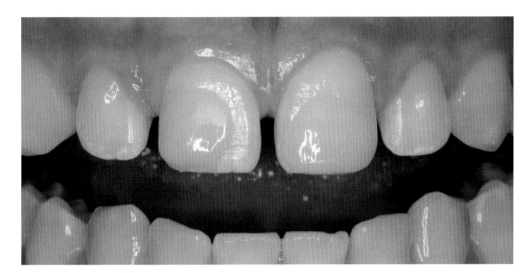

Fig. 4.15 Perhaps the best way to determine the colour of the restoration is to test the selected resin composite on the tooth to be treated, without the use of acid etching. Polymerization and polishing to judge the final colour are mandatory.

original tooth positions. This procedure will be discussed in detail in the clinical section later (see Chapter 5.2, Figs C5.2.9–C5.2.15).

DIRECT ANTERIOR ESTHETICS

The orthodontic correction of anterior mal-occlusions is often considered the least invasive treatment option. However, several aspects of orthodontic treatment require careful consideration.

Orthodontic treatment involves bone remodelling and often a movement of teeth through the alveolar bone. The increased activity of osteoclasts should be considered invasive at a cellular level, as any excessive, uncontrolled activity can lead to excessive bone loss or root resorption.[18,19] Furthermore, patients' discomfort over the duration of fixed orthodontic treatment, and the lack of maintenance and/or effectiveness of patients' oral hygiene procedures, due to the position of orthodontic brackets and retention wires, are often underestimated detrimental factors. The adverse consequences of reduction in oral hygiene compliance during orthodontic treatment are the resulting white-spot carious lesions, which occur in areas of plaque stagnation around brackets, and the associated gingival or periodontal pathologies that need to be managed long after the removal of orthodontic brackets.[20]

Due to extensive research and development of strong and durable dental adhesives and esthetic restorative materials, resin composites can be used for the visual camouflage of abnormally positioned teeth as a direct, minimally invasive alternative to some orthodontic and prosthodontic treatment options. Moreover, direct restorative procedures involving resin composite restorations are often necessary as an adjunct to orthodontic treatment, to complete the final, often more subtle, esthetic results.[21]

The cases described in this chapter were treated with Filtek Supreme XTE layered resin composite system (3M ESPE, USA). This material was heated to 50°C in a composite heater (Ease-it, Rønvig, DK) to reduce its viscosity and thus increase its physical adaptability to the tooth surface during placement. The optical properties of Filtek Supreme XTE are excellent and in most cases the desired colour and translucency were reached using the reddish hue (A), medium value/chroma (2) and the body phase (B) of the composite. This phase of the resin composite has a moderate translucency and is more heavily filled than the enamel phase. That is why the value remains relatively unchanged when the thickness of the material increases. This is a very important quality, especially when varying thicknesses of resin composite need to be added to adjacent teeth. The highly translucent enamel phase (E) was not used frequently by the authors because of the high influence of its thickness on the total value of the restoration. The phenomenon whereby the value of the restoration falls when the thickness of a translucent phase of composite increases has been well described in the dental literature.[22,23] In cases where the whole tooth thickness is to be restored (Class IV), the enamel phase as well as the dentine phase (opaque version) of the resin composite can be very useful. The dentine phase is used to build up the mamelons and the enamel phase to accentuate the presence of mamelons in the incisal region of the treated tooth (Fig. 4.16A–G).

Professionals must be aware of the critical optical behaviour of translucent materials, where colour value decreases with increased material thickness.[22,23] Therefore, it is often not sufficient to use only the thin enamel tab provided by the manufacturer to determine the translucency of the tooth (Fig. 4.16B). It is advisable to make an individualized colour tab, trying out different thicknesses and phases of resin composite until the optimal result is found. The ideal optical result with Filtek Supreme XTE, according to the authors in the cases discussed, was achieved with the moderate translucent, medium opacity resin composite (A2B) on the vestibular (labial) tooth surface, and the highly translucent resin composite added only between the mamelons.

Direct placement of esthetic resin composites can be useful in the minimally invasive management of some clinical cases of tooth wear. Where only anterior teeth are worn, the necessary space for restoration can be achieved by increasing the distance between the antagonist teeth (Dahl principle). Thanks to this well-described phenomenon, selective invasive tooth reduction can be avoided in many cases.[24–26]

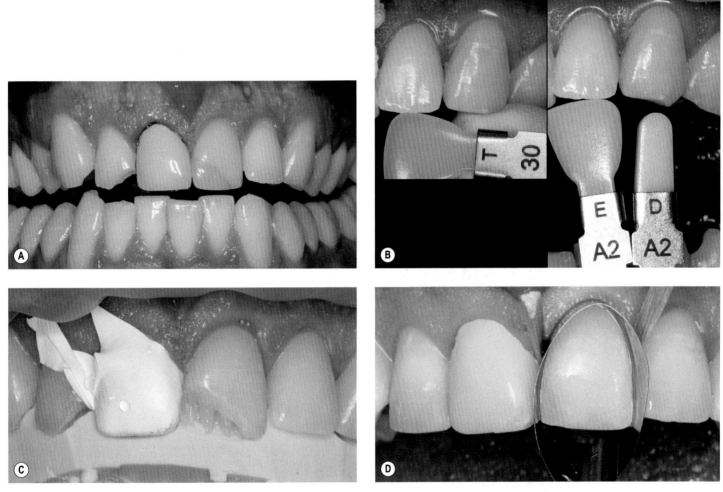

Fig. 4.16 This 30-year-old male patient was not satisfied with the appearance of his crown (#11). He also wished to have his lateral and other central incisor restored with crowns so that his smile would look more harmonious. (A) After clinical evaluation and having discussed all the possible consequences of different treatments, a minimally invasive, pragmatic esthetic solution to restore the lateral and central incisors (#21 and #12) with direct resin composite layering followed by a porcelain crown on #11 was advised and agreed with the patient. (B) Teeth #22 (translucent) and #23 (chromatic) were used to determine the colour and translucency for the Class IV restorations of #21 and #12 using the manufacturer's shade tabs (Ivoclar Vivadent). The transparent tab served to establish the level of transparency in the thinnest incisal portion of the tooth. (C) In this case, a palatal putty impression was used to make an individualized mould/index to aid the direct build-up of the Class IV restorations. The incisal part of the mould was cut out to prevent any interference from the putty index with the shaping process of the mamelons. Teflon tape was used to provide isolation from the adjacent teeth. The mamelon build-ups were accomplished using opaque dentine shade, while the enamel (translucent phase) was applied between them. (D) After the Class IV restoration was completed, the veneering procedure on #21 was facilitated using an AutoMatrix band which served to isolate the tooth from its adjacent neighbours.

Continued

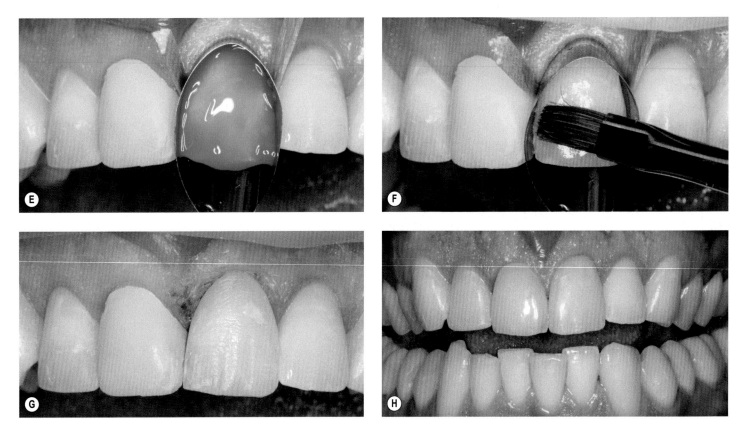

Fig. 4.16 *Continued*   (E) With the AutoMatrix band in place, the bonding procedure was repeated. (F) After etching, rinsing and drying, the adhesive was applied. (G) After the direct resin composite layering procedure, the matrix was removed and the veneer shaped using fine diamond burs. (H) The final appearance of the restored dentition after the veneering of the #12, polishing and replacing the crown on #11.

In a past study of 1007 patients it was observed that 22% had more than 10% of their teeth surfaces worn to an unacceptable degree.[27] The authors therefore concluded that the excessive wear in the younger age group (20–30 years) was due mainly to dental erosion. Above this age, wear was the result of more generalized attrition due to clenching and grinding habits.

In cases of severe tooth wear the treatment rationale must be additive. Resin composite may be the material of choice as it adheres to any tooth surface, which has been shaped by the characteristic wear type. Contrary to this, dental porcelain is a brittle material that needs more tooth preparation to establish smooth and rounded surfaces for support. This makes porcelain a less than adequate material for the minimally invasive treatment of wear, despite its sublime optical properties. This pragmatic approach to the treatment of tooth wear, involving resin composite adhesion to enamel and dentine, has been well described in the literature.[25]

A drawback of the minimally invasive direct resin composite approach is the uncertainty of long-term restoration retention and esthetics, which will be dependent upon the patient's diet, smoking habits, dental hygiene and chewing habits. Therefore, treatment with resin composite cannot be considered as final. Dentists need to review and monitor their patients over subsequent years, continuing non-operative preventive care, oral hygiene advice, and periodic polishing or refurbishment/repair of any damaged or worn restoration surfaces. However, the reparability of resin composites and the fact that treatment is reversible should be considered as advantageous. Moreover, a restoration that can be adjusted simply as many times as needed and with an instant, predictable result that is relatively inexpensive, may be considered the ideal restorative option.[25]

ESSENTIALS

- Due to excellent adhesion and nature-emulating optical properties, resin composites can be used to build up naturally looking restorations directly in the mouth. Some indirect techniques, which are more invasive and more expensive, can therefore be avoided or postponed.

- Handling properties of contemporary resin composites allow for direct shaping and re-shaping in order to mimic the esthetic smile values. Patients who do not wish for an invasive procedure or prolonged orthodontic treatment can be managed successfully with this approach.

- Building up teeth with resin composite is a reversible and constantly optimizing, dynamic process. Other operative techniques are therefore not excluded. If age or wealth of patients is an important issue, restoring with resin composite can provide a very good substitute, prior to planned implant surgery or more invasive, fixed prosthodontics.

PATIENTS' FAQs

Q. How well are resin composite restorations fixed to my teeth? Will they fall off when I chew vigorously?

A. Adhesion of contemporary composites to enamel and dentine is excellent if applied judiciously. Only heavy biting forces could cause chipping of the composite. It is the responsibility of the dentist to establish a correct occlusion and articulation, but it is the patient's responsibility to avoid extreme forces, e.g. nail biting, Sellotape tearing, etc.

Q. Does the appearance of these restorations deteriorate over time and how long will it be before I would need new ones?

A. Resin composites will abrade and stain over time depending on the material type and patients' habits. When an adequate resin composite is chosen and thorough instructions are given to patients, it is the author's experience that the esthetics can remain acceptable up to 10 years or more.

Q. If I decided to have the resin composite removed and to have porcelain restorations or to undergo orthodontic treatment, would this still be possible?

A. If necessary, resin composites can be easily removed from tooth surfaces, leaving healthy tissue underneath. The tooth surface is still suitable for bonding procedures with porcelain and also with new resin composite material and bonding of orthodontic brackets.

Seminal literature

Burke FJT, Kelleher GDM, Wilson N, Bishop K. Introducing the concept of pragmatic esthetics, with special reference to the treatment of tooth wear. J Esthet Restor Dent 2011;23(5): 277–93.
This article shows that resin composite restorations, bonded using a three-step bonding procedure, provide reliable restorations for worn teeth. The esthetic result might not conform to the highest principles of dental esthetics, but represents an effective way of protecting teeth from further tooth surface loss while improving patient-perceived esthetics.

Gresnigt MM, Kalk W, Özcan M. Randomized controlled split-mouth clinical trial of direct laminate veneers with two micro-hybrid resin composites. J Dent 2012;40(9):766–75.
In this article different micro-hybrid composite materials were used to test the survival rate on intact teeth and on teeth with existing restorations. After sandblasting with Co Jet (3M ESPE) there was no significant difference between the two groups.

Rosa M, Zachrisson BU. Integrating space closure and esthetic dentistry in patients with missing maxillary lateral incisors: further improvements. J Clin Orthod 2007;61(9):563–73.
This article describes how one can further improve clinical esthetic results, using orthodontic space closure along with cosmetic finishing using composite materials in patients with missing incisors.

Further reading

Dozic A. Capturing Tooth Color. Electronic Tooth Color Measurement. Thesis, ACTA Dental School, Amsterdam University; 2005.
In order to select the appropriate colour of the resin composite, it can be valuable to measure the colour spectrum of the teeth.

Goldstein CE, Goldstein RE, Garber DA. Imaging in Esthetic Dentistry. Improving Visualization in your Practice. Chicago: Quintessence Publishing; 1998. p. 7–18.
Standardized digital imaging can be used as an effective visualization tool in dentistry.

Kloet de H. Esthetische Tandheelkunde met Facings van Composiet Materiaal. Acta Qual Pract 2006;1(5):26–37.
The patient's expectations should be managed at a safe and realistic level using grades to describe the appearance of the smile before and after actual treatment.

Kois DE, Schmidt KK, Raigrodski AJ. Esthetic templates for complex restorative cases: rationale and management. J Esthet Restor Dent 2008;20:239–50.
Resin composite mock-ups are an excellent method for trying out the shape of the new restorations directly in the mouth.

Talarico G, Morgante E. Psychology of dental esthetics: dental creation and the harmony of the whole. Eur J Esthet Dent 2006;(4):302–12.
Proper care planning is essential for patient satisfaction of the esthetic outcome.

Villarroel M, Fahl N, De Sousa AM, De Oliveira OB. Direct esthetic restorations based on translucency and opacity of composite resins. J Esthet Restor Dent 2011;23:73–88.
Resin composite itself can be used to determine the appearance of planned restorations.

REFERENCES

1. Maio G. Being a physician means more than satisfying patient demands: an ethical review of esthetic treatment in dentistry. Eur J Esthet Dent 2007;2(2):147–51.

2.   Talarico G, Morgante E. Psychology of dental esthetics: dental creation and the harmony of the whole. Eur J Esthet Dent 2006;1(4):302–12.

3.   Kloet de H. Esthetische Tandheelkunde met Facings van Composiet Materiaal. Acta Qual Pract 2006;1(5):26–37.

4.   Bengel W. Mastering Digital Dental Photography. Reproducible Conditions. London: Quintessence Publishing Co; 2006. p. 110–15.

5.   Goldstein RE, Garber DA. Improving aesthetic dentistry through high technology. J Californian Dent Assoc 1994;22(9):23–9.

6.   Goldstein CE, Goldstein RE, Garber DA. Imaging in Esthetic Dentistry. Improving visualization in your practice. Chicago: Quintessence Publishing; 1998. p. 7–18.

7.   Dozic A, de Kloet de H. Improving aesthetics in a narrow jaw with composite, Part I. Dent Today 2011;30(6):108–11.

8.   Dozic A, de Kloet H. Improving aesthetics in a narrow jaw with composite, Part II. Dent Today 2011;30(7):118–22.

9.   Kois DE, Schmidt KK, Raigrodski AJ. Esthetic templates for complex restorative cases: rationale and management. J Esthet Restor Dent 2008;20:239–50.

10.   Roeters J, Kloet de H. Handboek Esthetische Tandheelkunde. Nijmegen: STI; 1998. p. 14–18.

11.   Dozic A. Capturing Tooth Color. Electronic Tooth Color Measurement. Thesis, ACTA Dental School, Amsterdam University, Amsterdam; 2005. p. 23–33.

12.   Chu SJ, Trushkowsky RD, Paravina RD. Dental color matching instruments and systems. Review of clinical and research aspects. J Dent 2010;38(2):2–16.

13.   Baratieri LN, Araujo E, Monteiro S Jr. Color in natural teeth and direct resin composite restorations: essential aspects. Eur J Esthet Dent 2007;2(2):172–86.

14.   Magne P, So WS. Optical integration of interproximal restorations using the natural layering concept. Quintessence Int (Berl) 2008;39(8):633–43.

15.   Dietschi D. Optimizing smile composition and esthetics with resin composites and other conservative esthetic procedures. Eur J Esthet Dent 2008;3(1):274–89.

16.   Vanini L, Mangani F, Klimovskaia O. Conservative Restoration of Anterior Teeth, Part I. Viterbo Italy: ACME English edition; 2005.

17.   Villarroel M, Fahl N, De Sousa AM, De Oliveira OB. Direct esthetic restorations based on translucency and opacity of composite resins. J Esthet Restor Dent 2011;23:73–88.

18.   Pizzo G, Licata ME, Guiglia R, Giuliana G. Root resorption and orthodontic treatment. Review of the literature. Minerva Stomatol 2007;56(1–2):31–44.

19.   Brezniak N, Wasserstein A. Orthodontically induced inflammatory root resorption. Review of the literature. Angle Orthod 2002;72(2):175–84.

20.   Ardu S, Castioni NV, Banbachir N, Krejci I. Minimally invasive treatment of white spot enamel lesions. Quintessence Int (Berl) 2007;38(8):633–6.

21.   Rosa M, Zachrisson BU. Integrating space closure and esthetic dentistry in patients with missing maxillary lateral incisors: further improvements. J Clin Orthod 2007;61(9):563–73.

22. Schmeling M, Meyer-Filho A, Andrada MAC, Baratieri LN. Chromatic influence of value resin composites. Oper Dent 2012;35(1):44–9.

23. Schmeling M, Andrada MAC, Maia HP, Araujo EM. Translucency of value resin composites used to replace enamel in stratified composite restoration techniques. J Esthet Restor Dent 2012;24(1):53–8.

24. Reis A, Higashi C, Loguercio AD. Re-anatomization of anterior eroded teeth by stratification with direct composite resin. J Esthet Restor Dent 2009;21:304–17.

25. Burke FJT, Kelleher GDM, Wilson N, Bishop K. Introducing the concept of pragmatic esthetics, with special reference to the treatment of tooth wear. J Esthet Restor Dent 2011;23(5): 277–93.

26. Mizrahi B. The Dahl principle: creating space and improving the bio-mechanical prognosis for anterior crowns. Quintessence Int (Berl) 2006;37:245–51.

27. Smith BGN, Robb ND. The prevalence of tooth wear in 1007 dental patients. J Oral Rehabil 1996;23:232–9.

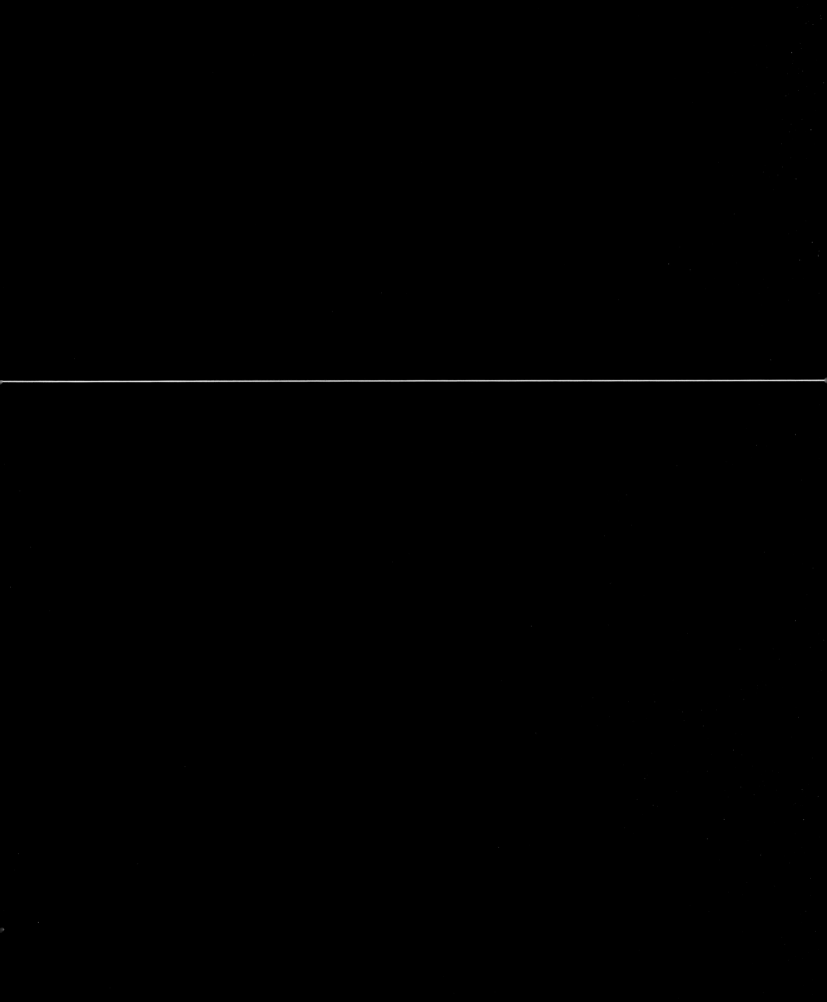

CHAPTER 5

Direct Esthetics: Clinical Cases

H. DE KLOET, A. DOZIC

INTRODUCTION

In this chapter, the technical minimally invasive operating principles discussed in Chapter 4 are illustrated in a series of four clinical cases. In each, the interaction between the patient and the dentist is paramount in managing patient expectations and perceived outcomes. The clinical techniques depicted, although requiring significant levels of manual dexterity and skill, can be gained through practice and attendance on postgraduate master class courses.

CLINICAL CASE 5.1

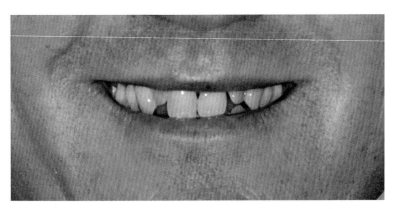

Fig. C5.1.1 A 43-year-old male complained of the poor appearance of his smile and the uneven distribution of his front upper teeth. This affected him adversely to the extent that he was reluctant to smile in public.

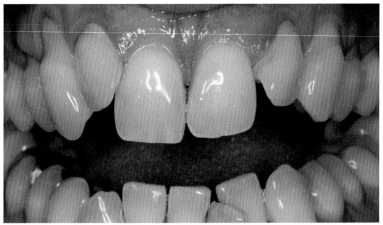

Fig. C5.1.2 After a full assessment of the patient and explanation of the decision making process and potential outcomes, it was clear that direct resin composite restorations would be adequate to fulfil his needs and expectations. In this case it was necessary to remove minimal but sufficient quantities of dental tissue, which would otherwise interfere with achievement of an ideal esthetic result.

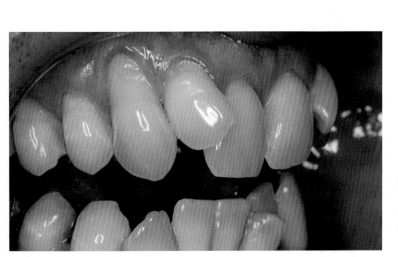

Fig. C5.1.3 In this Class II Division II case, the mesio-labial aspect of the lateral incisors had to be removed. Building up neighbouring teeth is preferable whenever possible to grinding down healthy tooth tissue, but there are situations in which some selective and minimal tooth removal is inevitable. Another reason not to remove tooth substance is the risk of introducing occlusal discrepancies, e.g. labial veneers on lower teeth or in crossbite situations.

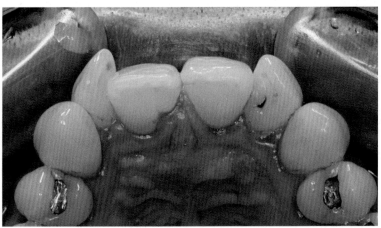

Fig. C5.1.4 An occlusal view which shows clearly the arch length discrepancy in the maxillary central incisor region.

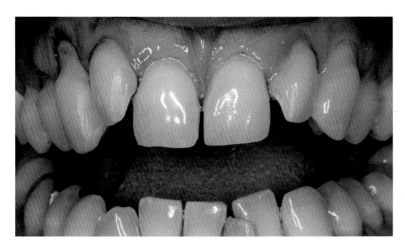

Fig. C5.1.5   The lateral incisors have been ground selectively, guided by the continuing presence of enamel. During this process no local anaesthesia was administered, permitting the patient to discern between enamel and dentine.

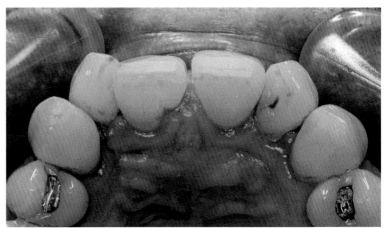

Fig. C5.1.6   Existing restorations that are of good quality, opacity and colour can be maintained and air-abraded preceding the adhesive procedure.[1,2] Insufficient or questionable restorations should be removed, and carious lesions should be managed minimally invasively with suitable excavation procedures. Insufficient restorations located cervically should be maintained in this stage, as they facilitate the placement of rubber dam isolation.

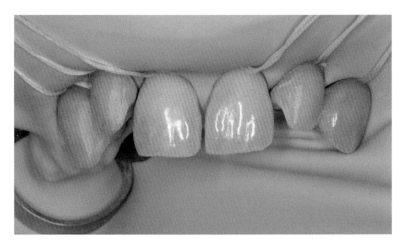

Fig. C5.1.7   For controlled working conditions, rubber dam isolation is advisable in this phase. The prepared teeth can be checked with gingivae retracted, without bleeding or saliva contamination, which compromise visibility and an efficient bonding procedure. Etching and bonding can be performed for all surfaces in one step and there is no danger of contamination of gingivae or mucosa with potentially hazardous chemicals. A prerequisite for reliable bonding is a clean substrate that can be achieved by air abrading with aluminium oxide (27 μm alumina) powder.

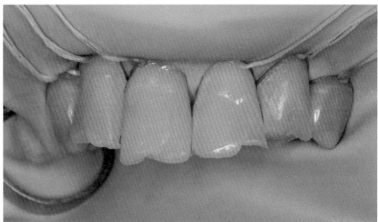

Fig. C5.1.8   A rubber dam clamp is placed on a distally positioned premolar or molar to create a 'dump' where it is easy to perform suction. The tooth surface (enamel and dentine) can be etched effectively or treated with a self-etch bonding system. It is of utmost importance to follow precisely the clinical instructions for the specific product.

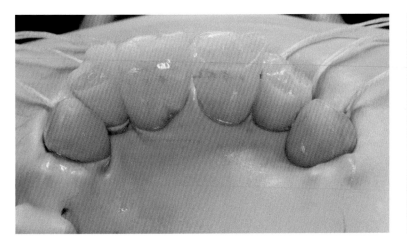

Fig. C5.1.9   Using clear matrix strips (Directa, Sweden), the palatal, incisal and proximal surface restorations are built up incrementally using a strong hybrid resin composite. Diastemata and interdental black triangles are closed and the position/level of the incisal edges established. The excess material is guided towards the incisal edge, where it can be removed more easily. Special care is taken to avoid overhangs in the cervical region. Sometimes it is advisable to make a putty mould/index for the construction of the palatal surface (Chapter 4, Fig. 4.16C), but in most cases a free-hand technique using custom matrices is sufficient. Indeed, in some instances, the rubber dam may prevent the putty index from seating fully, so precluding its use.

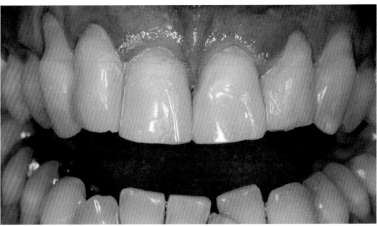

Fig. C5.1.10   Once the basic framework of the restorations has been placed, the restoration contours can be adjusted to the correct length and labial profile. This can best be done after the removal of the rubber dam.

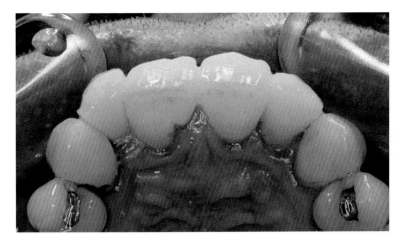

Fig. C5.1.11   Finally, occlusion and articulation are checked. At this stage, any pre-existing insufficient cervical restorations can be removed and the gingival cavities can be modified as necessary.

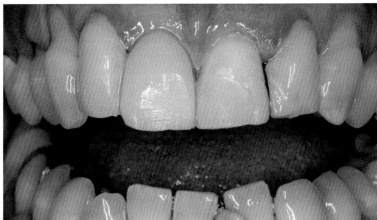

Fig. C5.1.12   The direct resin composite veneers can be placed. A free-hand method is only possible when partial coverage of the labial surface is required. When the planned direct laminate veneer restoration extends to gingival or sub-gingival level, a matrix can be of great help in avoiding contamination during the bonding procedure.

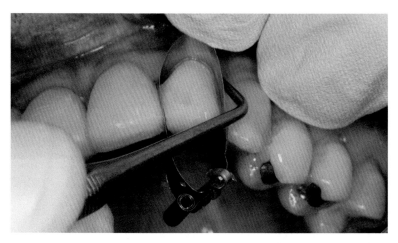

Fig. C5.1.13 A clear matrix (e.g. Contour-Strip, Ivoclar Vivadent) or a stiffer metal matrix used in this case (e.g. AutoMatrix, Dentsply), that can be curved to follow the cervical contour of the tooth to be treated, should be placed carefully using fine flat plastic instruments to guide the matrix into place without traumatizing the gingival tissues.

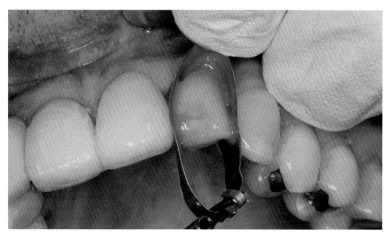

Fig. C5.1.14 The matrix can be supported inter-proximally by wedges or with polymerized resin placed on the outer surface of the matrix. Within the matrix, the bonding procedure is performed once more. In this case, a three-step etch-and-rinse system (Type 1, 4th generation) is used.

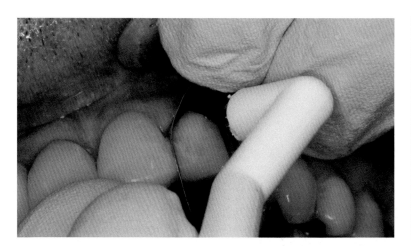

Fig. C5.1.15 Primer and resin are applied separately and polymerized. At this stage, a grey tint can be used in the incisal area to offer a level of translucency. A final composite layer covers the tint so the translucency stays in the depth.

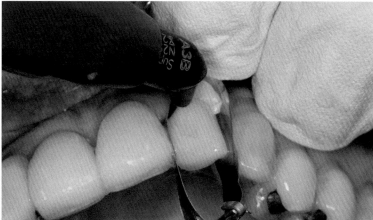

Fig. C5.1.16 The resin composite is ejected slowly and with great care, depending on its viscosity, taking care not to displace the matrix. A high viscosity composite can be heated (e.g. Ease-it composite heater, Rønvig) to make syringing less hazardous. A better flow of resin composite will facilitate its adaptation on the tooth surface and helps prevent the inclusion of air voids.

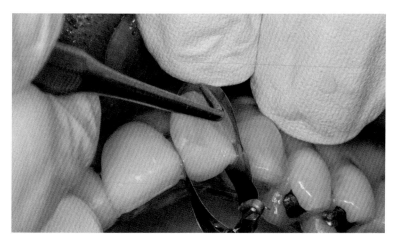

Fig. C5.1.17   The resin composite is spread over the labial surface and adapted in the shallow space between the surface and the matrix with clean metal instruments.

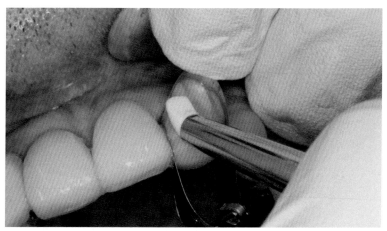

Fig. C5.1.18   The final modelling can be performed with silicone tips (e.g. TPEN2, Micerium). In the cervical part a high chroma, opaque material is adapted and polymerized; in the middle third a shade with less chroma is applied and to the incisal area a more translucent, higher value shade is advisable. The different shades are placed in incremental layers over each other like roof tiles to enable a smooth transition from one to another.[3,4]

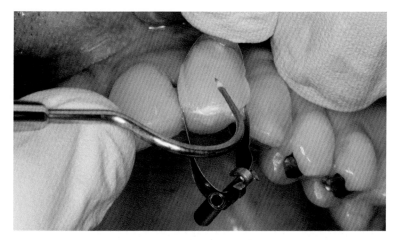

Fig. C5.1.19   If required, special characteristics can be built in with white tints to create chalky spots and cracks; the same can be done with brown and ochre characterizers.

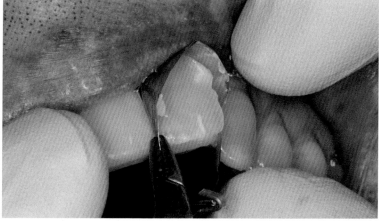

Fig. C5.1.20   After polymerization the matrix is removed, the facing is again photo-polymerized and contoured coarsely to the correct shape. Then the next tooth is veneered.

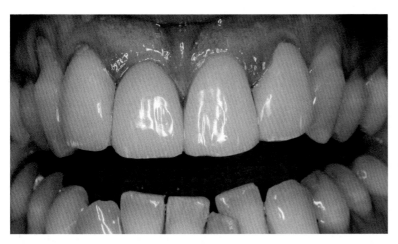

Fig. C5.1.21   Finally, all restorations are sculpted with fine diamond finishing burs, creating surface texture and natural looking incisal edges and embrasures. The polishing is performed using Sof-Lex (3M ESPE) and Politip-P green polishers (Ivoclar Vivadent). The patient is instructed to perform effective oral hygiene.[5]

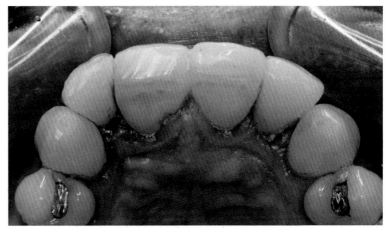

Fig. C5.1.22   The occlusal view reveals the harmonious continuity of the labial surface profile, utilizing the space available.

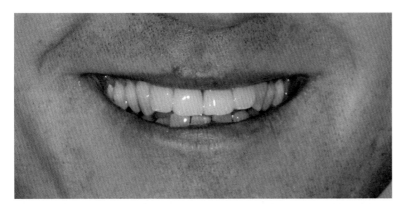

Fig. C5.1.23   The esthetic result was acceptable to the patient and his social boundaries were lifted. It is advisable to recall the patient within 2–3 months to re-assess the patient's preventive behaviour, including checking his oral hygiene/motivation and gingival condition, and to review the restorations and perform any necessary adjustments in shape and to complete the final polishing.

CLINICAL CASE 5.2

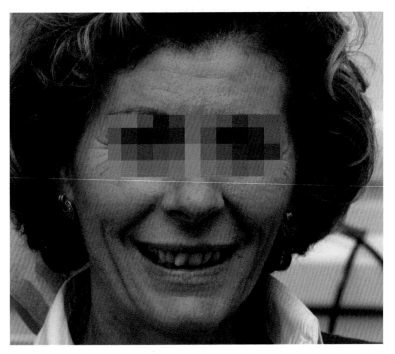

Fig. C5.2.1   Portrait view of a 56-year-old female who was not satisfied with the appearance of her upper front teeth, 2 years after periodontal surgery was completed.

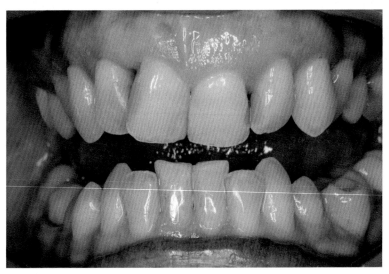

Fig. C5.2.2   Patient's esthetic complaints were related to the unevenness of the gums, the colour of the old restorations, the crowding and the rotated position of the maxillary central incisors.

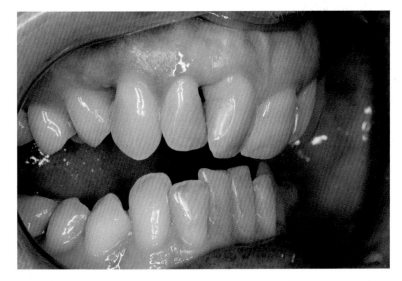

Fig. C5.2.3   Lateral view of the upper front teeth illustrated the rotation and retroclination of the maxillary central incisors.

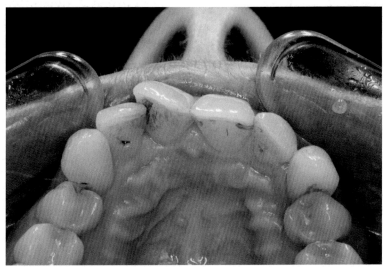

Fig. C5.2.4   Occlusal view of the maxillary front teeth shows clearly the arch length discrepancy.

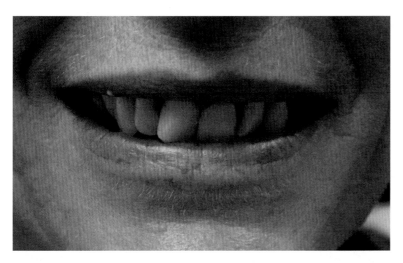

Fig. C5.2.5   Ambient light photograph of the patient's smile where the effects of incident light and casting shadows are visible.

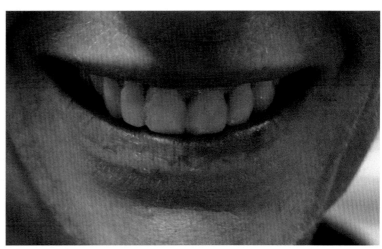

Fig. C5.2.6   Direct mock-up using unbonded resin composite to evaluate the change in shape, thickness and colour. Patient can see and feel the difference.

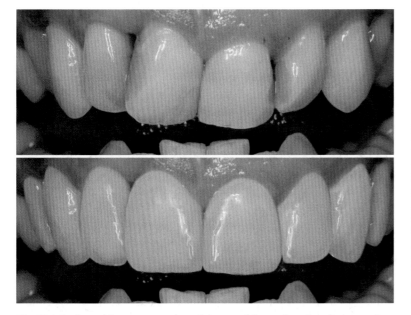

Fig. C5.2.7   Dental image processing of the possible results, after the correction of discrepancies to meet the patient's wishes and expectations, enhances the communication between the two parties about various management options, their risks and potential outcomes.

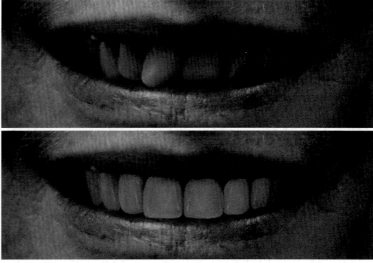

Fig. C5.2.8   Dental image processing using ambient light to show the change in the light and shadow areas.

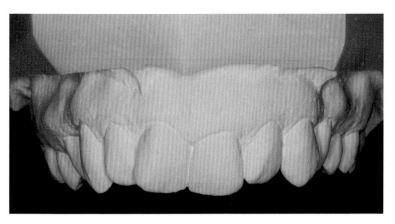

Fig. C5.2.9   In this case it was decided to fabricate a direct resin composite build-up first on a duplicate plaster model.

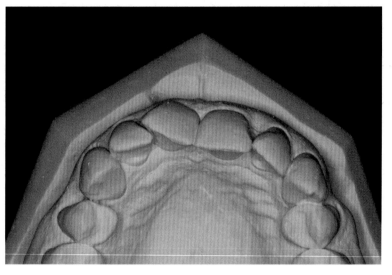

Fig. C5.2.10   Plaster model of the original clinical situation, incisal view.

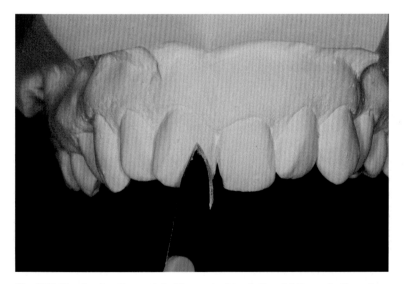

Fig. C5.2.11   Carving the model with a scalpel to distinguish the reduction of thickness.

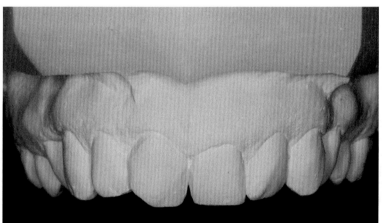

Fig. C5.2.12   The model is prepared for the addition of the material (resin composite 'wax-up'), frontal view.

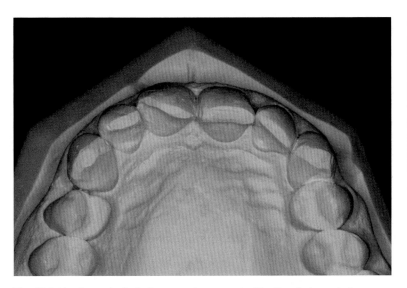

Fig. C5.2.13   From the incisal aspect, the amount of tooth substance to be removed is visible clearly.

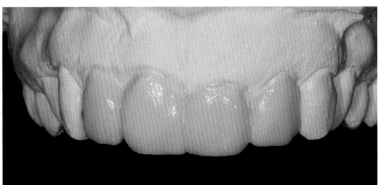

Fig. C5.2.14   The model is 'waxed-up' using a low viscosity resin composite.

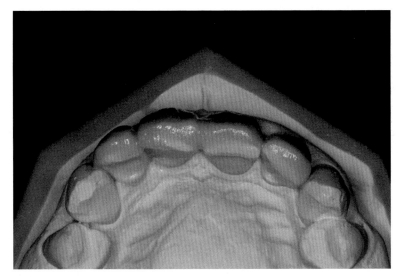

Fig. C5.2.15   The incisal view shows the alteration in the position of the new labial tooth surfaces.

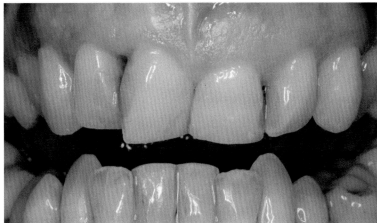

Fig. C5.2.16   A minimal reduction in tooth substance, guided by the carved plaster model as shown in Figures C5.2.12 and C5.2.13.

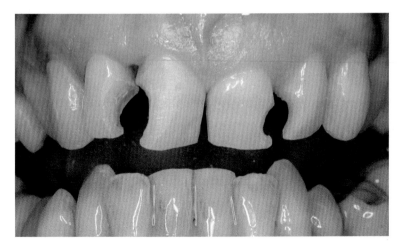

Fig. C5.2.17 The poor quality restorations are removed and the teeth inspected for the presence of secondary caries.

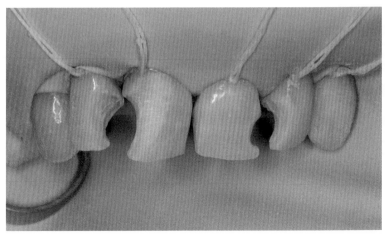

Fig. C5.2.18 Rubber dam isolation is achieved using ligatures of waxed dental floss to assure a dry working field and clear access to the cervical regions of the teeth.

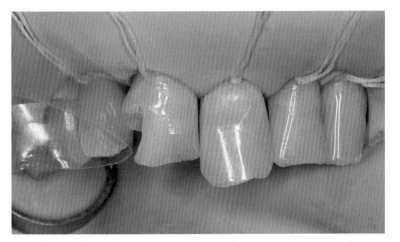

Fig. C5.2.19 The mesial, distal and incisal direct resin composite build-ups are created using a three-step (Type I) bonding procedure with clear matrix strips (Directa), inter-proximally.

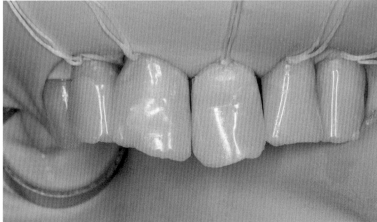

Fig. C5.2.20 The restorations are completed and ready for contouring.

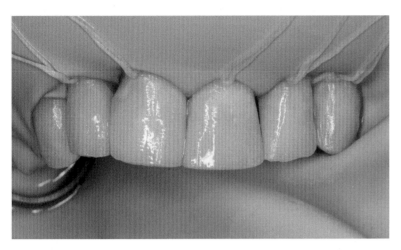

Fig. C5.2.21 The teeth are shaped with fine grit diamonds to establish the basic labial contours and profiles.

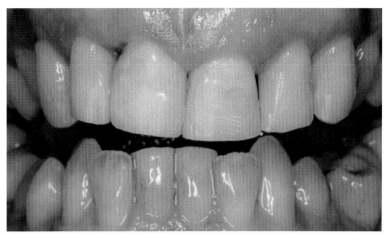

Fig. C5.2.22 After removing the rubber dam the occlusion was checked, the length of the incisors and the position of the incisal edges were determined.

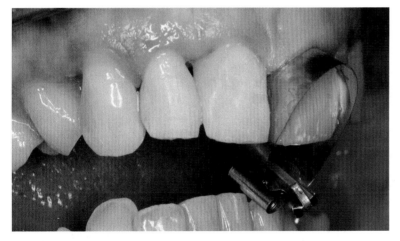

Fig. C5.2.23 The placement of the direct resin composite facings is facilitated by using the AutoMatrix MR (Dentsply) as shown in the previous case.

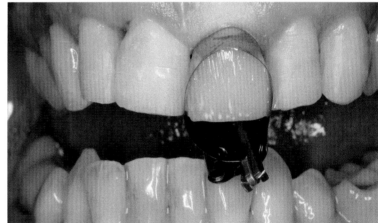

Fig. C5.2.24 The AutoMatrix is positioned just sub-gingivally in the cervical area, at an angle of 45° to help create a natural emergence profile. Chalky spots and microcracks are imitated using white characterizer (Kolor + Plus, Kerr).

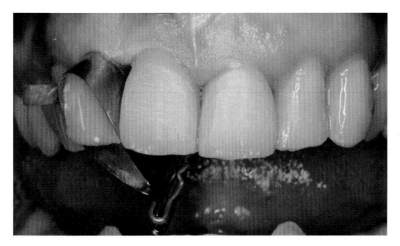

Fig. C5.2.25 Consecutively, the four maxillary incisors were veneered using the same procedure described above.

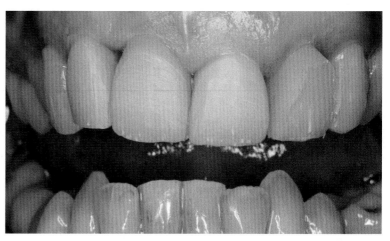

Fig. C5.2.26 The AutoMatrix on tooth #22 was removed. The final labial contour of this tooth has still to be established.

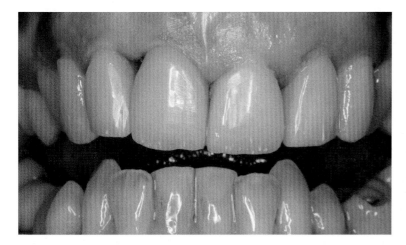

Fig. C5.2.27 All teeth are polished using fine diamond burs and silicone rubber Politip-P green cups (IvoclarVivadent).

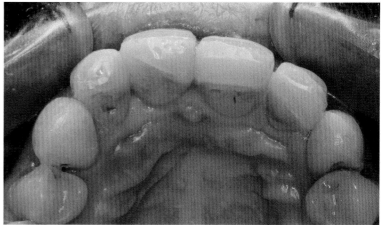

Fig. C5.2.28 The occlusal view clearly demonstrates the amount of added material in the incisal aspect.

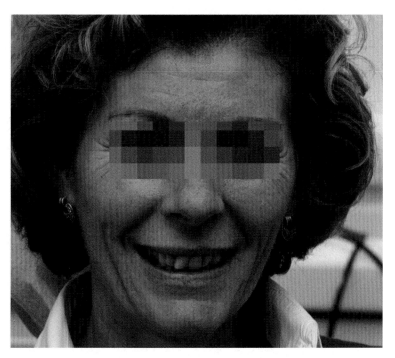

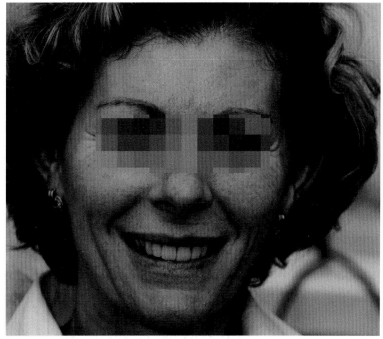

Fig. C5.2.29 Portrait before treatment (ambient light with fill-in flash).

Fig. C5.2.30 Portrait with reshaped and resin composite treated teeth.

CLINICAL CASE 5.3

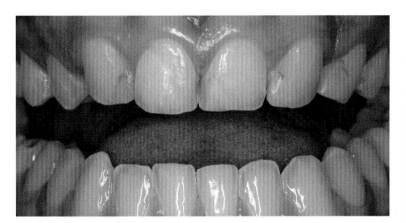

Fig. C5.3.1 Frontal view of the maxillary anterior teeth of an 18-year-old female suffering from missing lateral incisors. Five years ago, upon completion of the orthodontic treatment (aimed to close the diastemata), her dentist tried to camouflage the missing teeth with composite build-ups on teeth #11, #21, #13, #23, #14 and #24.

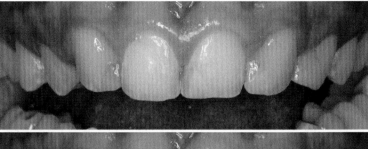

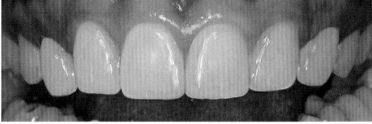

Fig. C5.3.2 The treatment proposed, using Paint Shop Pro image processing software (Corel), gives the patient the opportunity to appreciate the alterations that could be made and give adequate, informed feedback.

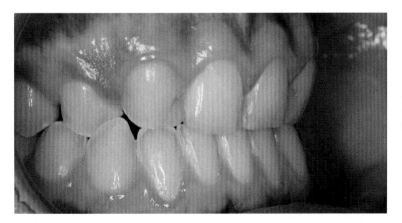

Fig. C5.3.3 Lateral view shows the cross-bite between teeth #14 and #43 and the retroclination of both the maxillary and mandibular anterior teeth.

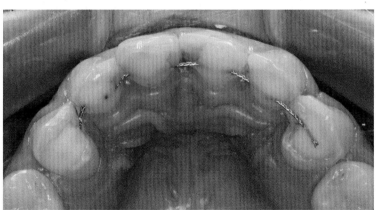

Fig. C5.3.4 Permanent palatal orthodontic retention wire had to be removed prior to the commencement of treatment.

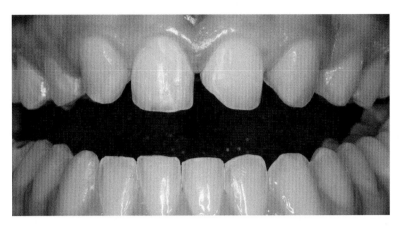

Fig. C5.3.5   From this image it is clear that after removing the original resin composite masking restorations by the previous dentist, the labial curvature of the canines has been flattened somewhat to transform them into a more lateral incisor labial profile.

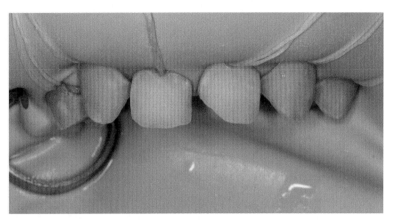

Fig. C5.3.6   After placing the rubber dam as described previously, the teeth are air-abraded with alumina powder to aid the bond of new resin composite to any residual resin composite left on the teeth after the previous restorations were removed.

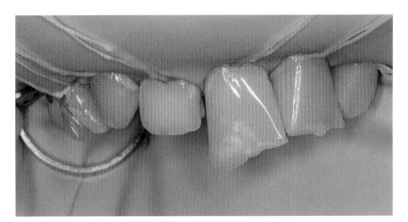

Fig. C5.3.7   The resin composite restoration framework (mesial, distal and incisal) is constructed using Directa Clear Matrix inter-proximally with special attention given to the midline position.

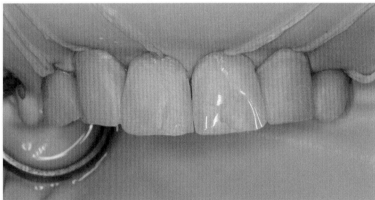

Fig. C5.3.8   After removal of the excess resin composite, the new incisal level is determined.

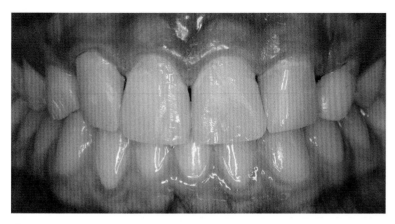

Fig. C5.3.9 This frontal image shows that the cross-bite shown in Figure C5.3.3 has been corrected successfully.

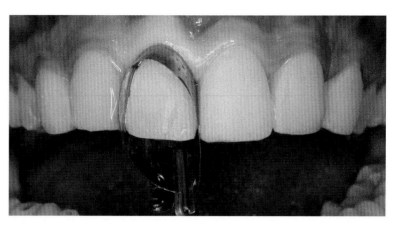

Fig. C5.3.10 The new, more pronounced position of the labial surfaces was achieved with the use of AutoMatrix NR.

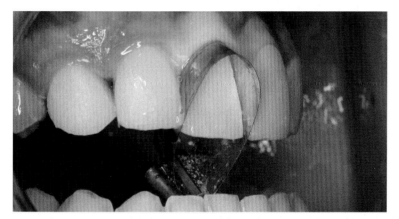

Fig. C5.3.11 The high-value body composite shade was applied to enhance the reflection of the light from the labial surface line angles, suggesting an even more protruded tooth position.

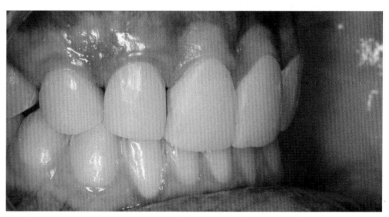

Fig. C5.3.12 After contouring, it is clear that the emergence profile, achieved with the direct labial veneers, is natural and that the vertical axes of the maxillary anterior teeth appear more natural than in the original situation.

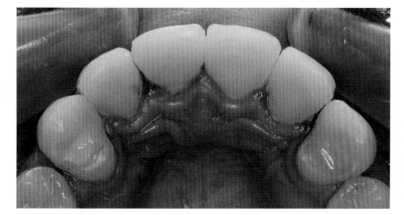

Fig. C5.3.13 Viewing occlusally, the central incisors appear wider than the canines, because they were transformed successfully into lateral incisors.

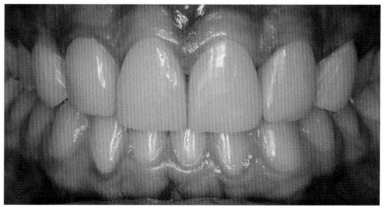

Fig. C5.3.14 Directly after the treatment, the teeth are polished with special attention given to the labial surface texture and form, recreating importantly the reflective line angles mesially, distally, cervically and incisally, thus providing an acceptable natural-looking result.

CLINICAL CASE 5.4

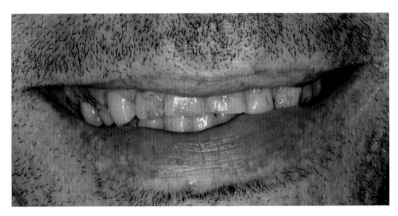

Fig. C5.4.1 A 37-year-old male patient displaying only a few millimetres of his central incisors during a tight-lipped smile. Clearly, he is embarrassed to show his upper front teeth.

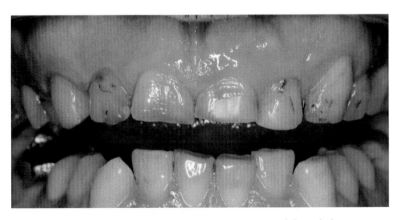

Fig. C5.4.2 The wear of his upper front teeth is severe and the existing restorations are discoloured.

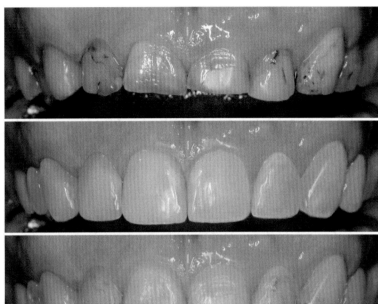

Fig. C5.4.3 Image processing with Paint Shop Pro software (Jasc) showing the original situation, the proposed treatment using minimally invasive direct resin composite restorations and the projection of the proposed changes on the original situation to estimate the necessary lengthening of the teeth. This process helps communicate clearly to the patient the operative treatment options, the risks and the final results, and helps match the restorative outcome to the patient's expectations.

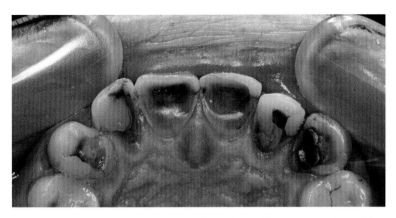

Fig. C5.4.4   Occlusal view of the initial situation showing the extreme wear of the palatal surfaces and the exposure of dentine that has become stained over time.

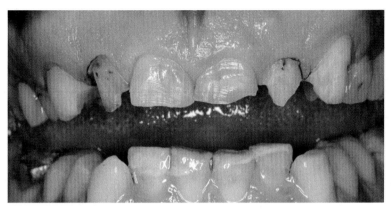

Fig. C5.4.5   Frontal view after partial removal of the existing poor quality resin composite restorations.

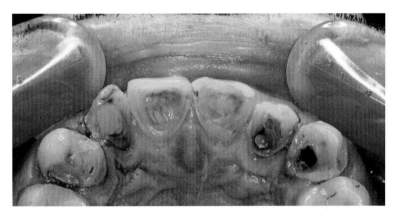

Fig. C5.4.6   Occlusal view shows the minimal removal of tooth substance, enough to create space for the direct resin composite build-ups to follow.

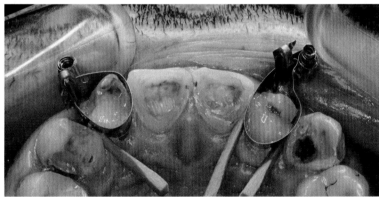

Fig. C5.4.7   The first step was the construction of new palatal surfaces on teeth #12 and #22, using a free-hand direct technique described in the previous cases. An alternative technique in this type of case might have been to wax-up the palatal surfaces on a plaster model and manufacture a clear rigid acrylic palatal splint from the laboratory. This splint could then be used to help guide and position clinically the placement of resin composite.

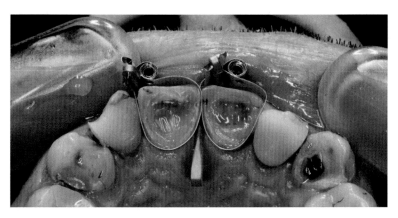

Fig. C5.4.8   After the palatal surfaces of the two lateral incisors were created, the central incisors are then built up, also using AutoMatrix NR.

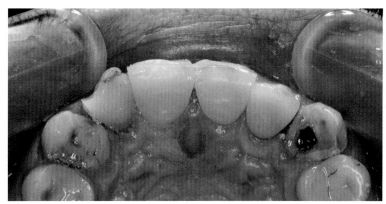

Fig. C5.4.9   The main reason to begin the procedure with the palatal build-ups is to help position and retain the rubber dam for controlled working conditions and defining initial pre-determined occlusal stops.

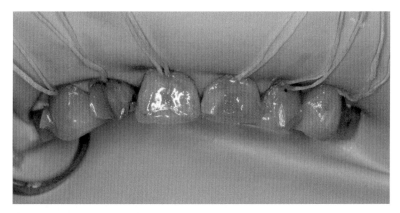

Fig. C5.4.10   The rubber dam with ligatures in situ; this provides protection to the adjacent teeth and soft tissues from air-abrasion, acid etching and applying the bonding agent.

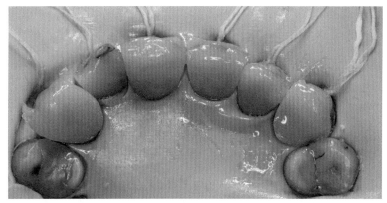

Fig. C5.4.11   The palatal aspect of the canines is constructed with free-hand direct placement of resin composite and the teeth are ready for lengthening.

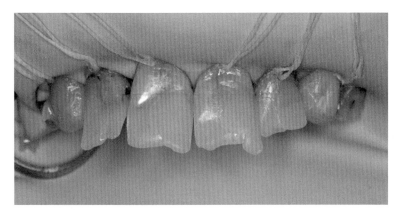

Fig. C5.4.12　The second step is to establish the exact proportions/dimensions of the teeth and the position of the midline.

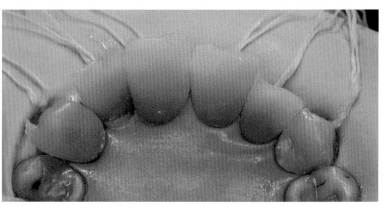

Fig. C5.4.13　The join between the palatal restorations and the incisal resin composite is checked from the occlusal aspect. This should be seamless as fresh increments of resin composite fuse on photo-polymerization due to the presence of the undisturbed air-inhibited layer on the palatal composites.

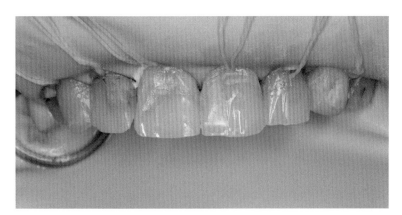

Fig. C5.4.14　The altered contours of the teeth are visible clearly after the removal of the excess composite.

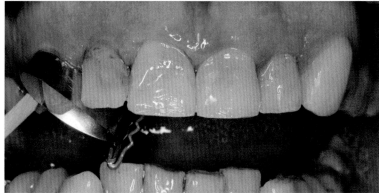

Fig. C5.4.15　The third step (placement of the direct labial resin composite veneers) commenced after the removal of the rubber dam and the establishment of occlusion and articulation.

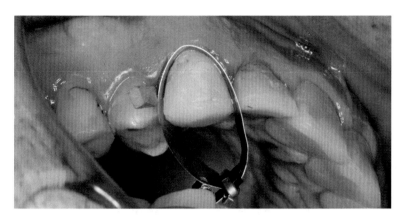

Fig. C5.4.16   This image shows how effectively the labial surface of the canine is isolated and defined with an AutoMatrix and a wooden wedge. Within the matrix, the bonding procedure is performed as described previously.

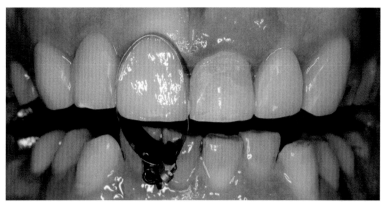

Fig. C5.4.17   The procedure continued with labial incremental layering of flowable resin composite with respect to the shade map assessed for the teeth. Cervical part mostly A3.5B (chromatic and less translucent body composite), mid-labial part A3B and the incisal part A2B (higher value, less chroma and moderate translucency).

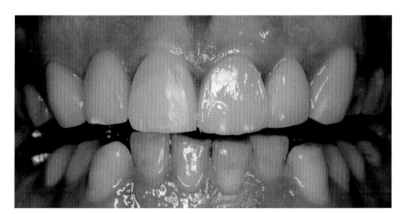

Fig. C5.4.18   In the incisal area, chalky spots and microcracks are added using white characterizer (Kolor + Plus, Kerr). After removal of the matrix the labial surfaces are shaped using a flame-shaped diamond bur (Horico FG249U010) and the palatal surfaces are contoured using a pear-shaped diamond bur (Komet FG379EF023lg).

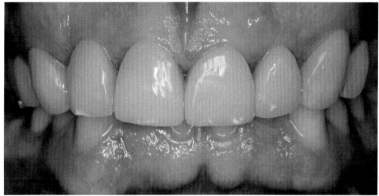

Fig. C5.4.19   Finally, the surfaces are polished with Soflex (3M ESPE) discs (coarse to fine) and polishing cups (Politip P green, Ivoclar Vivadent).

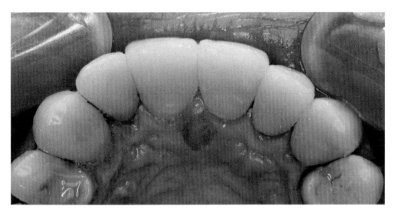

Fig. C5.4.20 The labial composite surface profiles are distributed naturally and harmoniously within the available space.

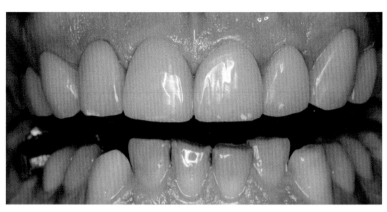

Fig. C5.4.21 The 3-month review of the patient shows excellent gingival health, natural surface luster and texture of the restorations. The patient reported excellent function and was not disturbed by a slight change of overbite caused by the lengthening of the maxillary anterior teeth.

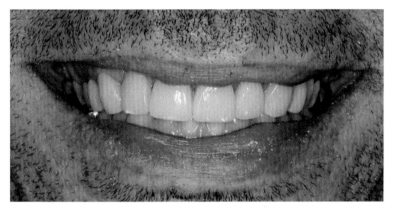

Fig. C5.4.22 The post-treatment image shows natural looking incisal edges, the incisal translucency and the chalky, 'hypoplastic' spots. The final result is satisfactory to the patient.

REFERENCES

1. Özcan M. The use of chairside silica coating for different dental applications: a clinical report. J Prosthet Dent 2002;87:469–72.

2. Gresnigt M. Clinical and Laboratory Evaluation of Laminate Veneers. Netherlands: Thesis, Dental School Groningen University; 2011.

3. Dozic A, de Kloet H. Improving aesthetics in a narrow jaw with composite. Part I. Dent Today 2011;30(6):108–11.

4. Dozic A, de Kloet H. Improving aesthetics in a narrow jaw with composite. Part II. Dent Today 2011;30(7):118–22.

5. Meijering ACH. A Clinical Study on Veneer Restorations. Netherlands: Thesis, Dental School Radboud Nijmegen University; 1997.

CHAPTER 6

Direct Posterior Esthetics:
A Management Protocol for the Treatment of
Severe Tooth Wear with Resin Composite

J. HAMBURGER, N. OPDAM, B. LOOMANS

INTRODUCTION

Tooth wear is a concern in dentistry but diagnosis is often difficult due to its multi-factorial aetiology. The main causes for tooth wear (tooth surface loss) are a combination of both erosion (more common in the younger population) and attrition (bruxism, found more commonly in the older population). During the early stages further tooth wear may be prevented by reducing acid consumption or prescribing an acrylic occlusal nightguard to prevent attrition due to bruxism. When tooth wear is more severe, leading to extensive loss of tooth substance, restorative operative treatment is required and general dental practitioners can feel less confident in managing these patients. Sometimes a total rehabilitation including increasing the occlusal vertical dimensions and re-organizing the occlusion has to be performed. In this chapter a minimally invasive, tooth tissue preserving and direct operative reconstruction protocol with relatively low costs, good predictability and sufficient longevity is outlined and discussed.

TREATMENT OPTIONS

Whenever a patient visits a dental practice with severe tooth wear or is referred to a specialist, a comprehensive verbal history (anamnesis) must be obtained to help elucidate the patient's needs, hopes and expectations of the dental care requested. Does the patient experience tooth wear as a problem or is it just the referring dentist who is concerned about the state of the patient's dentition. Functional problems causing patients' suffering and resulting from severe tooth wear include sensitivity, problems with mastication and/or problems with the resulting esthetics. In situations where no direct treatment is requested by the patient, the need for restorative intervention must be questioned, especially if the dentist feels that postponing any treatment will not result in a more extensive or complicated operative care plan in the future. In those cases it may be advisable to monitor and review the condition, with study models and intra-oral photographs, to see if there is any continued active progression, as well as focussing non-operative preventive patient care on eradicating all aetiological factors. Several indices (for example, BEWE [basic erosive wear examination] or TWI [tooth wear index]) exist to help dentists with this. With the BEWE index, the surface affected most severely in each sextant is recorded using a four-level score and the cumulative score is classified and matched to risk levels which guide the management of the condition.[1] This scoring system is straightforward but its main disadvantage is that it is designed for erosive wear alone. Because tooth wear often has a multi-factorial aetiology, this index alone might be insufficient for monitoring purposes. Another more general index is the Smith and Knight TWI.[2] Several others are described, but unfortunately none are accepted internationally as the gold standard method for measuring and monitoring tooth wear. Moreover, patients suffering from severe tooth wear are often classified in the highest categories within these indices. This, in turn, makes the indices less helpful for monitoring and deciding when is the best moment to intervene operatively. For this purpose, sequential dental study casts are the simplest method used to compare tooth wear stages over time. Wear progression and patients' expectations of treatment are important factors in deciding the right moment to commence restorative work. The possible disadvantages of restorative options and the limited longevity of every invasive restorative treatment should be explained clearly to the patient. During this informed and well-documented consent, a mutual decision can be made concerning whether to start restorative intervention or continue with the monitoring process.

When the decision to commence operative treatment is made, there are several options to choose from. A brief overview of the options follows, but it should be noted that, to date, no treatment technique is properly evidence based or supported by ample high-quality clinical studies/trials.

INDIRECT OPTIONS

Indirect treatment implies the use of restorations that are manufactured outside the patient's mouth and cemented to the tooth to gain retention. Restorations include crowns, bridges, porcelain facings/veneers and indirect resin composite restorations. The dental technician models the morphology of the restorations instead of the dentist. From case reports, there are considerable variations in the materials used which include glass-ceramic, gold and porcelain fused to metal crowns.[3–5] The disadvantages of this indirect approach include the relatively high cost, the invasive nature of the care and the increased risk of potentially catastrophic failures in the medium to long term.[6,7]

Indirect resin composite restorations are also an option used to treat patients with severe wear. Positive treatment outcomes[8] are described as well as negative results.[9] Advantages of indirect resin composite restorations compared to crowns in the treatment of patients with severe tooth wear include a reduced susceptibility to fracture and the reduced overall initial financial outlay.

DIRECT OPTIONS

Direct resin composite restorations can be used to treat patients with severe tooth wear. Resin composite has been proven to be a restorative material delivering good long-term results;[10–14] however, none of the quoted references describe the treatment of patients with severe tooth wear. Promising clinical results in patients with severe tooth wear treated with direct resin composite are described in several case reports.[15-19] However, in a randomized clinical trial in 2006, the authors concluded that the use of composites for restoring worn posterior teeth was contraindicated given the high failure rate after 3 years.[9] In contrast, however, promising clinical results were reported in a case series of a non-invasive technique for posterior vertical bite reconstructions using direct resin composite.[20-21] A study in 2011, with a mean observation time of 4 years, showed minimal failure and high patient satisfaction.[7] In this study, patients were treated according to the method described later in this chapter.

Treating patients with severe tooth wear operatively can be demanding technically for general dentists. Treatment success is highly dependent on the clinical skills of the operator and their appreciation of the biological and mechanical considerations of the particular case. Modelling the anatomy of teeth directly in the mouth can be difficult and time consuming. Until now, a formal treatment protocol for using direct resin composites to restore severely worn teeth at an increased vertical dimension has not been described in the literature. Past case reports do not provide much more information other than that teeth are adjusted in occlusion.[22] A method using a semi-direct technique includes restoring the anatomy by means of a pre-fabricated template.[20,21]

THE NIJMEGEN 'DIRECT SHAPING BY OCCLUSION' APPROACH

In this section, the treatment protocol used in the Department of Dentistry of the Radboud University Medical Center in Nijmegen (The Netherlands) will be described,[7] and the aim is to show the essentials of this management protocol as it differs from other, more standard procedures. The approach described here includes minimal preparation of teeth, reduced costs and increased outcome predictability. A novelty in this technique's protocol is the 'direct shaping by occlusion' (DSO) technique. The principle behind DSO is to obtain an occlusion at the new increased vertical dimension by getting the patient to close into the soft uncured resin composite prior to its polymerization, using pre-determined and pre-fabricated putty occlusal stops to guide the new vertical dimension.

When a patient is referred to the Department of Dentistry of the Radboud University Medical Center in Nijmegen, the first appointments include taking an extensive verbal history (anamnesis) and a comprehensive dietary analysis. Moreover, intra-oral clinical pre-operative photographs, bitewing and dental panoramic radiographs and impressions for study casts are made (Figs 6.1–6.3).

A patient-centred care plan, including emphasis on managing the causes of the ongoing tooth wear, as well as the expected costs of treatment, is discussed with the patient. After mutual, documented initial approval, non-bonded resin

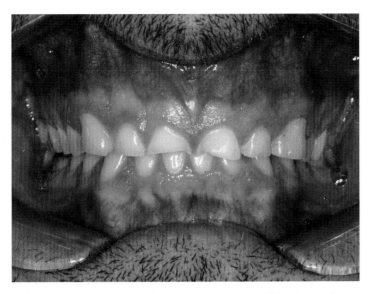

Fig. 6.1 Anterior, frontal view (teeth in intercuspal position [ICP]) of a patient with severe tooth wear.

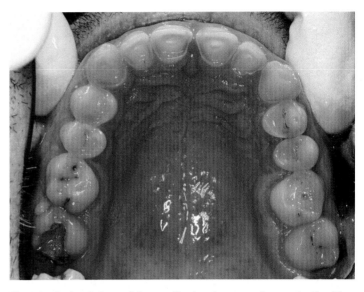

Fig. 6.2 Occlusal views of the maxilla showing severely worn teeth with multiple areas of exposed dentine.

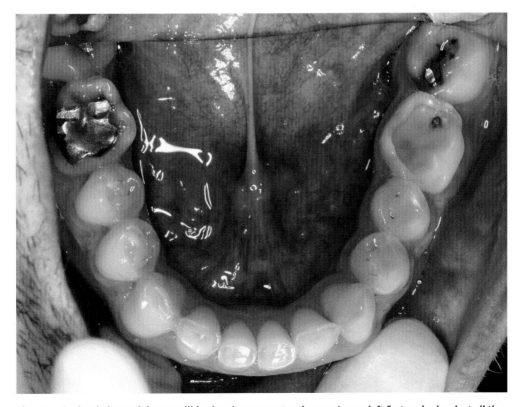

Fig. 6.3 Occlusal views of the mandible showing severe tooth wear. Lower left first molar has lost all the enamel on the occlusal surface.

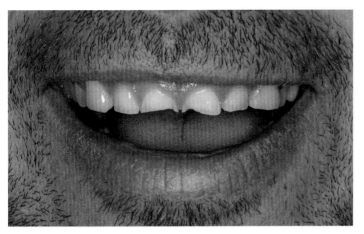

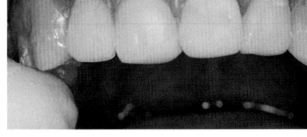

Fig. 6.5 Direct, non-bonded resin composite mock-ups placed on teeth #13–23.

Fig. 6.4 An esthetic concern existed because the anterior teeth were markedly shortened and irregular, so affecting adversely the patient's appearance.

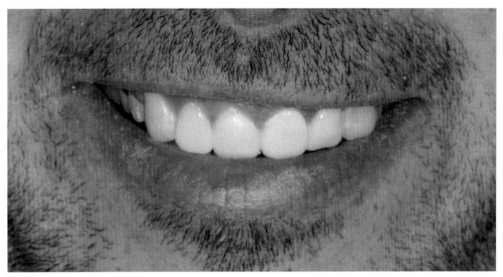

Fig. 6.6 The patient evaluated the esthetic appearance of these mock-ups directly in situ.

composite mock-ups overlying the maxillary anterior teeth (#13–23) are placed directly and evaluated with the patient to establish the desired esthetic appearance (Figs 6.4–6.6).

After the comprehensive clinical assessment of the severity of the tooth wear and documented discussions about the realistic treatment outcomes and potential concerns, consent is gained and the increase in occlusal vertical dimension (OVD) is determined, with the use of a dental semi-adjustable articulator with maxillary and mandibular casts mounted in maximum intercuspal position (ICP). The space required for the restoration of functional anatomy and the esthetics of the dentition are the primary factors in deciding the amount by which to increase the OVD. Another factor taken into consideration is the minimum vertical space required to accommodate an adequate thickness of the restorative material, in order to ensure the intrinsic strength/fracture toughness of the final restoration is maximized.

This newly determined vertical dimension is transferred to the patient's mouth using silicone occlusal stops. These stops are manufactured on the study casts mounted in the dental articulator. After separation of the casts with petroleum jelly, two small portions of heavy bodied silicone or putty are applied to the occlusal surfaces in the molar regions and the articulator is closed, at the increased vertical dimension, until the silicone is set fully. The silicone stops are adjusted with a scalpel blade to permit freedom of mandibular movement in the horizontal plane when occluding at the increased vertical dimension. Subsequently, these occlusal stops are placed in the mouth. Using a guided closure technique, the retruded contact position is determined using impression material.[23] Bite registration is then used to remount the casts in centric relation at the new increased vertical dimension. Two new silicone stops in the posterior area are then made and used intra-orally to copy the desired new relationship in the mouth.

The restorative procedure starts with the lower anterior teeth (#33–43) after which the upper anterior teeth are reconstructed. A metal matrix band (Tofflemire nr. 11) is positioned and secured with wooden wedges, from the palatal side, and is adjusted using a high speed bur so that the band is not in contact with the lower anterior teeth when the patient closes their mouth with the stops in situ. Subsequently, the adhesive procedure (preferably using a three-step etch and rinse system) is performed. Before the first layer of hybrid resin composite is placed, a thin layer of flowable resin composite can be applied and left uncured to improve adaptation at the outline (snow-plough technique).[24] For larger defects the resin composite is placed incrementally but the final occlusal layer of composite should be applied in bulk. The lower anterior teeth are coated thinly with petroleum jelly and the patient is asked to close their mouth into the silicone stops, after which the composite is cured from the buccal side. After 40 seconds, the patient can open their mouth and the photocuring is continued from the occlusal surface. Subsequently a labial veneer restoration is made using a suitable anterior resin composite. The veneer restoration consists of a dentine shade and an enamel shade, and finally a translucent incisor shade is used to mimic incisal translucency. The finishing procedure of the restoration must be delicate in order not to disrupt the already established morphology and esthetic appearance. Sequentially, all maxillary anterior teeth (#13–23) are treated according to the same procedure.

To ensure the curve of Spee is maintained, the maxillary first premolars are built up in line with the canines, without making occlusal contact with the lower teeth. Using the DSO technique, the lower premolars are restored into contact with the upper first premolars (Figs 6.7–6.10).

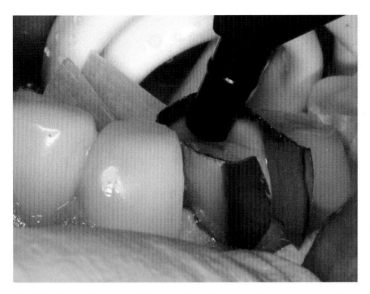

Fig. 6.7 After placement of the matrix and wedges, the resin composite is applied.

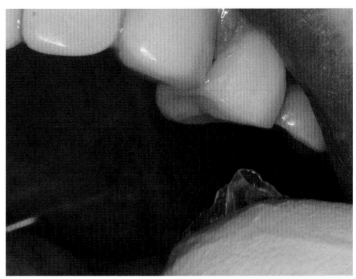

Fig. 6.8 The antagonist teeth are separated with a thin layer of petroleum jelly.

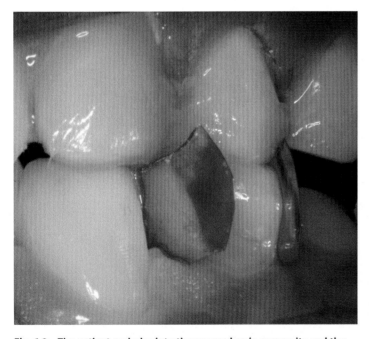

Fig. 6.9 The patient occludes into the uncured resin composite and the vertical relationship is guided by the restored anterior teeth.

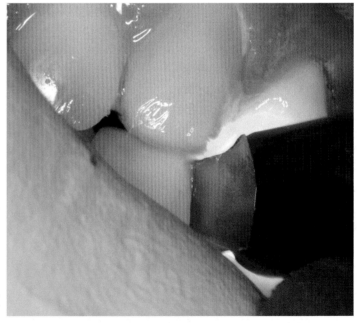

Fig. 6.10 Initial photocuring of the resin composite is performed in occlusion.

After the premolars have been restored, the mandibular posterior teeth are shaped and completed using hand instruments. The silicone stops are now not required as the new OVD is stabilized by the newly reconstructed anterior teeth and premolars. Finally, the remaining upper posterior teeth are treated following the same described technique (Figs 6.11–6.13).

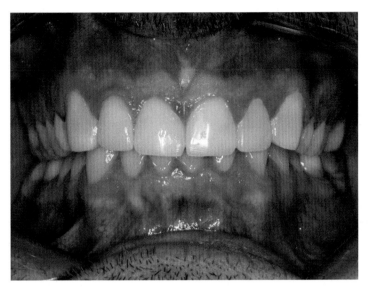

Fig. 6.11 An anterior view of the final restored dentition.

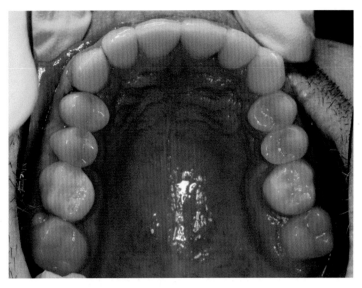

Fig. 6.12 Final result for the maxillary teeth after direct minimally invasive DSO treatment.

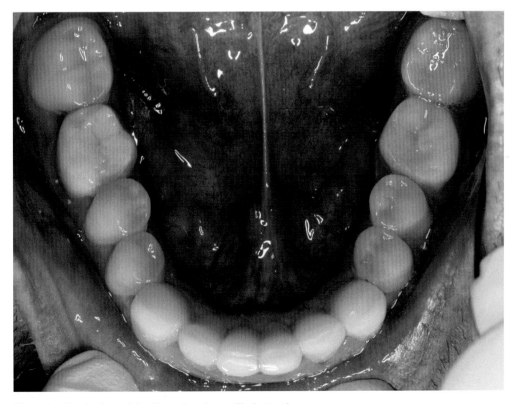

Fig. 6.13 The final result for the restored mandibular teeth.

BOX 6.1
ADVANTAGES AND DISADVANTAGES OF THE DSO TECHNIQUE

Advantages

- Occlusion achieved in a simple and predictable way

- Generally, cuspal lateral guidance occurs naturally using this treatment technique because of the anatomy and the inter-digitation of teeth

- Maximum thickness of resin composite is achieved resulting in an increased strength of the final restorations

- As this is a minimally invasive technique, biological damage is reduced to a minimum

- The DSO technique falls within the remit of techniques dentists can learn and use in their general daily practice. The method by which teeth are treated sequentially using a matrix and wedges to separate them is similar to the standard techniques used to restore teeth with conventional resin composites. The finishing and polishing are also relatively easy when the matrices and wedges are placed properly

Disadvantages

- As the occlusal morphology has to be modelled directly intra-orally, this method compared to an indirect technique could be clinically more time consuming and challenging to the operator

- When using the DSO technique, rubber dam isolation is not possible. Its presence would prevent the patient from occluding or using the silicone stops for creating the measured increase in occlusal vertical dimension. Thus, care is required to expel as much intra-oral moisture as possible using cotton wool rolls, absorbent cellulose pads and careful suction

The treatment order is not rigid and can be adapted according to the patient's situation. There might be cases in which the mandibular front teeth are not worn down severely. In that case, lower front teeth are not restored and the treatment starts with the maxillary anterior teeth. For advantages and disadvantages of the DSO technique, see Box 6.1.

EVIDENCE

The DSO technique has been used for several years in the Department of Dentistry of the Radboud University Medical Center in Nijmegen and the results are promising;[7] however, this paper by Hamburger et al does not describe the DSO technique implicitly, but in all the reported cases, this technique was used. Therefore, it can be concluded that this well controlled step-by-step technique of treating patients with severe tooth wear could be a reliable method of direct management.

PATIENTS' FAQs

Q. Is it a painful treatment option?

A. Fortunately, in general it is not a painful treatment method. As mechanical tooth preparation is limited to only producing a bevelled finishing margin or some minimal resistance form, teeth are not sensitive and the biological integrity of the pulp is not put at risk when compared to more invasive indirect restorative treatments.

Q. How much time does a general case take?

A. It takes between 3 and 5 sessions, each of 3–4 hours duration, to restore a full dentition.

Q. What is the longevity of the direct restorations?

A. Long-term results are not yet available and have to be determined by a prospective clinical study. This is currently being undertaken at the Radboud University Medical Center in Nijmegen. Based on initial experiences, life expectancy of these direct, minimally invasive restorations is between 10 and 15 years. Thereafter, refurbishment/repair can be carried out as required. Reasons for treatment failure may be related to the initial cause of the tooth wear which must be elucidated and treated primarily before any operative care is undertaken. It is conceivable that patients with tooth wear wear mainly caused by mechanical aspects like bruxism may exhibit failures sooner than patients with tooth wear mainly due to chemical aspects like erosion. These causes, as well as the direct restorative care offered, must be carefully managed.

Seminal literature

Bartlett D, Sundaram G. An up to 3-year randomized clinical study comparing indirect and direct resin composites used to restore worn posterior teeth. Int J Prosthodont 2006; 19(6):613–17.

Hamburger JT, Opdam NJ, Bronkhorst EM, et al. Clinical performance of direct composite restorations for treatment of severe tooth wear. J Adhes Dent 2011;13(6):585–93.

REFERENCES

1. Bartlett D, Ganss C, Lussi A. Basic erosive wear examination (BEWE): a new scoring system for scientific and clinical needs. Clin Oral Investig 2008;12(Suppl. 1):S65–8.

2. Smith BG, Knight JK. An index for measuring the wear of teeth. Br Dent J 1984; 156(12):435–8.

3. Dahl BL. The face height in adult dentate humans. A discussion of physiological and prosthodontic principles illustrated through a case report. J Oral Rehabil 1995;22(8):565–9.

4. Fradeani M, Bottachiari RS, Tracey T, et al. The restoration of functional occlusion and esthetics. Int J Periodontics Restorative Dent 1992;12(1):63–71.

REFERENCES

5. Stewart B. Restoration of the severely worn dentition using a systematized approach for a predictable prognosis. Int J Periodontics Restorative Dent 1998;18(1):46–57.

6. Groten M. Complex all-ceramic rehabilitation of a young patient with a severely compromised dentition: a case report. Quintessence Int 2009;40(1):19–27.

7. Hamburger JT, Opdam NJ, Bronkhorst EM, et al. Clinical performance of direct composite restorations for treatment of severe tooth wear. J Adhes Dent 2011;13(6):585–93.

8. Magne P, Stanley K, Schlichting LH. Modeling of ultrathin occlusal veneers. Dent Mater 2012;28(7):777–82.

9. Bartlett D, Sundaram G. An up to 3-year randomized clinical study comparing indirect and direct resin composites used to restore worn posterior teeth. Int J Prosthodont 2006;19(6): 613–17.

10. Chrysanthakopoulos NA. Placement, replacement and longevity of composite resin-based restorations in permanent teeth in Greece. Int Dent J 2012;62(3):161–6.

11. Da Rosa Rodolpho PA, Donassollo TA, Cenci MS, et al. 22-Year clinical evaluation of the performance of two posterior composites with different filler characteristics. Dent Mater 2011;27(10):955–63.

12. Nikaido T, Takada T, Kitasako Y, et al. Retrospective study of the 10-year clinical performance of direct resin composite restorations placed with the acid-etch technique. Quintessence Int 2007;38(5):e240–6.

13. Opdam NJ, Bronkhorst EM, Loomans BA, et al. Longevity of repaired restorations: a practice based study. J Dent 2012;40(10):829–35.

14. van Dijken JW. Durability of resin composite restorations in high C-factor cavities: a 12-year follow-up. J Dent 2010;38(6):469–74.

15. Belvedere PC. Full-mouth reconstruction of bulim ravaged teeth using direct composites: a case presentation. Dent Today 2009;28(1):126, 128, 130–1.

16. Bernardo JK, Maia EA, Cardoso AC, et al. Diagnosis and management of maxillary incisors affected by incisal wear: an interdisciplinary case report. J Esthet Restor Dent 2002;14(6): 331–9.

17. Reis A, Higashi C, Loguercio AD. Re-anatomization of anterior eroded teeth by stratification with direct composite resin. J Esthet Restor Dent 2009;21(5):304–16.

18. Stephan AD. Diagnosis and dental treatment of a young adult patient with gastroesophageal reflux: a case report with 2-year follow-up. Quintessence Int 2002;33(8):619–26.

19. Tepper SA, Schmidlin PR. Technique of direct vertical bite reconstruction with composite and a splint as template. Schweiz Monatsschr Zahnmed 2005;115(1):35–47.

20. Attin T, Filli T, Imfeld C, et al. Composite vertical bite reconstructions in eroded dentitions after 5.5 years: a case series. J Oral Rehabil 2012;39(1):73–9.

21. Schmidlin PR, Filli T, Imfeld C, et al. Three-year evaluation of posterior vertical bite reconstruction using direct resin composite – a case series. Oper Dent 2009;34(1):102–8.

22. Reston EG, Corba VD, Broliato G, et al. Minimally invasive intervention in a case of a noncarious lesion and severe loss of tooth structure. Oper Dent 2012;37(3):324–8.

23. Wilson PHR, Banerjee A. Recording the retruded contact position: a review of clinical techniques. Br Dent J 2004;196:395–402.

24. Opdam NJ, Roeters JJ, de Boer T, et al. Voids and porosities in class I micropreparations filled with various resin composites. Oper Dent 2003;28(1):9–14.

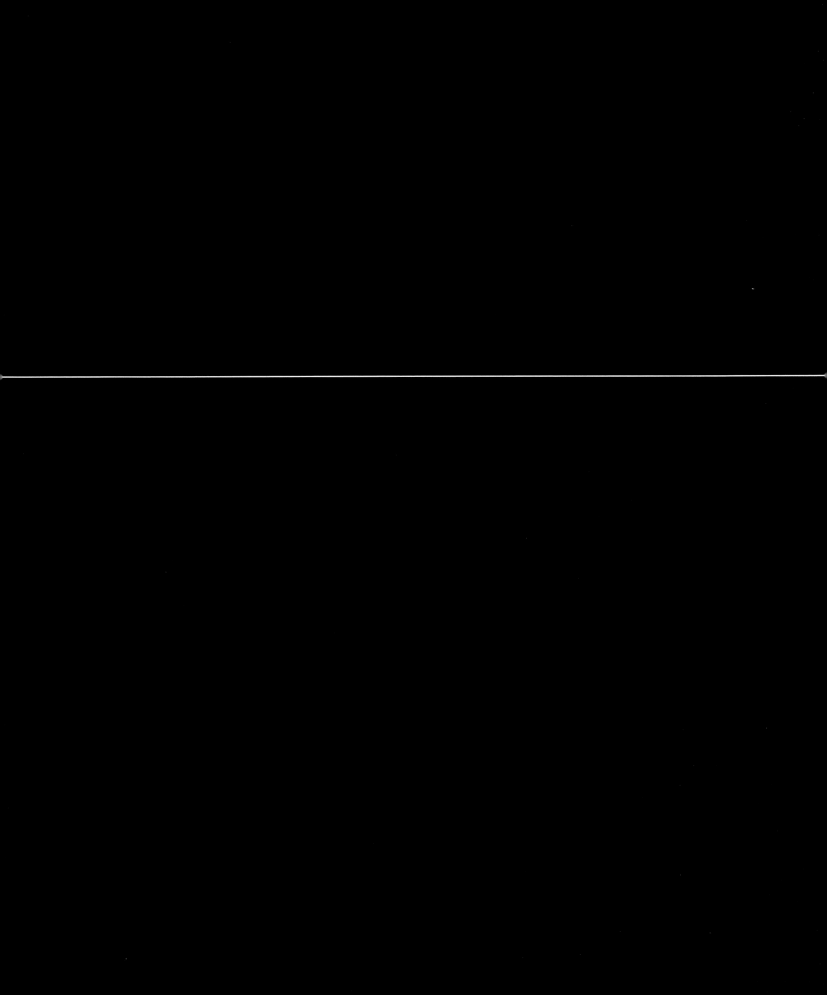

CHAPTER 7

Direct Posterior Esthetics: Clinical Case

J. HAMBURGER, N. OPDAM, B. LOOMANS

INTRODUCTION

This chapter illustrates a case of severe generalized tooth wear in a young patient, where the Nijmegen approach to direct resin composite reconstruction was used successfully. Here again, as previously mentioned, the clinical assessment of the patient and detailed scrutiny of the patient's wishes and expectations played a significant role in helping to decide on the minimally invasive (MI) approach to rebuilding his teeth. This MI approach will only work in cases where patient motivation is high and long lasting for maintaining their oral health and eliminating causative factors that have led to tooth destruction.

CLINICAL CASE

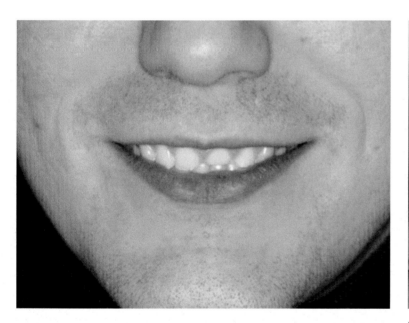

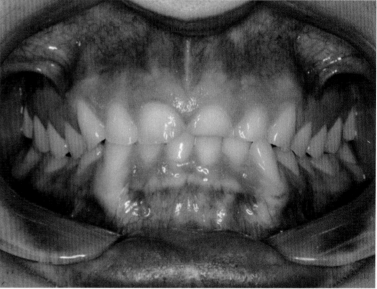

Fig. C7.1 A 25-year-old man was referred to the Department of Dentistry of the Radboud University Medical Center in Nijmegen (The Netherlands) to the restorative clinic specializing in the management of tooth wear. During the examination severe tooth wear was observed. History revealed that normal function was restricted due to pain from cold food and drinks, touching and chewing, especially sweets. The patient is a chef in a high-class restaurant and suffers professionally due to his clinical restrictions during food tasting.

Fig. C7.2 The verbal history showed that the patient often experiences gastro-oesophageal reflux disease (GORD). The appearance of the tooth wear was erosive and, therefore, the most likely aetiology was established as GORD. The patient was advised to contact his physician who prescribed omeprazol 20 mg. After 2 weeks, but before the actual dental treatment had started, this already resulted in a reduction of tooth sensitivity, less thirst during the night, improved general welfare and a better taste.

Due to the tooth wear, an esthetic problem existed because his anterior teeth were markedly shortened. Oral hygiene was good, a healthy periodontium was present and caries risk was established as low.

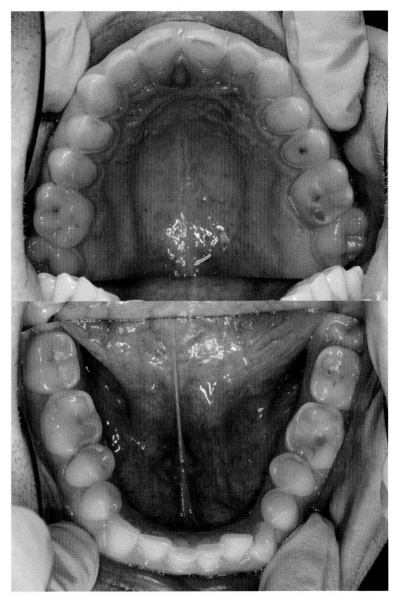

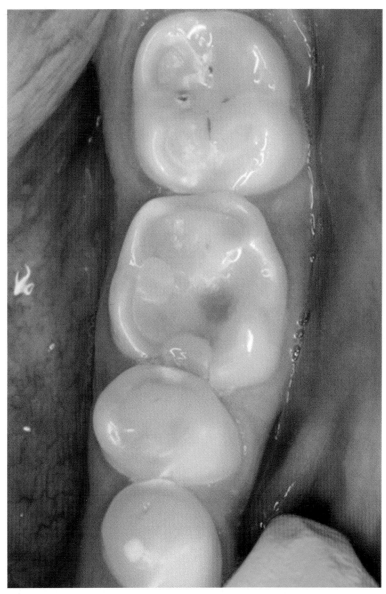

Fig. C7.3   Occlusal views of the mandible and the maxilla. From 16 to 26 the palatal cusps and the occlusal surfaces have been severely damaged. Palatal cusps of the upper premolars have totally disappeared, resulting in multiple dentine exposures. In the lower molars most of the occlusal enamel has already disappeared. (BEWE score = 18.)

Fig. C7.4   Intra-oral view of the lower left quadrant. The tooth wear extends into dentine at several locations. Typical for erosive tooth wear, the resin composite restorations in tooth 36 stand proud from the occlusal surface.

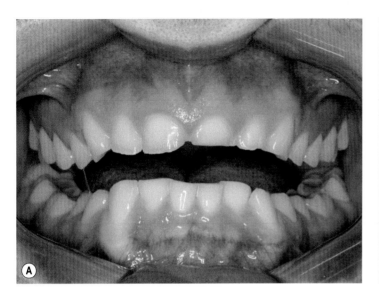 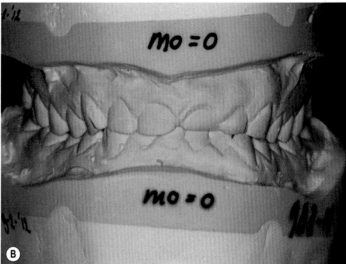

Fig. C7.5A,B Anterior view in and out of occlusion showing extruded mandibular anterior teeth, due to erosive wear of the palatal surfaces of the maxillary teeth. Tooth 21 shows a marked decrease in crown length.

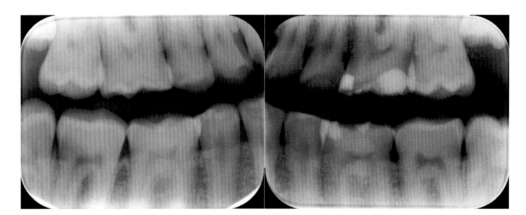

Fig. C7.6 Bitewing radiographs confirm the low caries risk and good periodontal status. Considerable wear on the occlusal surfaces can be observed.

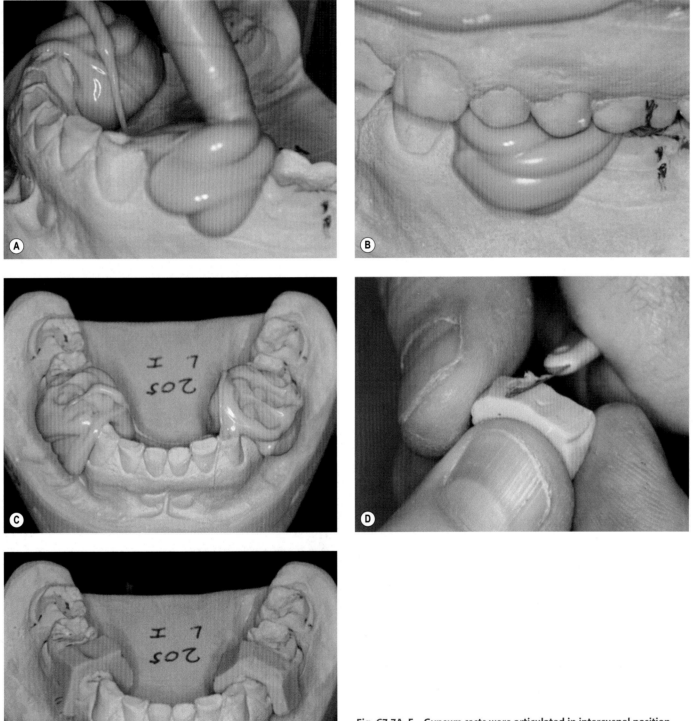

Fig. C7.7A–E Gypsum casts were articulated in intercuspal position using an Artex articulator (Girrbach Dental, Germany). The vertical dimension was raised 4.5 mm by adjusting the articulator's incisal pin and using a hydrophilic vinyl polysiloxane registration material (Star VPS, Danville, USA), bilateral stops registering this new vertical dimension were made in the posterior region. These stops were removed from the casts and flattened on their occlusal surfaces.

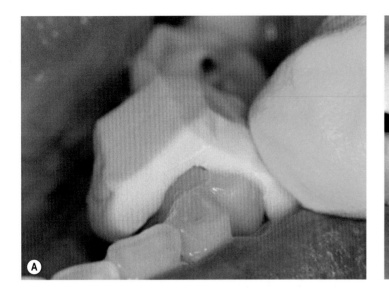

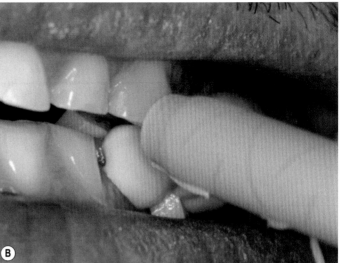

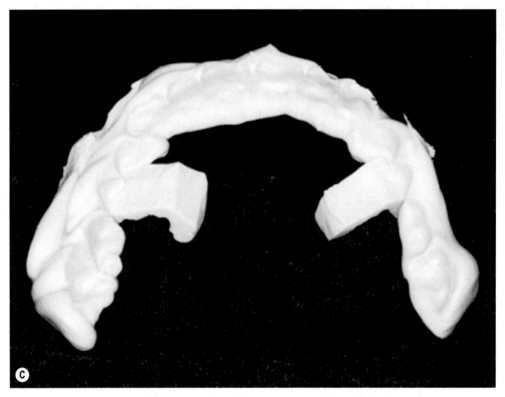

Fig. C7.8A–C   Both stops were placed in the patient's mouth to replicate the new occlusal vertical dimension (OVD) position clinically. To fix the new occlusal relation in intercuspal position or retruded contact position the stops were 'relined' with registration material.

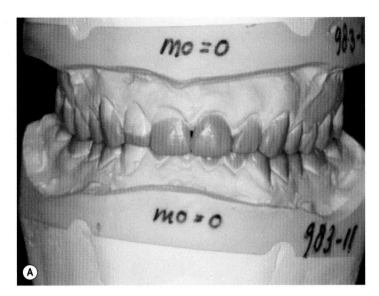

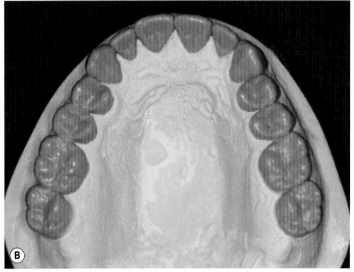

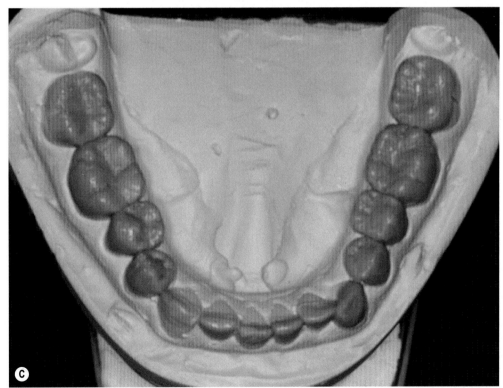

Fig. C7.9A–C   Based on this bite registration and a direct mock-up on teeth 13–23, a diagnostic wax-up model was made to get an understanding of the new dental relationship.

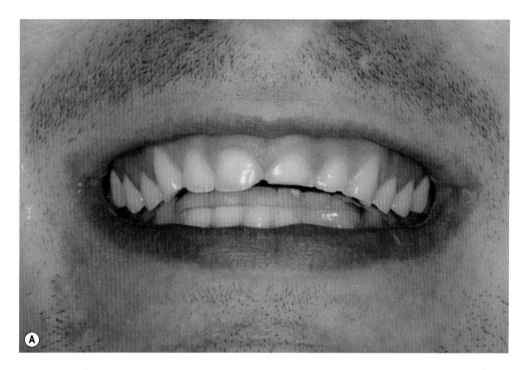

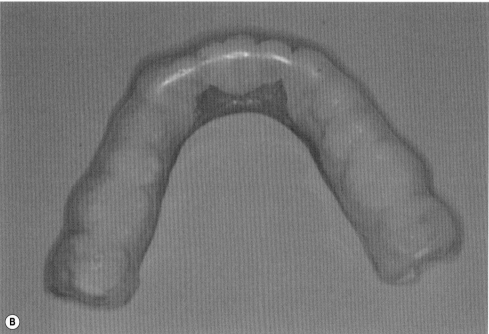

Fig. C7.10A,B A rigid occlusal splint was manufactured to test the increase in OVD for a period of 3 weeks. The splint was placed on the lower teeth.

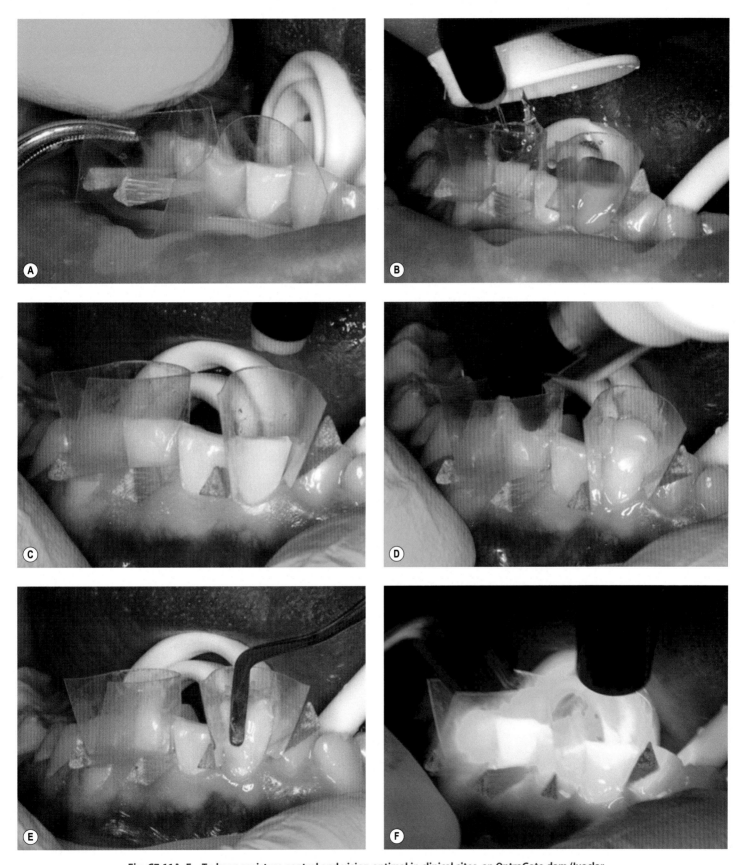

Fig. C7.11A–F   To keep moisture control and vision optimal in clinical sites, an OptraGate dam (Ivoclar Vivadent, Liechtenstein) was placed, including a tongue shield on the lingual aspect. The restorative process commenced with building up the mandibular anterior teeth. The morphology was shaped according to the situation in the wax-up.

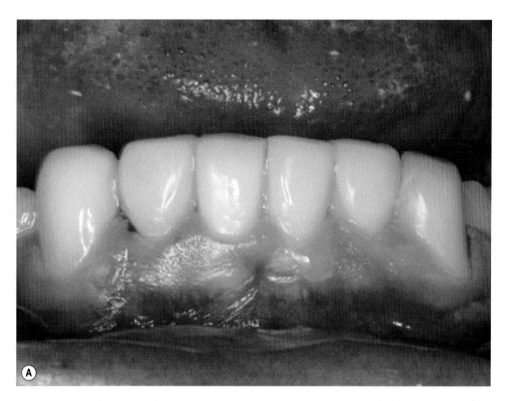

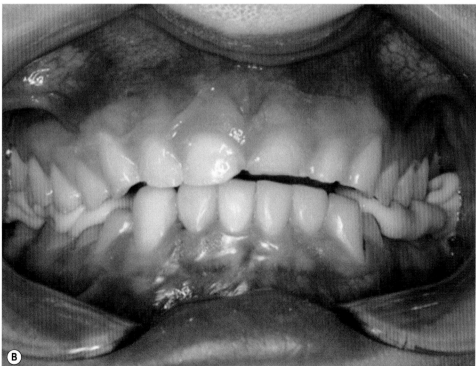

Fig. C7.12A,B   The lingual aspect of the mandibular anterior teeth was restored using Clearfil AP-X (A2, Kuraray Ltd), and the labial side with direct composite veneers (Empress Direct [A2E, Ivoclar Vivadent]). Using the silicone stops, the mandibular teeth were checked to be out of occlusion with enough vertical space remaining to restore the maxillary anterior teeth.

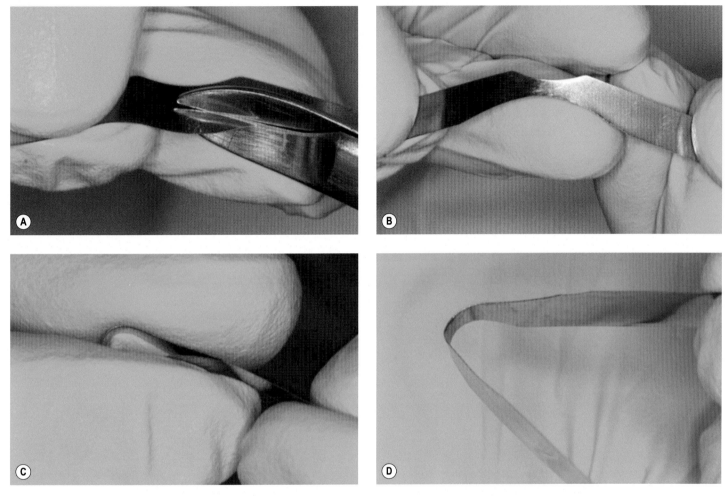

Fig. C7.13A–D A metal matrix band (Tofflemire 11) was used to restore the palatal morphology of the maxillary anterior teeth. The matrix was adjusted and preformed so that it adapted well to the palato-cervical region.

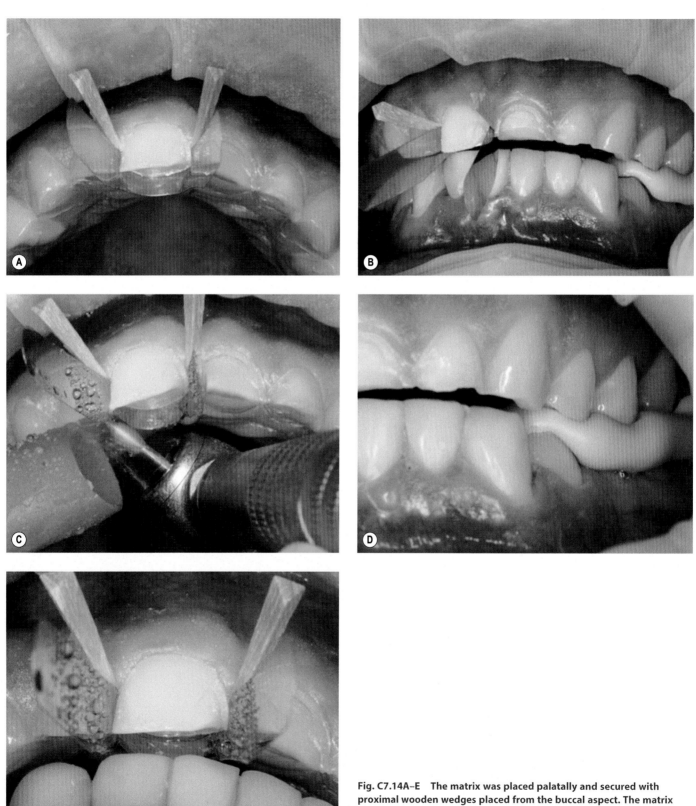

Fig. C7.14A–E The matrix was placed palatally and secured with proximal wooden wedges placed from the buccal aspect. The matrix was adjusted so that it was possible for the patient to occlude into the silicone stops without interference from the matrix band.

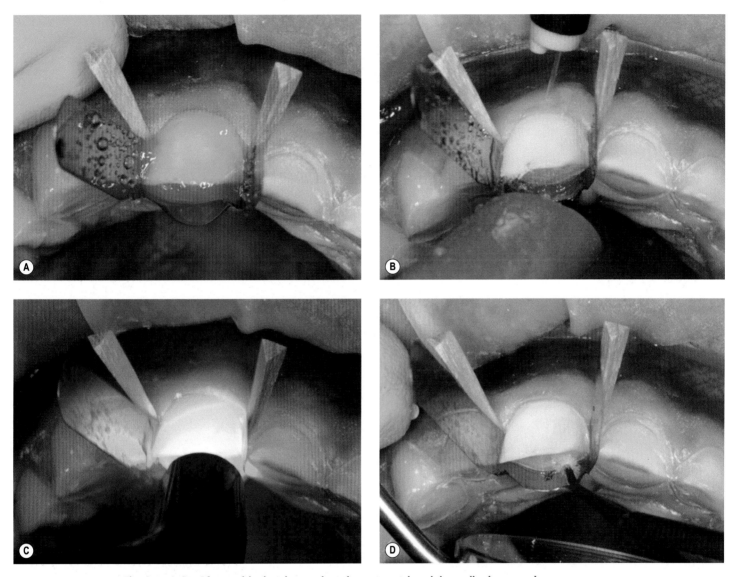

Fig. C7.15A–D After positioning the matrix, a three-step etch and rinse adhesive procedure was performed. The 37% phosphoric acid was applied for 15 seconds, rinsed thoroughly and gently air-dried. The primer was then applied and gently dried. Finally, the bonding agent was applied, gently dried and light cured for 15 seconds.

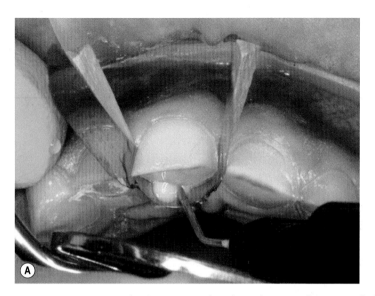
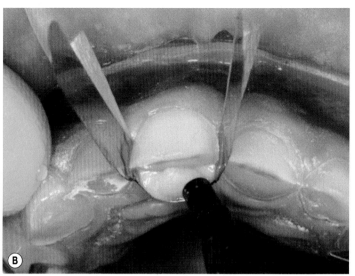

Fig. C7.16A,B   Before the resin composite was applied, a thin layer of flowable resin composite (Clearfil Majesty Flow, Kuraray) was placed palato-cervically. This layer was not photocured separately. Subsequently, Clearfil AP-X (Kuraray) was extruded directly from the compule, pushing the flowable composite and resulting in optimal marginal adaptation (the 'snow-plough technique'). After adaptation with instruments, this first layer of resin composite was photocured

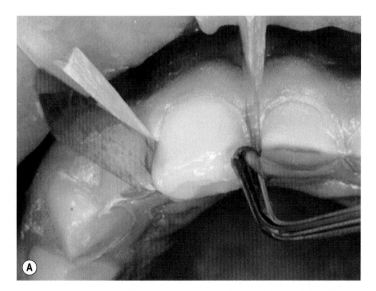
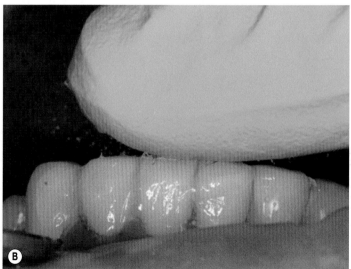

Fig. C7.17A,B   When the superficial occlusal increment of resin composite was applied, the palatal surface was shaped using a hand instrument (ASH 49) and the mandibular anterior teeth were coated in petroleum jelly.

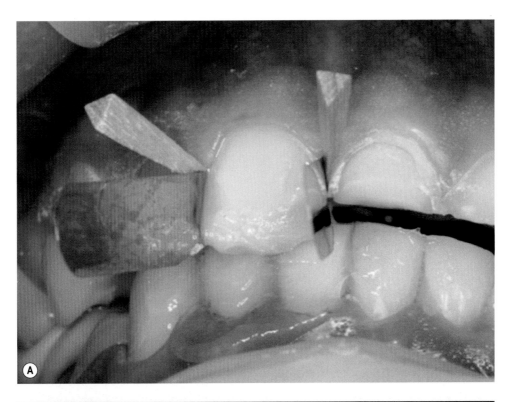

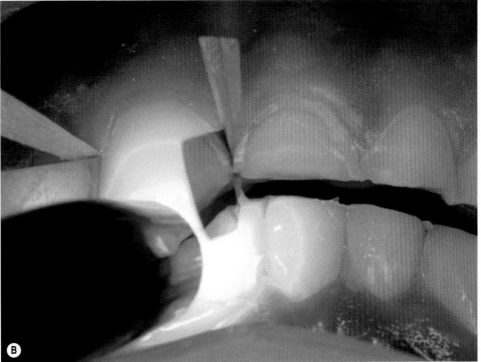

Fig. C7.18A,B With the silicone stops in situ, the patient occluded into the uncured final increment of resin composite. Maintaining this position, the resin composite was photocured for 20 seconds from the buccal aspect. The patient was asked to open his mouth and the material was photocured for a further 20 seconds from the palatal aspect. This is called the DSO (direct shaping by occlusion) technique.

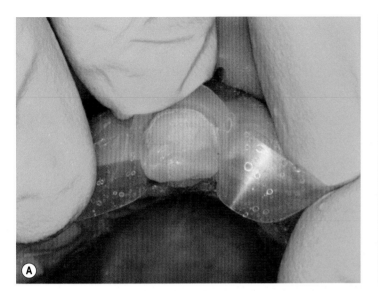

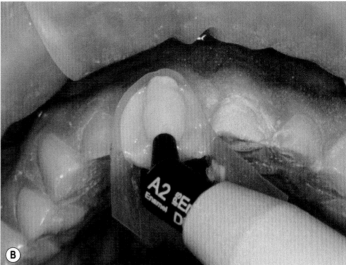

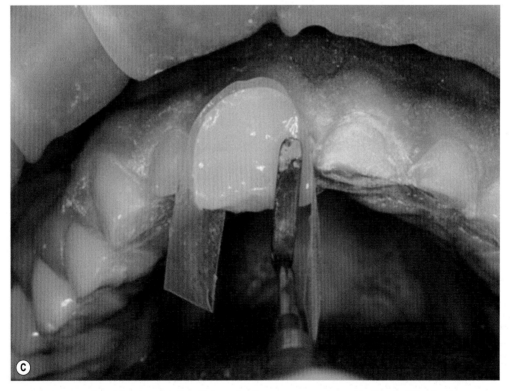

Fig. C7.19A–C After this gross shaping of the palatal contour, a contour strip (Ivoclar Vivadent) was placed and a direct resin composite labial veneer restoration was placed. Firstly, a dentine-coloured composite (A2 Dentin, Empress Direct, Ivoclar Vivadent) was applied, shaped and photocured. Secondly, an enamel shade (A2 Enamel, Empress Direct) and, finally, the incisal shade (Opal, Empress Direct) were applied incrementally.

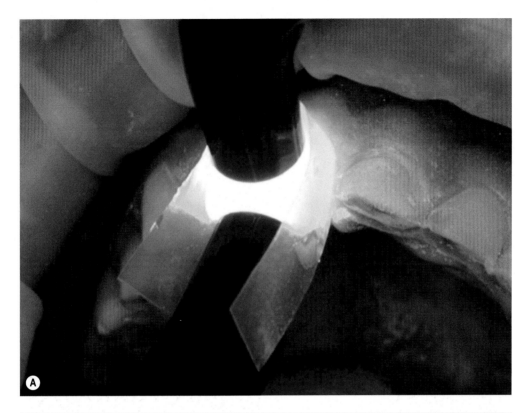

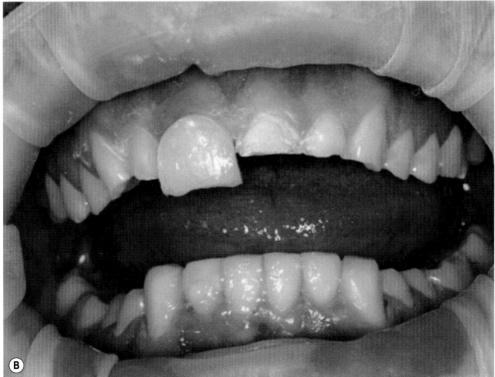

Fig. C7.20A,B   After application of the final increment of resin composite, the restoration was photocured from both the buccal and palatal aspects.

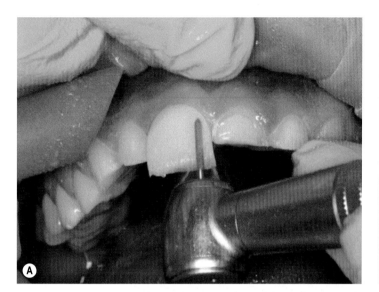
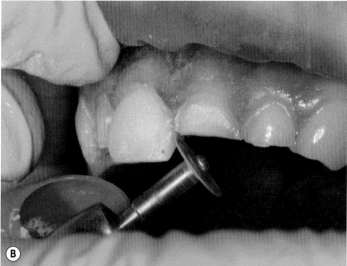
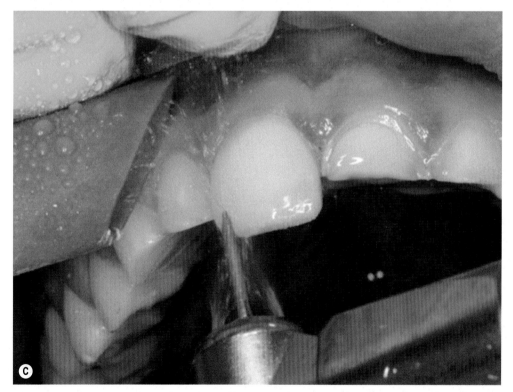

Fig. C7.21A–C   The restoration was shaped and finished using diamond burs and Sof-Lex discs (3M ESPE).

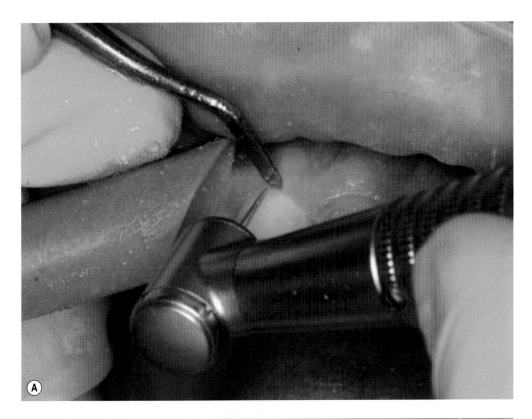

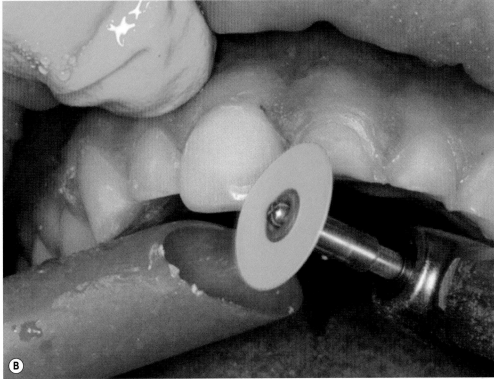

Fig. C7.22A,B While finishing the cervical margin, the gingival area was protected using a hand instrument. Finally, fine Sof-Lex discs were used to polish the restoration.

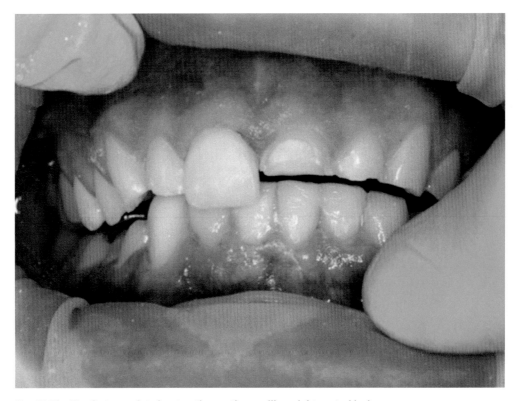

Fig. C7.23   The first completed restoration on the maxillary right central incisor.

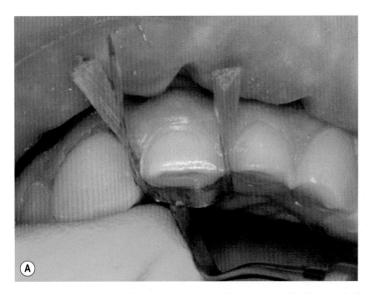

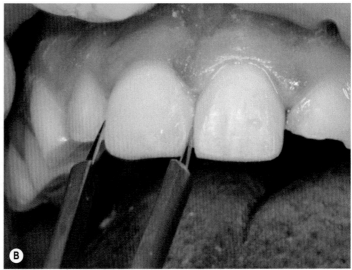

Fig. C7.24A,B   The adjacent central incisor was built up using the same procedure. During shaping and finishing, orthodontic dividers were used to check the width:length ratios of the resin composite restorations.

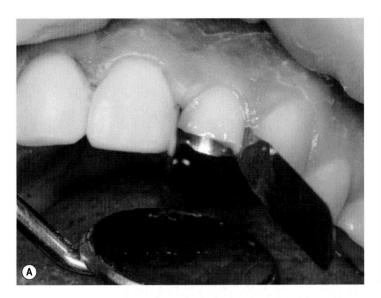

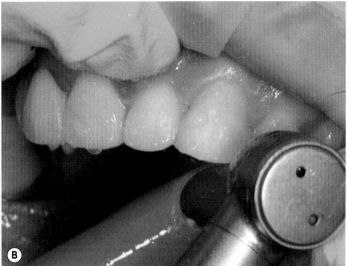

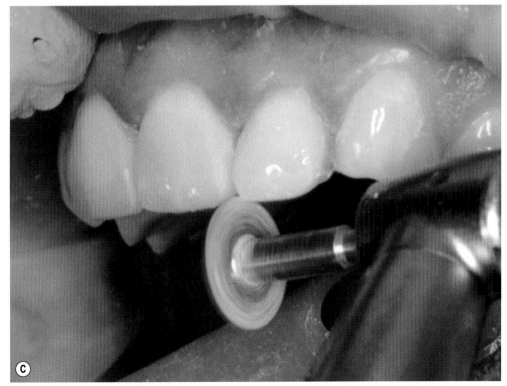

Fig. C7.25A–C   Following the same DSO technique, all maxillary anterior teeth were built up in the same way.

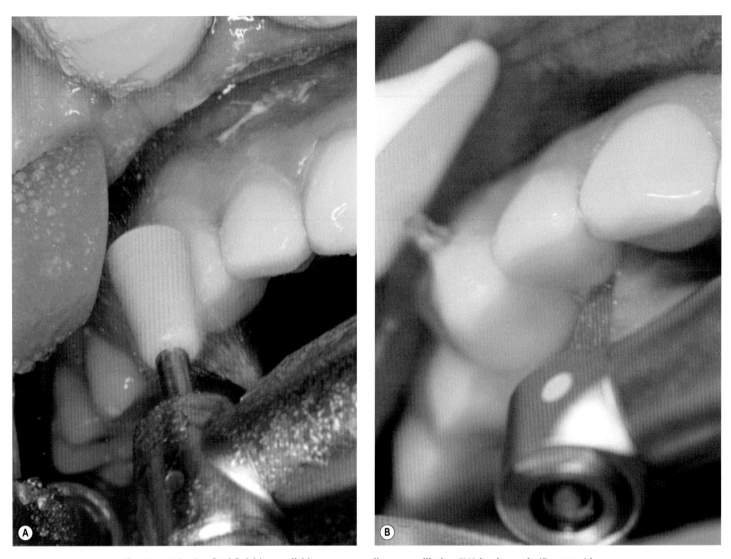

Fig. C7.26A,B   For final finishing, polishing cups as well as an oscillating EVA lamineer tip (Dentatus) in a 61LC handpiece (KAVO) (for sub-gingival margins) were used.

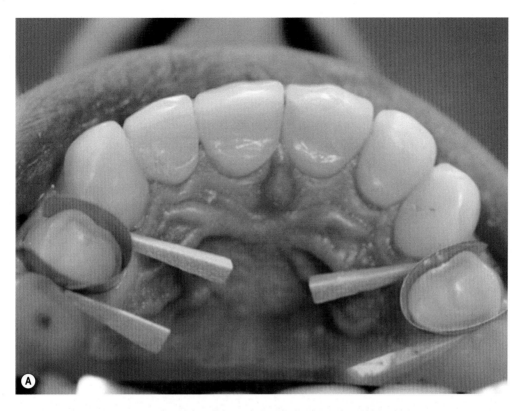

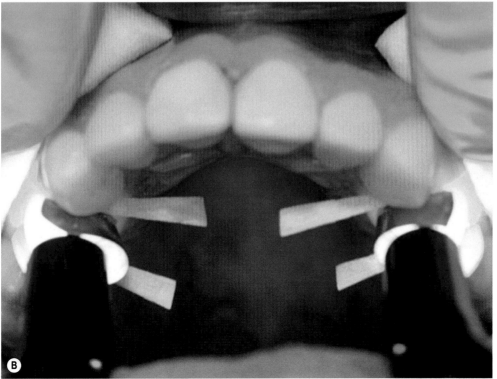

Fig. C7.27A,B   Next, the maxillary premolars were restored. No preparation was necessary because teeth were free of restorations or caries. Two metal matrices (Hawe Neos 1001-C Tofflemire matrices) were placed and secured with wedges.

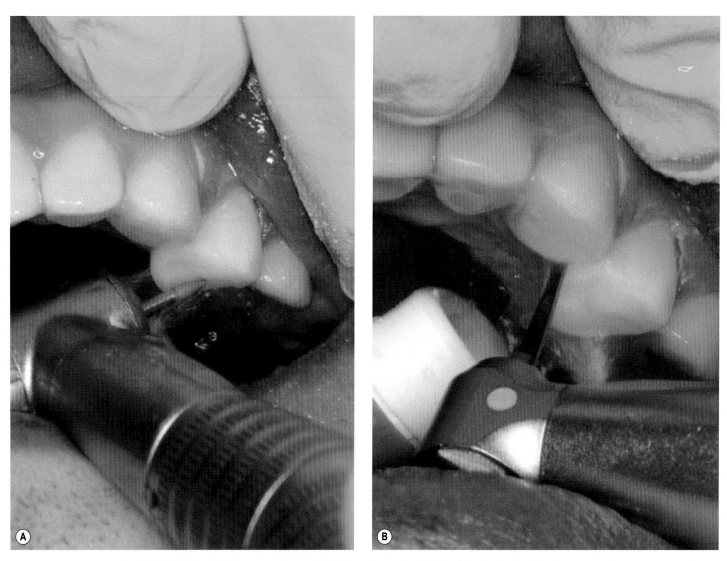

Fig. C7.28A,B   The finishing procedure was similar to those described previously. Occlusal surfaces were modelled into the desired form so that the curve of the maxilla was optimized esthetically.

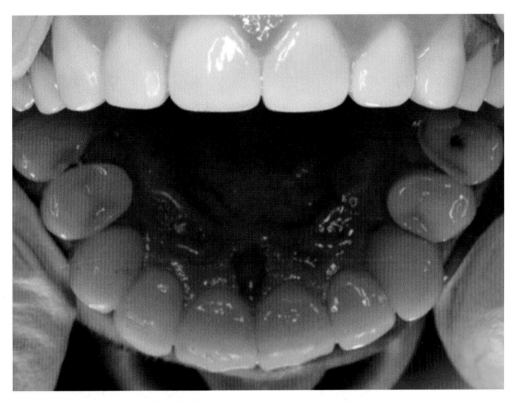

Fig. C7.29 **The maxillary teeth to the first premolars were now restored to the correct catenary curve. Palatally, the occlusal contact areas with the lower incisors can be seen. From now on the silicone stops became redundant, as the restored teeth established the new OVD and canine guidance.**

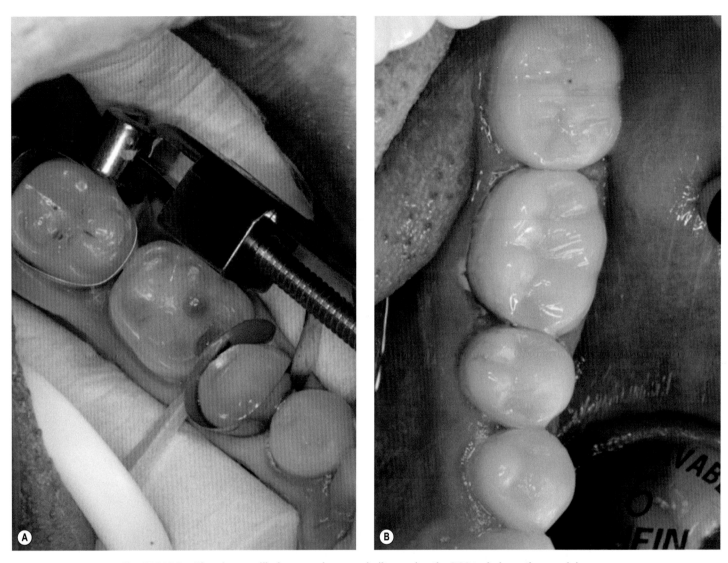

Fig. C7.30A,B   After the mandibular premolars were built up using the DSO technique, the remaining posterior teeth were restored in accordance with the established occlusal plane.

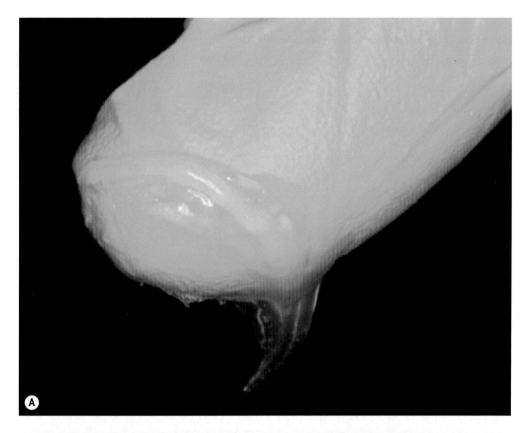

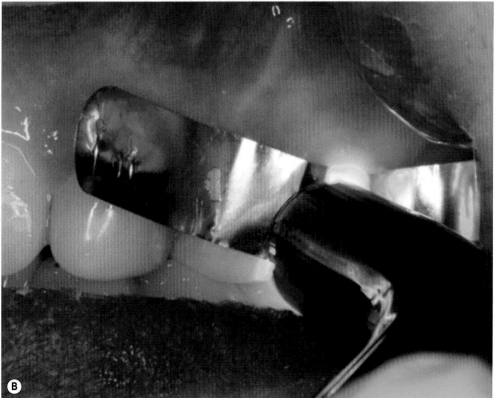

Fig. C7.31A,B Next, the maxillary second premolars and molars were restored using the DSO technique. The antagonists were separated with a thin layer of petroleum jelly before the patient occluded into the uncured resin composite. Initial photocuring of the resin composite was performed in occlusion, after which the restorations were photocured from the palatal aspect.

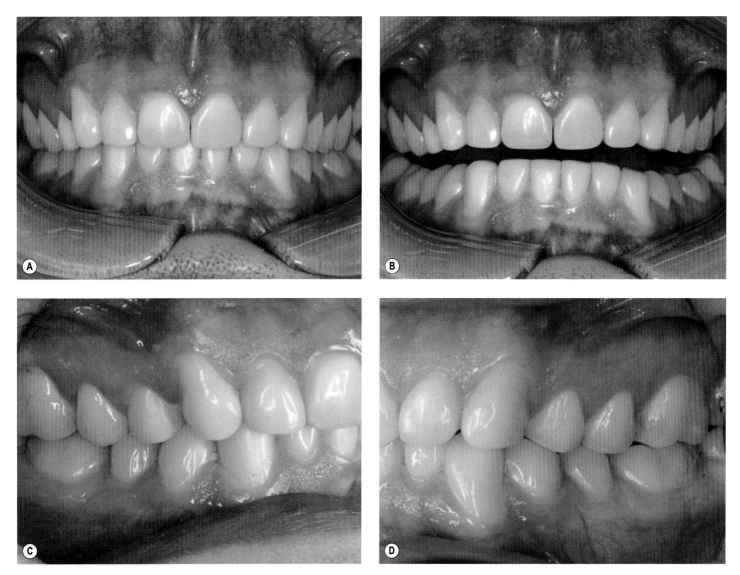

Fig. C7.32A–D   The final result of the direct minimally invasive (MI) treatment can be seen. A suitable occlusion and intercuspation were achieved.

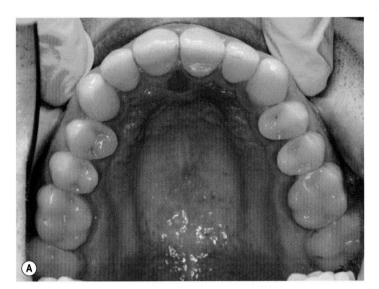

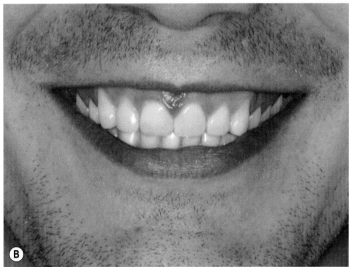

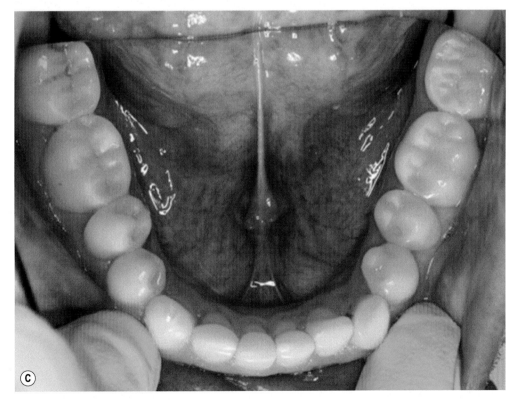

Fig. C7.33A–C   As with Figure C7.32, the final result of the direct MI treatment can be seen. A suitable occlusion and intercuspation were achieved.

MATERIALS USED

OptraGate (Ivoclar Vivadent)

Star VPS (Danville) bite registration material

Tofflemire matrix 11, Hawe Neos 1001-C

Plastic contour matrix (Ivoclar Vivadent)

Phosphoric acid 37% (DMG)

Clearfil SA Primer (Kuraray)

Clearfil Photo Bond (Kuraray)

Clearfil AP-X (Kuraray): for occlusal and palatal/lingual surfaces

Empress Direct (Ivoclar Vivadent): for buccal surfaces in the esthetic zone

Sof-Lex discs (3M ESPE)

Polishing cups (Ivoclar Vivadent)

EVA lamineer tip (Dentatus) in a 61LC handpiece (KAVO)

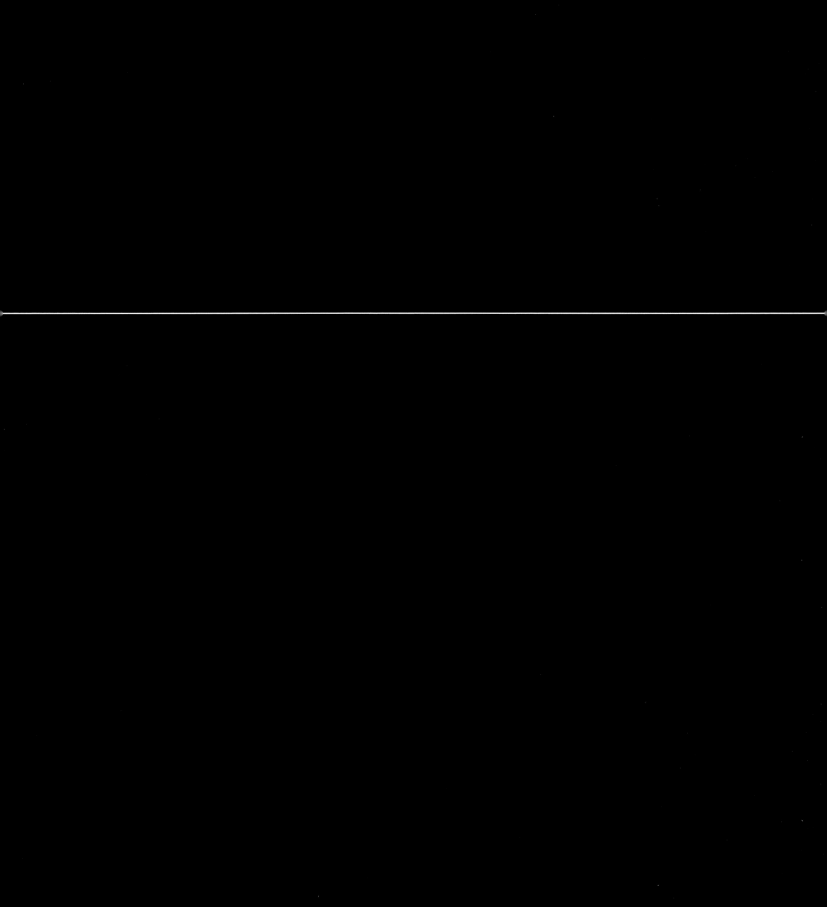

Minimally Invasive Replacement of Missing Teeth: Part 1

L. MACKENZIE

INTRODUCTION

The average person will not retain their complete adult dentition for a lifetime and while the automatic replacement of missing teeth with a fixed or removable appliance is often unnecessary, tooth loss in the esthetic zone is of serious concern in most societies. Many patients will seek restorative treatment and judge the outcome on the basis of esthetics rather than function.

Contemporary prosthodontics offers a range of options for the replacement of lost or absent teeth, but with each one there is a biological cost to pay for the remaining natural dentition and the supporting periodontal tissues.

This chapter and Chapter 9 describe the relative merits of minimally invasive prosthodontics for tooth replacement with emphasis on those techniques that preserve the maximum amount of healthy tooth tissue.

PREVALENCE OF TOOTH LOSS

Adult dental health has shown a continuous improvement since the 1960s and for younger adults the prospect of retaining a considerable number of healthy teeth throughout a long life has never been higher. Tooth loss, however, remains commonplace. The latest extensive survey from the United Kingdom[1] reveals that the average adult has between 27 and 32 teeth (and approximately 18 sound, unrestored teeth). While the prevalence of caries and periodontitis continues to reduce, extensive disease persists (Fig. 8.1) and is concentrated in a relatively small proportion of adults.[1]

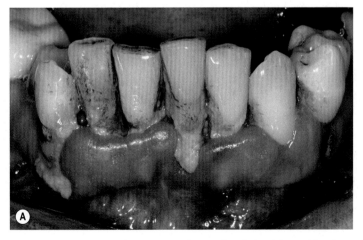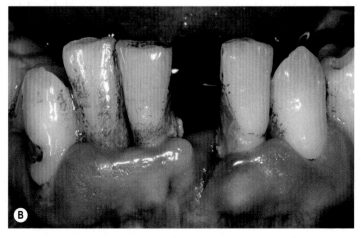

Fig. 8.1A,B   Advanced periodontitis resulting in tooth loss presents numerous management difficulties.

AETIOLOGY OF TOOTH LOSS

While teeth may be lost due to trauma or be missing for developmental reasons, the vast majority of teeth lost in adulthood are as a result of caries, periodontitis or extraction at the end of a cycle of restoration replacement and repair that is sometimes referred to as the 'dental countdown'.

In this respects it is hopeful that preventive strategies and the wide range of modern minimally invasive operative techniques will help reduce the incidence of tooth loss in future generations.

REASONS FOR REPLACING LOST TEETH

The aim of contemporary MI dentistry is to help patients maintain healthy oral tissues for a lifetime. However, it is a well-reported fact that many traditional restorative procedures have the opposite effect, especially in the case of tooth replacement.[2,3]

To reduce the risk of shortening the lifespan of an abutment or adjacent/opposing teeth, it is essential for practitioners to consider carefully the risks and benefits of intervention. The most commonly cited reasons for restoration of a missing tooth are based on:

- Esthetics

- Function

- Psychological factors

- Phonetics

- Prevention of tooth movement.

ESTHETICS

Methods for cosmetic tooth replacement date back over 2000 years[4] and in modern dental practice, patient demand for esthetic tooth-coloured restorations has never been higher. Tooth loss in the esthetic zone may seriously affect a patient's appearance and most will enquire about restorative options.[4,5] Contemporary dentistry offers a range of techniques using materials designed to blend inconspicuously with the patient's remaining dentition and practitioners must select the most appropriate, minimally invasive esthetic option for each individual case.

FUNCTION

Historically, tooth loss was often followed by 'reflex' replacement on the basis of restoring masticatory function. However, it is a well-documented fact that masticatory efficiency is possible with relatively few teeth[6] and therefore practitioners must exercise extreme caution when prescribing tooth replacement on a functional basis.

PSYCHOLOGICAL FACTORS

Prevention of tooth loss is one of the most commonly cited reasons for patients visiting their dentist and when gaps occur they can have a considerable impact on self-confidence.

PHONETICS

While tooth loss may have a reversible, short-term impact on speech patterns, it may also have a catastrophic effect on certain patients' abilities to play musical instruments.

PREVENTION OF TOOTH MOVEMENT

It is a commonly cited reason that tooth replacement should be prescribed to prevent unfavourable orthodontic movement resulting eventually from the sudden disequilibrium that follows tooth loss.[4] However, various studies have demonstrated that such changes may not occur[7,8] (Fig. 8.2) and that, even if they do, the clinical consequences are often negligible.

Before planning restorative treatment it is important to consider the evidence with regard to tooth movement. This information should be balanced with the possible deleterious consequences of over-eruption, tipping, drifting or rotation of teeth adjacent to or opposing a space (Boxes 8.1 and 8.2).

In summary, the routine restoration of edentulous areas should be avoided. Careful monitoring for potential problems and advice on oral hygiene protocols will avoid the provision of unnecessary restorative procedures.

OPTIONS FOR THE MANAGEMENT OF MISSING TEETH

The remainder of this chapter and Chapter 9 describe the range of options currently available for the management of lost or absent teeth (Box 8.3), with particular reference to the biological cost associated with each and emphasis

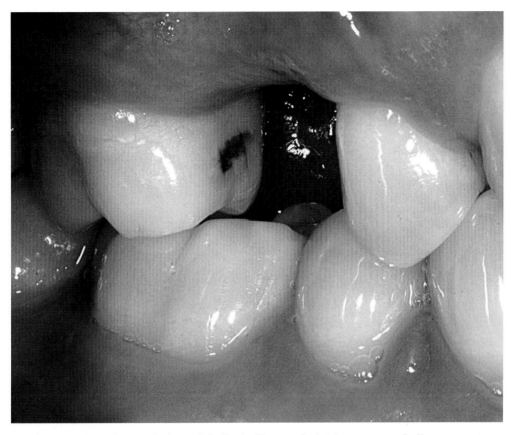

Fig. 8.2   Tooth loss often results in no clinically significant orthodontic movement of adjacent or opposing teeth.

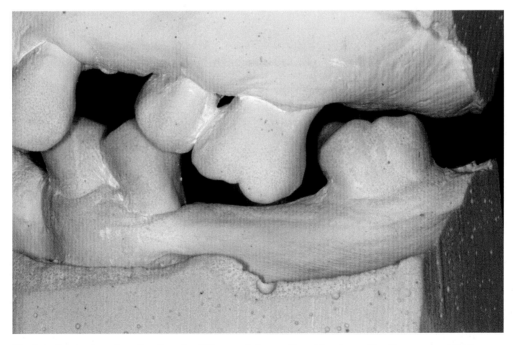

Fig. 8.3   Incomplete dental arches should be carefully monitored for signs of tooth movement that may complicate restorative treatment.

BOX 8.1
POSSIBLE NEGATIVE CONSEQUENCES OF TOOTH MOVEMENT FOLLOWING EXTRACTION

- Increased caries and periodontitis risk via plaque accumulation and food trapping
- Increased difficulty in oral hygiene measures
- Loss of esthetics
- Reduction in masticatory efficiency
- Loss of space for prospective restorative treatment (Fig. 8.3)
- Decreased support for axial loading/tooth mobility
- Loss of prospective fixed bridge abutments

BOX 8.2
EVIDENCE FOR TOOTH MOVEMENT FOLLOWING EXTRACTION

Over-eruption

- Some teeth show no sign of over-eruption[7]
- In the majority of cases, over-eruption is slight (<2 mm)[7,8]
- There is a lower risk of over-eruption if antagonist is lost in adulthood[8]

Tipping

- The majority of teeth (62%) show no signs of tipping[8]
- If movement has not occurred within 5 years of extraction, it is unlikely to occur[7]
- Tipping is more common where mesial rather than distal contacts are lost
- Tipping is more common in the mandible[8]
- Molar tipping of >15° is more common in the maxilla[8]

Mesial drift

- More likely if extraction occurs at <12 years of age[7]
- Reduced tendency if patient is >36 years of age[7]

given to those techniques that require the least or no tooth preparation at all. For each option the systematic, logical sequence of examination, diagnosis and care planning is implicit and described only when relevant.

NON-OPERATIVE MANAGEMENT

When patients present with incomplete dental arches, the number one consideration should be the preservation of their remaining teeth and they should be

BOX 8.3
MANAGEMENT OPTIONS FOR MISSING TEETH

- Non-operative management
- Re-implantation
- Wilkinson's extractions
- Orthodontics
- Transplantation
- Removable prosthodontics
- Implants
- Fixed prosthodontics
- Minimally invasive conventional bridges
- Metal–ceramic adhesive bridges
- Resin composite adhesive bridges
- All-ceramic adhesive bridges

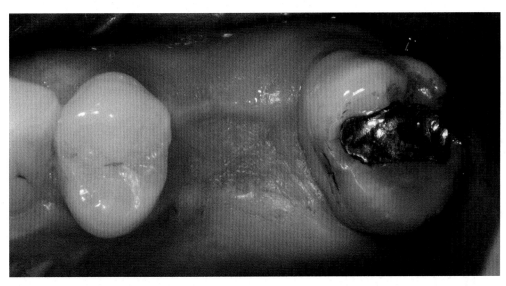

Fig. 8.4 Non-operative management should be the first consideration when assessing edentulous spaces.

informed thoroughly of the biological consequences of operative intervention.[5] Knowing when to choose 'masterly inactivity'[4] (Fig. 8.4) over operative dentistry for the long-term benefit of patients is a key skill in itself.

RE-IMPLANTATION

Even the latest restorative techniques have limitations in replicating accurately the complex anatomical, functional and optical properties of natural teeth. Therefore if a tooth is avulsed or rendered mobile (subluxed) following trauma, frequently the most esthetic and conservative treatment option is to try to preserve the natural tooth.

The complete displacement of the tooth from the socket may be considered as a true dental emergency. Management requires immediate tooth re-implantation as the prognosis is determined principally by the time elapsed since avulsion.

For case-specific information, including management details for subluxation, extrusion and intrusion, visit: http://dentaltraumaguide.org/[9]

EARLY EXTRACTIONS

First permanent molars are likely candidates for premature loss as they are affected commonly by caries, restorative procedures and developmental defects. If the long-term prognosis for these teeth is considered poor, they may be electively extracted allowing forward movement of the second permanent molars into their place. The timing of such procedures is critical to success:

- Lower first permanent molars of poor prognosis should be extracted when calcification of the inter-radicular dentine of the lower second molar is visible radiographically. (Dental age of 8–9 years.)

- For the upper first molars the timing of extractions is less critical and an acceptable result may still be obtained up to 11–12 years as long as molar crowding is present.

ORTHODONTICS

While employed commonly to correct crowded malocclusions, well-executed orthodontics is also an ideal minimally invasive option for space closure resulting from missing teeth. It may be used to close gaps completely or combined with other restorative techniques to optimize the esthetic outcome.

In this respect, orthodontics is useful in the anterior esthetic zone, for example in the management of hypodontia involving upper lateral incisors.

After third molars and mandibular second premolars, upper lateral incisors are the most common congenitally missing teeth.[10] Unfortunately, 'self-correction' by approximation of adjacent teeth is rare and operative treatment is often indicated. Figure 8.5 shows an acceptable esthetic outcome that used orthodontics and minimal enamel re-contouring to treat missing lateral incisors and an ectopic first premolar.

TRANSPLANTATION

This rarely used option involves the extraction of an unsaveable tooth and transplantation of a healthy replacement that has been extracted from elsewhere in

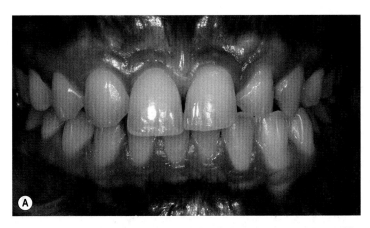
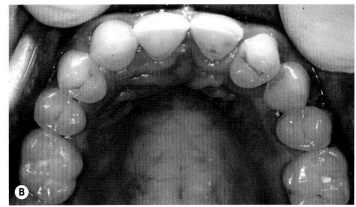

Fig. 8.5A,B   Minimally invasive management of hypodontia and an ectopic premolar using orthodontics and enamelplasty.

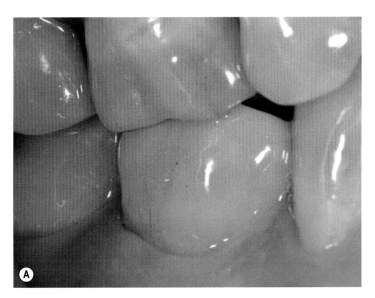
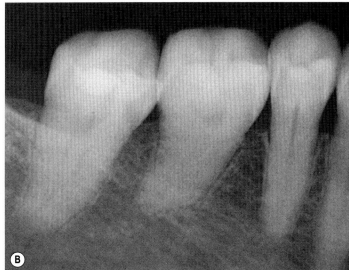

Fig. 8.6A,B   Clinical and radiographic images, taken 30 years post-operatively, of a lower third molar transplanted into a lower right first molar extraction socket. Courtesy of Dr J. McCubbin.

the mouth. Figure 8.6 shows a lower left third molar that was transplanted to replace an unrestorable lower right first molar 35 years previously.

REMOVABLE PROSTHODONTICS

Removable prosthodontics is the oldest method of tooth replacement[5] and is still employed widely, particularly for the restoration of longer spans. Removable partial dentures (RPDs) may be considered as one of the least invasive options for replacement of missing teeth, as long as they are designed carefully and maintained scrupulously. This is illustrated in Figure 8.7 where an upper canine,

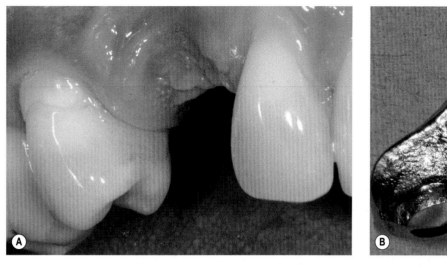

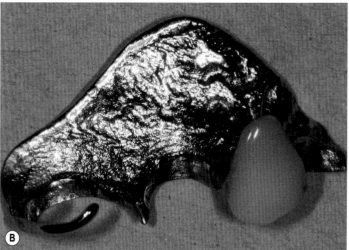

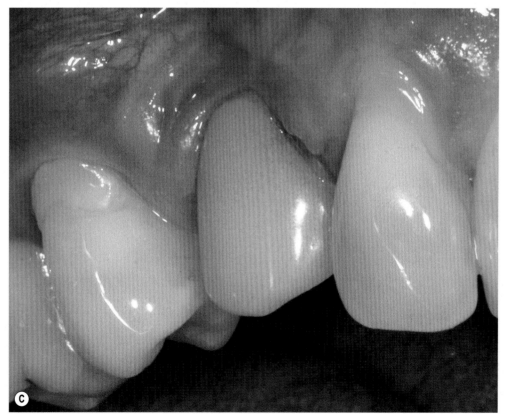

Fig. 8.7A–C   A 40-year-old cobalt–chromium, removable partial denture restoring a missing upper canine.

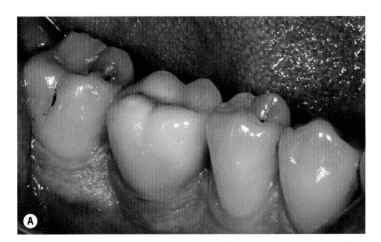 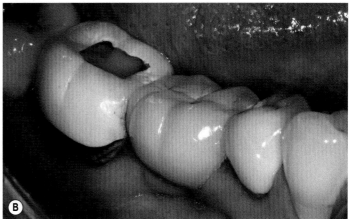

Fig. 8.8A,B   Implant-retained restorations (A) completely preserve adjacent teeth and carry a significantly better long-term prognosis than traditional prosthodontic techniques (B).

lost 40 years previously, has been replaced by an RPD worn continuously and removed only for cleaning (not to be recommended routinely!).

IMPLANTS

Implant-retained restorations may be considered as the treatment of choice for the esthetic restoration of missing teeth where surgical, restorative and economic factors permit.[5,11] With careful planning and operative techniques they have a good prognosis and often avoid completely the invasive treatment of other sound teeth (Fig. 8.8A).

FIXED PROSTHODONTICS

Fixed bridgework can carry an unacceptably high risk to the long-term health of a patient's dentition.[2–4] Therefore, the justification for restoring any space using fixed prosthodontics must be considered carefully and the potential for complications or irretrievable catastrophic failure assessed and outlined to the patient at the outset. In this respect, fixed/fixed bridgework may be singled out, as there are few procedures more destructive than the preparation of mutually parallel abutment teeth for conventional bridgework[4] (Fig. 8.8B).

SIMPLE CANTILEVER BRIDGEWORK

One method of minimizing potential complications associated with fixed prosthodontics is to utilize simple cantilever designs that require preparation of only

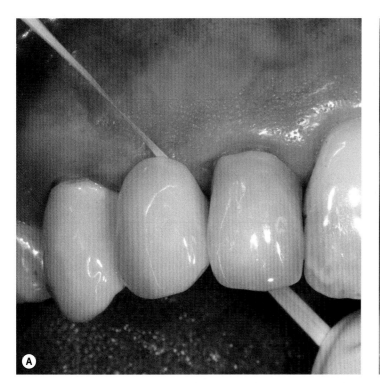
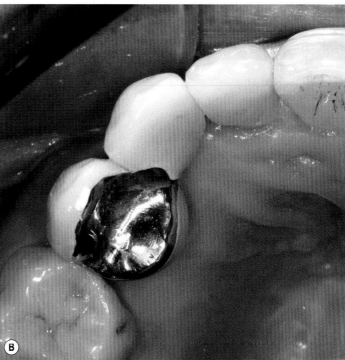

Fig. 8.9A,B (A) Simple cantilever bridges are esthetic and are easy to maintain. (B) Minimally invasive abutment preparation accommodates alloy only in areas that will not be seen.

one abutment tooth. In addition to avoiding the need for parallel abutments, simple cantilevers are considered to be:

- Easier to optimize esthetically[5]

- More amenable to plaque control (Fig. 8.9A)

- More amenable to failure detection if de-cementation occurs, and therefore repair.

Potential disadvantages relate to the application of leverage forces on abutments during function and these may be minimized by:

- Limiting span length to one pontic

- Selecting cases with reduced occlusal forces

- Avoiding pontic-only loading

- Designing to minimize non-axial loading

- Minimizing tooth reduction in areas where esthetic porcelain is unnecessary (Fig. 8.9B).

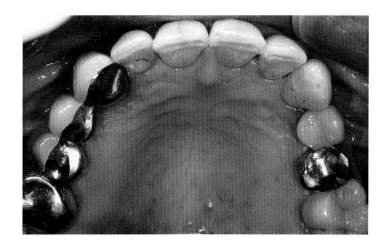

Fig. 8.10 Missing upper first premolars restored with bridges using traditional retainers (upper right) compared to a minimally invasive three-quarter gold retainer.

PARTIAL COVERAGE BRIDGE RETAINERS

This is probably the least used design for fixed bridge retainers,[5] which is unfortunate as it confers a number of advantages:

- More conservative tooth preparation (Fig. 8.10)

- Maintenance of enamel, therefore suitable for previously restored, weakened teeth

- Reduced involvement of gingival margins

- Margins are more accessible to oral hygiene measures

- Exposed axial tooth surfaces facilitate pulp testing

- Fit may be assessed readily

- Versatile path of insertion

- Simpler cementation technique.

These advantages must be weighed against potential disadvantages:

- Metal display (Fig. 8.11) may be unacceptable esthetically to some patients

- Less rigid casting is unsuitable for long spans

- Less retentive, therefore optimum axial length is essential.

The most common contemporary use of partial coverage retainers is for the fabrication of metal frameworks in metal–ceramic resin-bonded bridges.

METAL–CERAMIC RESIN-BONDED BRIDGES

The well-documented complications of aggressive tooth preparation have stimulated research, dating back over 40 years, into more minimally invasive

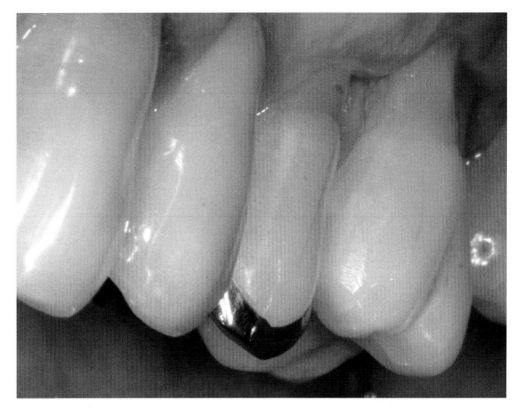

Fig. 8.11 Patients must be aware of the need for metal display when using this retainer design.

techniques for tooth replacement. In 1972, Alain Rochette was the first to describe a revolutionary 'non-mutilating', 'non-irritating' technique[12] suitable for tooth replacement that employed adhesive resin and required no tooth preparation.

While unperforated designs for definitive resin-bonded bridges (RBBs) are now favoured in virtually all published reports,[13,14] on occasion they may also deliver long-lasting restorations (Fig. 8.12).[13] RBB techniques have continued to evolve and offer significant advantages over traditional fixed prosthodontics[13,15] to such an extent that they may be considered as the next best option to dental implants for the predictable, esthetic restoration of short-span edentulous spaces where adjacent teeth are minimally, or completely, unrestored.[16]

ADVANTAGES OF RESIN-BONDED BRIDGES

Conservative

RBB design promotes minimally invasive tooth preparation compared to traditional techniques.[13,15,17] Preparations confined to enamel are functionally and biologically superior, particularly for young patients with relatively large pulps.[4]

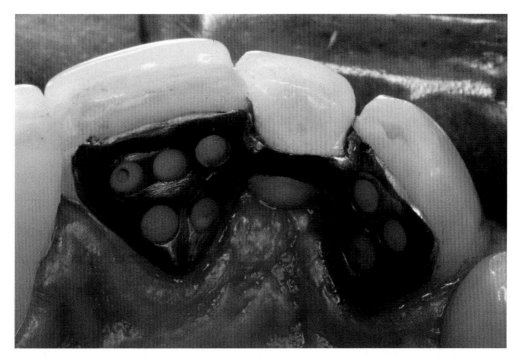

Fig. 8.12   Fixed/fixed resin-bonded bridge with Rochette design in continuous service for more than 30 years. Courtesy of Dr J. McCubbin.

When the occlusion is favourable, such as replacement of missing lower incisors (Fig. 8.13), tooth preparation may be avoided entirely.

Minimum long-term damage

Failure of RBBs is rarely catastrophic for abutment teeth, compared to traditional techniques.[11,13] In addition they are readily reversible[17] and may be employed as transitional restorations or as temporary prostheses prior to implant procedures.

Esthetics

RBBs have high patient satisfaction rates in esthetic terms[13] and, with careful case selection and designing, the optical properties of abutment teeth remain unaffected (Fig. 8.14).

Versatility

Although RBBs are frequently employed for replacement of anterior teeth, they have been shown to be successful for restoring posterior spaces in both maxillary and mandibular arches.[18]

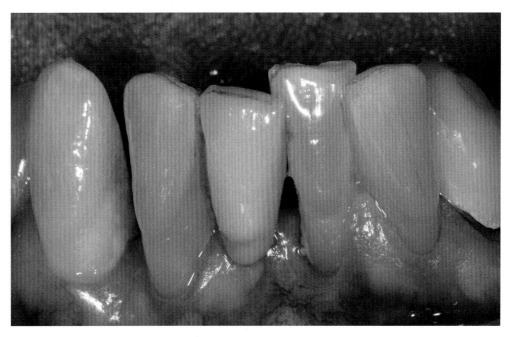

Fig. 8.13 Lingual resin-bonded bridge retainers on lower anterior teeth will often not be visible, allowing rigid retainer designs with minimal (or no) tooth preparation.

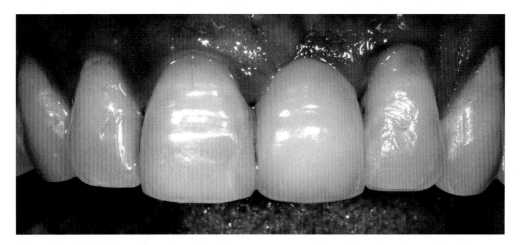

Fig. 8.14 Resin-bonded bridges are popular with patients and preserve the esthetics and integrity of abutment teeth.

Patient popularity

Minimal drilling confined to enamel is popular with patients[4] and often obviates the need for local anaesthetic[4] and provisional restorations. As well as minimal biological cost, if correctly prescribed and executed, RBBs have been shown to have a good cost/benefit ratio in financial terms.[13]

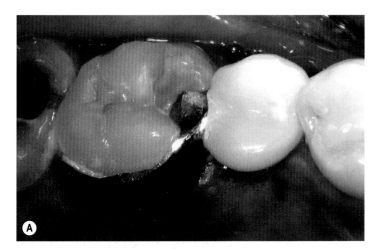
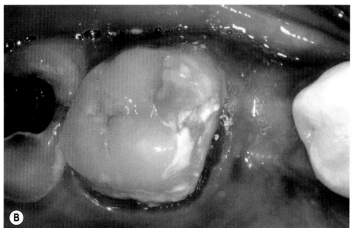

Fig. 8.15A,B   Sub-optimal design and technique will result in premature failure of resin-bonded bridges.

DISADVANTAGES OF RESIN-BONDED BRIDGEWORK

While they offer significant advantages over other modes of tooth replacement, it is an unfortunate fact that RBBs have not been accepted widely by all dental professionals. This may be a result of poor personal experience or from a general, undeserved[13,16,19] perception that they are unsuitable as long-lasting restorations. For practitioners to prescribe RBBs with confidence, it is essential to understand their limitations, contra-indications and potential disadvantages, as outlined in the following text.

Technique sensitivity

As with all adhesive procedures, successful long-lasting restorations will only result if case selection, design, preparation, manufacture and luting procedures are all optimized. Operator experience has been shown to have a significant effect on success[13] and high failure rate is the likely outcome of poor technique (Fig. 8.15). This will then result in loss of patient and operator confidence in this method of tooth replacement.[4,15]

Esthetics

While adhesive bridges made entirely from tooth-coloured materials (see Chapter 9) are increasing in popularity, most of the current long-term data pertains to metal–ceramic RBBs. In certain clinical situations, for example thin anterior teeth and occlusal surfaces of posterior teeth (Fig. 8.16A), metal display may be unacceptable to some patients. Furthermore, if abutment teeth are poor esthetically, RBBs offer little potential for changing their appearance (8.16B).[4,5,11]

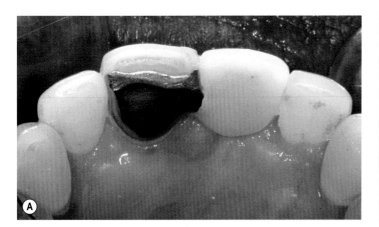 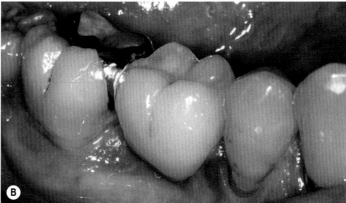

Fig. 8.16 Cantilever resin-bonded bridge replacing a lower first molar. When planning metal–ceramic RBBs patients must be informed well regarding retainer designs that will be visible.

Trial cementation and temporization

The nature of RBBs usually makes it impossible to cement restorations provisionally for diagnostic purposes and inter-appointment temporary restorations present challenges in fabrication and retention.

Longevity

Various studies report a wide range of failure rates for adhesive bridgework.[13,15,20] The reasons attributed most commonly to failure are:

- Poor case selection
- Inadequate retainer design
- Faulty bonding procedure
- Occlusal factors.

While general survival rates are not as encouraging as for some other indirect techniques, careful adherence to the following guidelines should result in predictability and deliver longevity rates enjoyed by routine users.

Regardless of restoration longevity rates, the biological advantages of RBB must be emphasized to patients, along with the fact that failure is rarely disastrous compared to conventional fixed prosthodontics.[13,16] Finally, if failure occurs (and restorations remain acceptable) they may often be re-cemented, increasing their functional longevity.[13,21]

GUIDELINES FOR SUCCESS WITH RESIN-BONDED BRIDGEWORK

Attention to detail is essential for successful RBBs.[5,13,17] While precise rules are lacking due to controversy among independent practitioners and researchers, careful study of four decades of evidence-based literature provides a set of general guidelines, which may be divided into:

- Patient factors

- Clinical factors

- Operator factors

- Laboratory factors.

PATIENT FACTORS

So that the patient can make an informed decision regarding RBB, detailed answers should be offered to the frequently asked questions in terms that are understandable for each individual patient. As the restoration appearance will be one of the patient's principal concerns,[4,5] the expected esthetic outcome should be communicated clearly at the outset. This may be facilitated by reference to photographic images of similar cases.

CLINICAL FACTORS

When selecting cases for RBBs, detailed assessment of the general state of the mouth should be carried out to include: the presence of other edentulous areas, risk of caries and periodontal disease and the necessity of restorative treatment elsewhere. Particular attention should be given to the following areas.

Abutment teeth

As quality adhesion is a prerequisite for success, sufficient enamel quality must be available for bonding. Case selection must not rely on heavily restored or mobile teeth, or on conditions where axial length is sub-optimal.[11,13,17] Clinical and radiographic assessment must reveal optimum periodontal and endodontic conditions and the need for replacement of existing restorations should be investigated.

Span length

Regardless of material, RBB retainers are thinner and more flexible than their full-coverage counterparts. Longer pontic spans will subject the casting and the adhesive bond to greater stresses and this situation will be exacerbated on mastication or parafunction.[4] Better long-term results have been demonstrated for RBBs that replace just one tooth with a single pontic.[4,13]

Pontic space

Where tooth movement has resulted in an unnaturally narrow or wide pontic space, adhesive bridges offer little scope for correction by modification of abutment teeth.[4,5]

Occlusal factors

For long-term success, RBB designs should not introduce occlusal interference[4] and the need to re-contour opposing or adjacent teeth should be considered. A diagnosis of severe parafunction generally precludes RBB techniques.[14]

Maintenance

As with all indirect restorations, long-term success will only result with optimal patient compliance regarding oral hygiene and avoidance of excessive loads. The importance of regular recall consultations should be stressed from the outset to allow careful monitoring, refinement and repair. The need for immediate assessment if failure is suspected should be emphasized. (Management protocols for RBB failure are described under 'Management of failure in resin-bonded bridgework' on p. 218.)

OPERATOR FACTORS

It is an accepted fact that the experience and technical skill of the dentist is the most important factor governing the success or failure of any adhesive procedure in dentistry. This is certainly the case for adhesive bridgework. For long-lasting, esthetic restorations, technique must be optimized with regard to the following:[4,13,16,17]

- Bridge design

- Pontic design

- Abutment preparation design

- Impression technique

- Cementation.

Bridge design

There is great variability of opinion regarding the design for adhesive bridges and most data refers to anterior bridgework, but research from various long-term clinical studies provides useful guidelines for maximizing success. As with conventional bridgework, retainer design may be divided into:

- Simple cantilever

- Fixed/fixed

- Fixed/movable

- Hybrid.

Simple cantilever design

Evidence suggests that cantilevers are recommended for anterior adhesive bridges, as increased failure rates have been demonstrated for fixed/fixed designs.[11,13,14,21]

For posterior adhesive bridges, evidence from well controlled clinical trials is lacking[19] but there is growing evidence that cantilever designs may be the treatment of choice for almost all RBBs.[11]

While cantilever designs will be subject to forces of higher magnitude in posterior segments and are contraindicated in parafunctional conditions,[4] they convey the same benefits as those for conventional cantilever bridges, i.e. more conservative, more cosmetic and easier to clean.[4]

Note that spring cantilever bridges are now of historical interest only and are not considered further.

Fixed/fixed designs

These have the advantage of increased resistance to occlusal loading and will resist orthodontic movement of abutment teeth;[13] however, this must be weighed carefully against their tendency for unilateral de-cementation, which is their most commonly reported mode of failure. Such de-bonds regularly go undetected (over 25% of cases)[13] and may result in destructive secondary caries (Fig. 8.17).

Other disadvantages of fixed/fixed designs:

- They are less conservative

- They are less esthetic

- It is difficult to visualize parallelism

- They are more difficult to manufacture

- They are more difficult to fit/cement.

Fixed/movable designs

As with conventional bridgework the incorporation of a movable joint offers a number of advantages:

- Allows independent movement of abutments, and redistributes stress more favourably on the framework and the adhesive bond[4]

- Allows abutments with different mobility characteristics to be united[4]

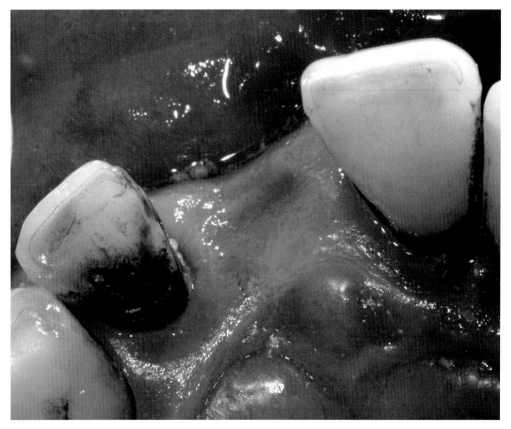

Fig. 8.17 Fixed/fixed designs are not recommended for anterior resin-bonded bridges as they have a tendency for unilateral de-bonds that often go undetected and may lead to secondary caries.

- Allows differing paths of insertion in non-parallel abutment teeth[4]
- Often allows more conservative tooth preparation.

Hybrid designs

Hybrid designs have a conventional retainer at one end and resin-bonded retainer at the other. They can be combined with fixed/movable design (Fig. 8.18) to avoid the potential hazards of differing retainer retention characteristics.[13]

Pontic design

Gingival surface

Modified ridge lap designs are used commonly for RBBs as they are esthetic and hygienic.[4,5]

Occlusal surface

It is recommended that pontics contact opposing teeth in intercuspal position, but have no guiding contacts in any excursions,[17] as repeated loads may dislodge

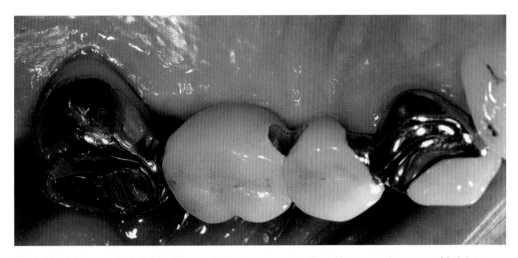

Fig. 8.18 A 25-year-old hybrid bridge replacing two upper teeth and incorporating a movable joint to reduce stress on the individual abutment teeth during loading. Courtesy of Dr J. McCubbin.

the restoration.[19] While it has been demonstrated that prescribed functional occlusal relationships are not maintained in 50% of patients,[13] the same study reported insignificant effects on restoration survival.[13]

Abutment preparation design

While RBBs may be employed successfully using a 'no-prep' technique[13] and 'textbook' designs are considered technically demanding to achieve, practitioners with highest RBB usage and success have been shown to be in favour of definite preparation.[19]

There is clear evidence that preparations modified with minimal resistance grooves, rest seats, guide planes and obvious finishing lines dramatically increase success rates,[14,11] as they convey the following benefits:[11,13,15,21]

- Increased surface area for retention

- Improved enamel/resin bond

- Improved resistance to displacement

- Limited stress on adhesive bonds

- Allow sufficient alloy thickness/rigidity and reduce stress on adhesive bond

- Easier to manufacture

- Precision seating ensured

- Restoration contours reduced

- Easier cementation.

RBB PREPARATION: GUIDELINES FOR SUCCESS (Figs 8.19 and 8.20)

- Abutment preparations should remain within enamel to avoid inferior dentine bonds[4,5,13,15,17]

- Preparations should cover as wide an area as possible, with outline form only limited by occlusal and esthetic constraints[11,13,17]

- Axial surfaces should be prepared for retainers that cover at least 180° of the abutment tooth circumference. This is termed the 'wrap-around' effect[17] and has been shown to improve restoration longevity significantly

- Proximal retainer margins should be extended as far as esthetics will allow and should be placed in cleansable positions

- Use of mutually parallel grooves can increase resistance form[14] significantly and compensate for situations where 'wrap-around' is sub-optimal

- Preparation features including resistance grooves simplify prosthesis location and cementation

- Posterior bridge retainers should incorporate occlusal coverage to resist the forces of displacement under load[14,17]

- Margin design should maximize axial height but should remain supra-gingival[17]

- Margins should be clear to the technician and placed in a cleansable position

- Chamfers are popular finishing lines[4] as they create room for alloys of sufficient rigidity and reduce the risk of over-contoured restorations[11]

- Existing restorations may be removed or modified to improve resistance form and increase framework rigidity[11,15,17]

- During preparation iatrogenic damage to adjacent teeth should be avoided

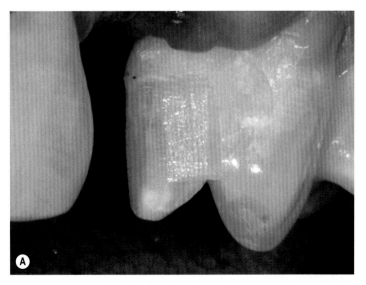
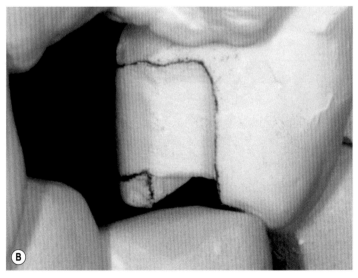

Fig. 8.19A,B Optimum preparation design for posterior resin-bonded bridges includes: preparation confined to enamel, occlusal coverage, supra-gingival margins and no occlusal contact on restoration margins.

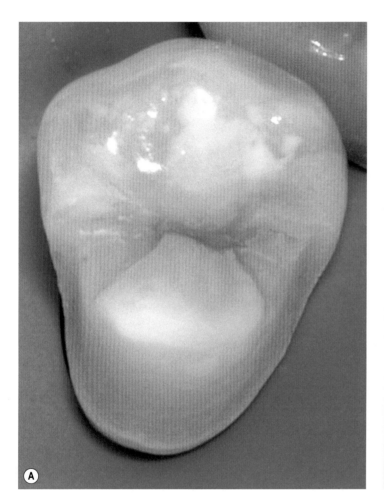
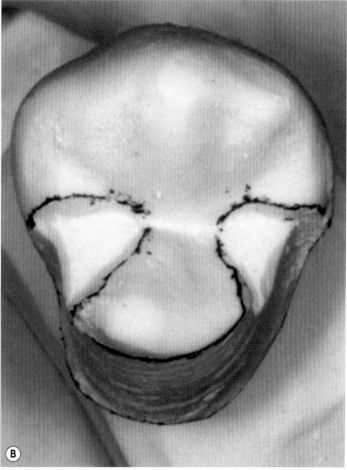

Fig. 8.20A,B Optimum preparation design for posterior resin-bonded bridges includes: preparation confined to enamel, occlusal coverage, supra-gingival margins and no occlusal contact on restoration margins.

Impressions

As precision fit is a fundamental requirement for successful RBBs, impression materials, equipment and technique should be optimized. Supra-gingival margin design often obviates the need for gingival retraction, but impressions should be checked carefully to ensure that all preparation features are captured accurately (Fig. 8.21).

Cementation

Moisture control is critical if the bridge is to bond properly to the tooth. Use of a rubber dam (Fig. 8.22) optimizes isolation, but careful technique is required to prevent it interfering with seating the prosthesis. Chemically active dual-cure luting cements are favoured for cementation of metal–ceramic RBBs and are described in Case 2 below.

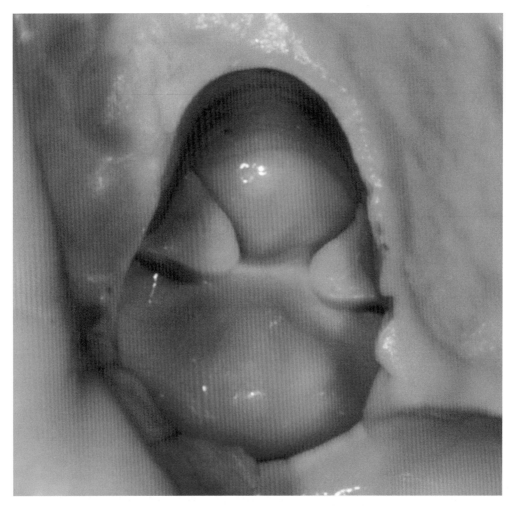

Fig. 8.21   Impressions should record RBB preparation details accurately.

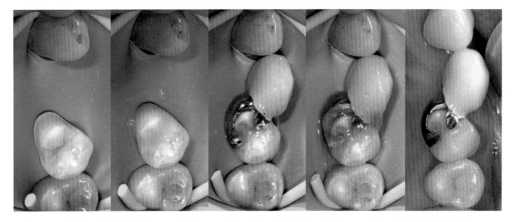

Fig. 8.22   Rubber dam isolation optimizes moisture control during all stages of resin-bonded bridge cementation.

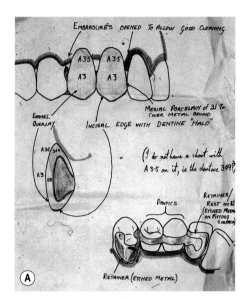
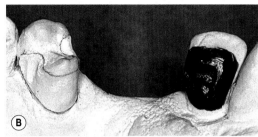
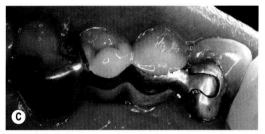

Fig. 8.23 Detailed laboratory prescriptions (A), trial preparations and diagnostic wax-ups (B) enhance communication between operator and technician. Restoration at 28 years after cementation (C). Courtesy of Dr J. McCubbin.

LABORATORY FACTORS

Communication

The versatility of RBBs often results in restorations with design features unique to each clinical case. Communication between operator and dental technician is paramount and may be enhanced by:

- Face-to-face contact
- Illustrated prescriptions[4] (Fig. 8.23A)
- Clinical photography
- Trial preparations
- Use of diagnostic wax-ups[4] (Fig. 8.23B)
- Margin marking and articulation checks by the operator.

Materials

High strength alloys are recommended for RBBs as they offer resistance to bending and wear, even in thin section.

CLINICAL TIPS

Thickness ≥0.5–0.7 mm should give sufficient RBB retainer rigidity for most alloys, but may reduce to approximately 0.3 mm in cervical areas to avoid over-contour.

Non-precious alloys are usually chosen as they:[4,13,15,17]

- Are more rigid (stiff) than precious alloys

- Optimize bonding and support for veneering porcelains

- Develop high bond strengths with chemically active luting resins, which may be further enhanced by surface treatments.

The predominant surface treatment for RBBs consists of air-abrasion with alumina particles (sandblasting/grit-blasting),[4,14,21] which increases the surface area for micro-mechanical bonding and promotes chemical interaction with luting resins.

MANAGEMENT OF FAILURE IN RESIN-BONDED BRIDGEWORK

When RBBs fail it is important to diagnose the aetiology to enable improvements in future procedures. De-cementation is the most common mode of failure observed for RBBs[13] and is caused predominantly by:

- Cohesive fracture within the luting cement layer[4,14]

- Adhesive failure of the cement bond to metal wings, leaving a cement layer on the tooth.[4]

Failure of cantilevers usually involves total de-bond with little or no warning. Patients should be made aware of this at the outset and if failure occurs the patient should be advised to:

- Retain the restoration in a safe place to avoid damage[13]

- Return immediately for diagnosis of the mode failure and assessment regarding the possibility of re-cementation following any necessary adjustments.[13]

RE-CEMENTING RESIN-BONDED BRIDGES

If failed RBBs are acceptable, they may be re-cemented to increase their functional life.[13,21] To optimize success, all traces of luting resin should be removed from the restoration[4] (ideally by sandblasting or occasionally by heat treatment) and from the tooth surface, which can be challenging and carries the risk of altering the prepared surface.[4] In addition, it should be expected that the lifespan of re-cemented restorations will be reduced and this requires communication to the patient.[14]

If bridges are unsuitable for re-cementation, they may be re-used as temporary restorations by converting metal wings to a perforated Rochette design.[4]

MANAGEMENT OF UNILATERAL DE-CEMENTATION

As the most prevalent mode of failure for fixed/fixed restorations is unilateral de-cementation which commonly goes unnoticed,[13] patients must be warned of the potentially serious consequences and made aware of the need for:

- Vigilant long-term maintenance[13]

- Regular attendance to enable early diagnosis.[13]

CLINICAL TIPS

Patients with fixed/fixed RBBs should return for immediate assessment if they:[13]

- Hear or feel breakage

- Feel an unfamiliar sharp edge

- Sense mobility

- Feel a 'squelching' sensation

- Experience a foul taste.

If unilateral de-cementation occurs, the simplest management option is to cut off the de-bonded wing and polish the sectioned connector[11] (Fig. 8.24). If RBB removal is required, it may be facilitated by application of a suitable sharp or ultrasonic instrument under the retainer, or the use of specialized bridge removal equipment.

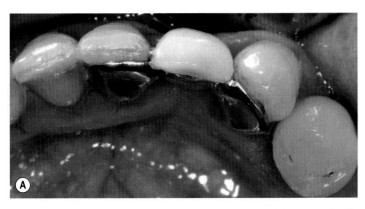
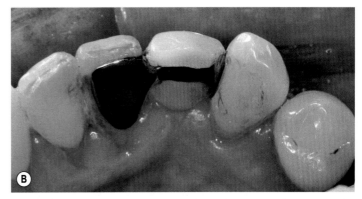

Fig. 8.24   Minimally invasive management of unilateral de-cementation of a resin-bonded bridge retainer.

CLINICAL CASE 8.1: MINIMALLY INVASIVE SIMPLE CANTILEVER BRIDGE

Assessment

A 50-year-old female patient presented with esthetic concerns regarding the appearance of the upper right posterior teeth. The area of main complaint comprised a missing second premolar with metal restorations in adjacent teeth. Active secondary caries was diagnosed at the mesial crown margin on the first molar. Special tests confirmed positive pulpal responses from all teeth and no signs of radiographic pathology.

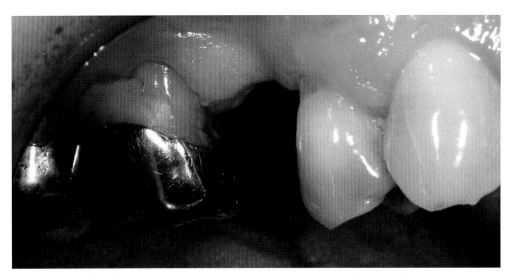

Fig. C8.1.1   Esthetic concerns resulting from missing second premolar and metal restorations.

Treatment opinions

The patient was informed of all of the various management options. A care plan was selected to restore esthetics using minimally invasive techniques and full written consent was gained for:

- Removal of the failed full veneer crown

- Restoration of the space using a metal–ceramic simple cantilever bridge after assessment and re-preparation of the first molar abutment.

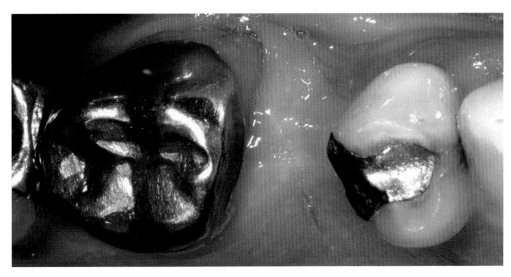

Fig. C8.1.2 Treatment plan: remove full veneer crown and replace with metal–ceramic simple cantilever bridge.

Preparation

Crown removal revealed distal secondary caries in addition to the mesial lesion (Fig. C8.1.3A). Minimal preparation was necessary to optimize the abutment tooth according to conventional design principles[22] with regard to:

- Occlusal convergence angles
- Axial height
- Margin placement
- Outline form
- Reduction for selected materials.

Buccal shoulder and chamfer margins elsewhere were all placed supra-gingivally and, following caries excavation, mesial and distal proximal boxes were prepared to enhance resistance and retention form (Fig. C8.1.3B).

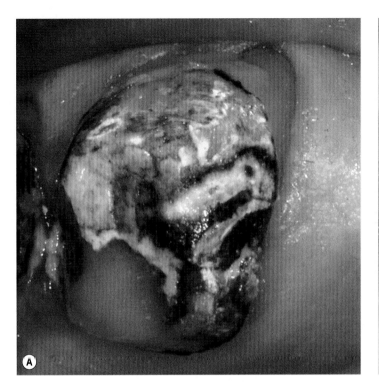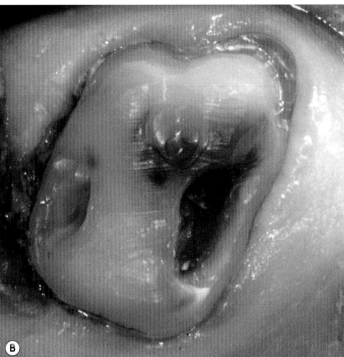

Fig. C8.1.3 (A) Crown preparation. (B) Preparation for simple cantilever bridge retainer.

Impression and temporization

Silicone and opposing alginate impressions were obtained along with the relevant occlusal records. A provisional crown was then fabricated in acrylic using a pre-operative template impression and cemented with a temporary style of cement.

Materials

The pre-existing preparation allowed sufficient room for both alloy and porcelain without the need for further occlusal reduction. The restoration was designed and constructed to:

• Maximize strength

• Maximize esthetics

• Minimize functional loads on the pontic during lateral excursions.

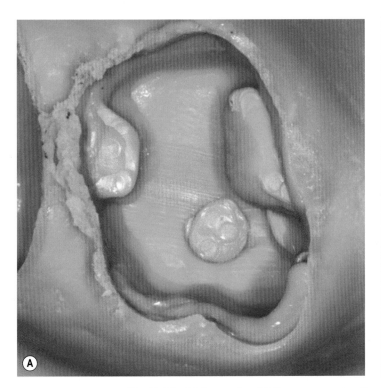

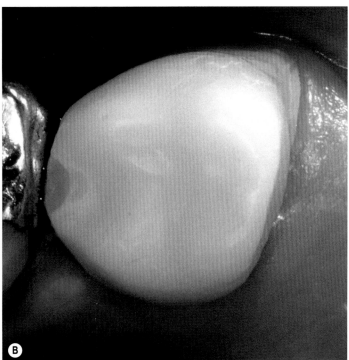

Fig. C8.1.4 (A) Impression. (B) Temporary restoration.

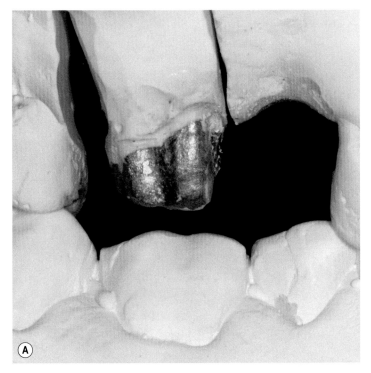

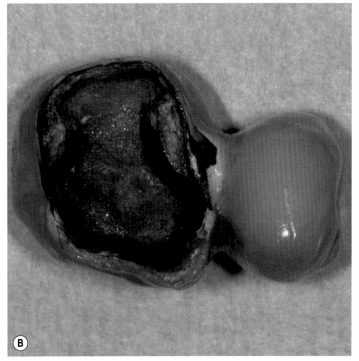

Fig. C8.1.5 (A) Articulated models. (B) Metal–ceramic simple cantilever bridge.

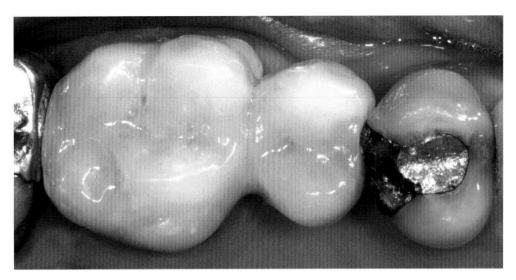

Fig. C8.1.6   Restoration complete.

Cementation

Following try-in, the restoration was cemented using zinc phosphate cement. The outcome was esthetically pleasing to the patient and at minimal biological cost to the residual dentition. Advice regarding maintenance was provided and an appointment made for review.

CLINICAL CASE 8.2: RESIN-BONDED BRIDGEWORK

Reason for attendance

A 40-year-old male patient attended the clinic with a retained upper right primary canine that had fractured and become painful to bite on. The permanent successor had failed to erupt and had been extracted during adolescence.

History, examination and diagnosis

A comprehensive history and examination were carried out. Special tests confirmed a positive pulpal response from teeth adjacent to the fractured primary tooth (Fig. C8.2.2A), and periapical radiography (Fig. C8.2.2B) allowed diagnosis of a mid-third fracture of its resorbing root and no pathology related to potential bridge abutment teeth. A detailed numbered list of the patient's esthetic requirements (following extraction of the unrestorable primary tooth) was made and intra- and extra-oral photographic images obtained to assist care planning.

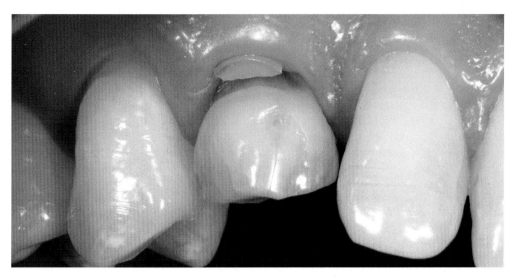

Fig. C8.2.1   Fractured, painful, retained primary canine.

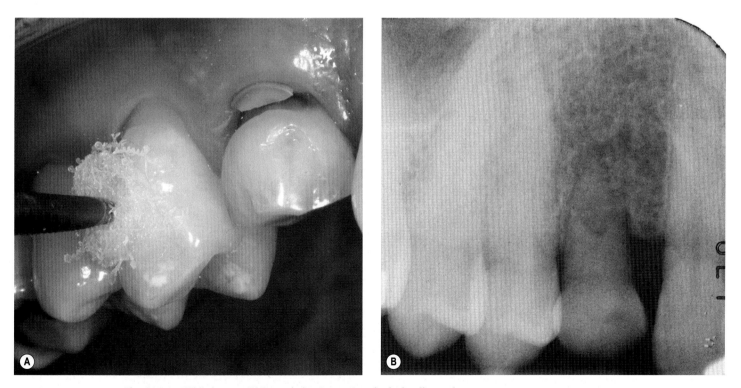

Fig. C8.2.2   (A) Pulp test. (B) Pre-existing (recent) periapical radiograph.

Occlusal examination

Intra-oral occlusal examination revealed:

- Stable intercuspal position between the intact maxillary and the mandibular arches

- Group function in both left and right lateral excursion

- Over-eruption of the opposing lower canine

- Upper right primary canine interfered with right lateral excursion

- Grade II mobility of the fractured primary tooth.

Facebow transfer, occlusal records and alginate impressions were obtained to allow fabrication and assessment of duplicate study models using a semi-adjustable articulator.

Occlusal registration may be supplemented by lateral and protrusive records and construction of an incisal guidance table, to increase accuracy when restoring anterior guidance.

Study models

The usefulness of study models should not be underestimated as they provide a 'technician's view' that is impossible to obtain clinically and allow:

- Detailed occlusal examination

- Planning of occlusal adjustments

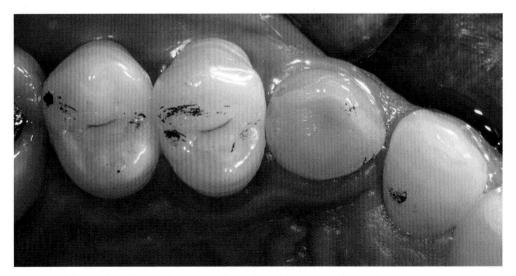

Fig. C8.2.3   Occlusal assessment.

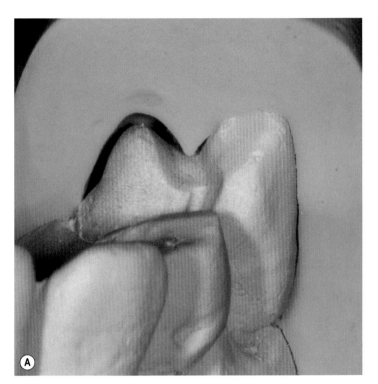 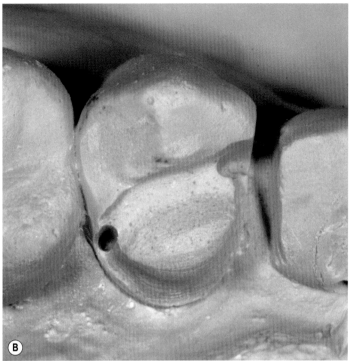

Fig. C8.2.4   (A) Tooth preparation index. (B) Trial preparation.

- Fabrication of a tooth preparation index (Fig. C8.2.4A)

- Diagnostic wax-up

- Trial preparations (Fig. C8.2.4B).

Treatment options

The patient was informed of the various management options available for the (immediate or delayed) restoration of space following extraction of the primary tooth, with respect to:

- Biological considerations

- Esthetic requirements

- Longevity estimation

- Financial implications

- Maintainance requirements.

As in any care plan it is essential that the patient's esthetic expectations of the final restoration are determined at the outset and that they are informed fully

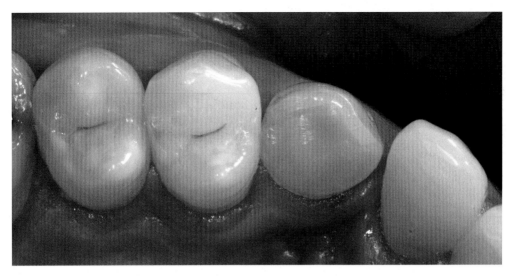

Fig. C8.2.5   All treatment options include extraction of the fractured primary canine.

of the planned appearance of each restorative option. This can present difficulties when RBBs that are planned as provisional/trial restorations are not usually an option and verbal descriptions are unlikely to give patients a clear perception of the outcome. This limitation may be partly overcome using:

- Diagnostic wax-ups

- Resin composite prototype

- Photographic images of other cases using similar restorations

- Image manipulation software.

If metal retainers form part of the proposed care plan, they may be excluded immediately in situations where metal display is unacceptable to the patient.

Care plan

In this case the patient gave informed written consent for:

- Preparation of upper right first premolar as an abutment tooth for an adhesive bridge retainer

- Enameloplasty of the opposing over-erupted canine and first premolar

- Extraction of the retained primary tooth

- Provision of an immediate replacement metal–ceramic resin-bonded cantilever bridge.

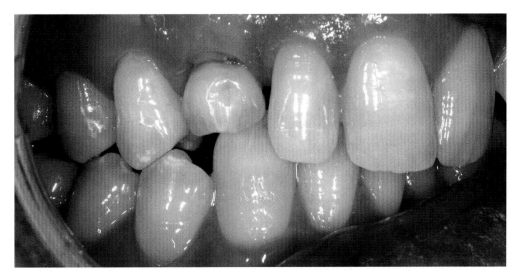

Fig. C8.2.6   Treatment plan: immediate replacement metal–ceramic RBB.

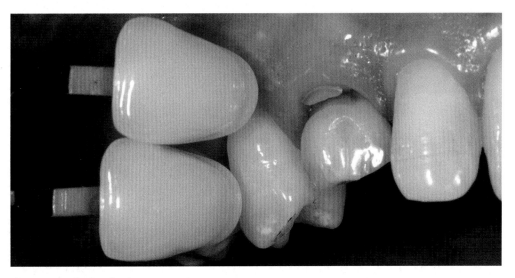

Fig. C8.2.7   Shade selection.

Shade and form selection

The desired shape and shade of the porcelain pontic was planned. Intra-oral and extra-oral photographs were taken from various angles to assist communication with the technician.

CLINICAL TIPS

When using metal retainers on thin anterior teeth, the alloy and opaque luting resin can affect the light transmission properties of the abutment tooth. When shade taking, it is recommended to place a cotton wool roll behind potential abutments to estimate their likely post-cementation appearance.

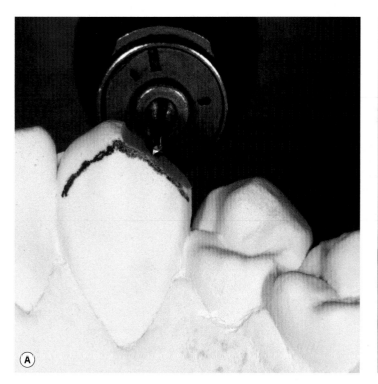 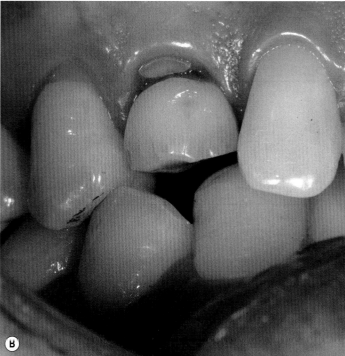

Fig. C8.2.8 (A) Trial preparation of over-erupted opposing teeth. (B) Enamelplasty informed by trial preparation.

Tooth preparation (opposing teeth)

Opposing teeth were adjusted following pre-operative measurements planned on the mounted study casts (Fig. C8.2.8A).

CLINICAL TIPS

Simulating adjustments to opposing (or adjacent) teeth simplifies operative intervention by:

• Providing views impossible to obtain clinically

• Allowing accurate reduction measurement

• Reducing the risk of undesirable dentine exposure.

Axial preparation

The retained primary tooth's distal surface was modified to prevent interference during abutment preparation, which was then carried out using a torpedo-shaped diamond bur.

During axial preparation, the adjacent premolar was protected using a metal sectional matrix (Fig. C8.2.9A). Preparation was confined to enamel and controlled with use of a silicone index (Fig. C8.2.9B).

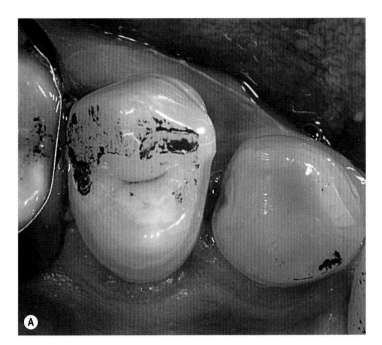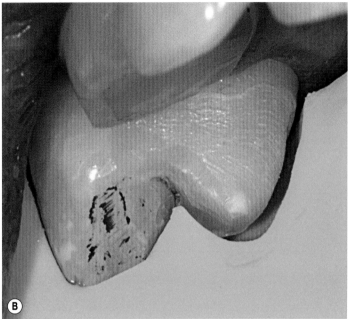

Fig. C8.2.9   (A) Axial preparation. (B) Silicone preparation index.

Suggested desirable features of axial preparation are:

• Supragingival chamfer margins

• Removal of undercuts from axial walls

• 180° 'wrap-around'

• Maximum proximal extension limited only to minimize metal display mesially and prevent damage to the adjacent tooth distally

• Margin placement in cleansable areas

• Adequate space for a rigid alloy retainer

• Preparation of near-parallel opposing mesial and distal surfaces.

CLINICAL TIP

Close-up photographic occlusal views assist assessment of axial convergence angles and reduce the risk of undercut and/or over-taper.

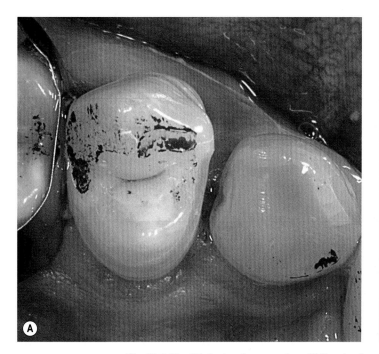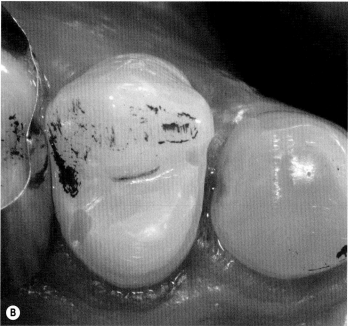

Fig. C8.2.10   (A) Occlusal preparation. (B) Proximal resistance grooves.

Occlusal preparation and proximal grooves

Occlusal preparation

The occlusal surface was reduced using the pre-operative trial preparation (Fig. C8.2.10B) as a guide. Preparation was:

- Confined to enamel

- Designed to cover the maximum area

- Limited only by esthetic considerations and occlusal restraints.

Proximal grooves

Parallel resistance grooves were prepared in opposing mesial and distal axial surfaces (Fig. C8.2.10B) using a thin tapered tungsten–carbide bur and confer the following advantages:

- Increased resistance form reduces stress on adhesive bond

- Increases rigidity of casting

- Precise location aids try-in and cementation

- Can compensate in conditions with sub-optimal wrap-around.

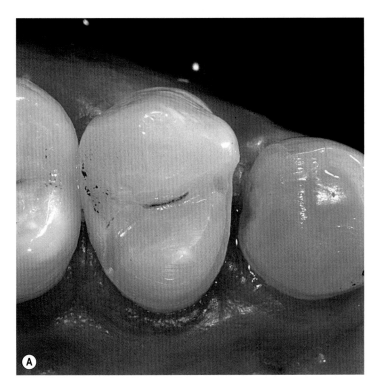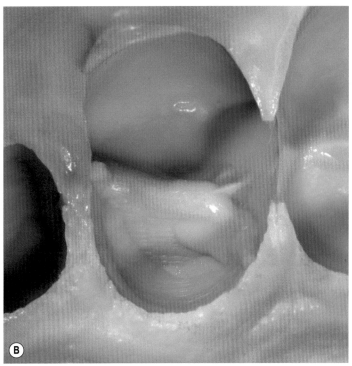

Fig. C8.2.11   (A) Preparation complete. (B) Impression.

Impression

The preparation was dried and examined. Supra-gingival margins obviated the need for gingival retraction. An impression was obtained using an addition-cured silicone material in a rigid metal tray with a one-stage putty/wash technique. The working impression was assessed for accuracy and an opposing alginate impression obtained to record the adjusted opposing teeth.

Temporization

This was carried out by application of flowable resin composite to the prepared abutment tooth and the retained primary canine. Relatively high volumetric shrinkage of conventional flowable resins allows retention on a temporary basis without the need for etching. The aims of temporization are to:

• Re-establish occlusal contacts where they have been removed

• Cover rough prepared surfaces

• Improve esthetics

• Reduce sensitivity in areas where the preparation has exposed superficial dentine.

CLINICAL TIP

Minimizing the interval between preparation and fitting will reduce the likelihood of deleterious occlusal changes.

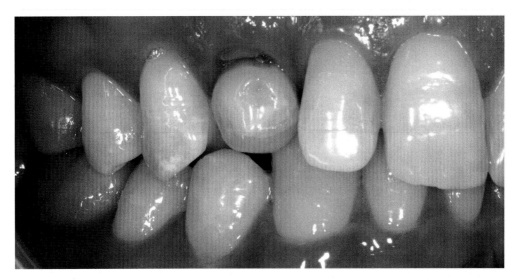

Fig. C8.2.12   Temporization with flowable composite.

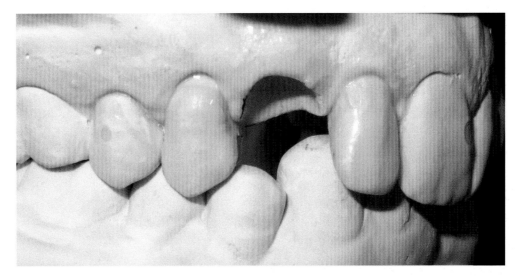

Fig. C8.2.13   Articulated models.

Model check

The articulated working models were returned to the operator to:

- Mark preparation margins

- Confirm accuracy of occlusal relationship

- Modify pontic area to estimate the correct form of the healed socket.

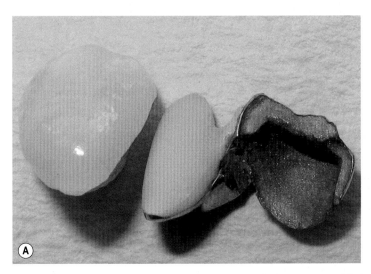 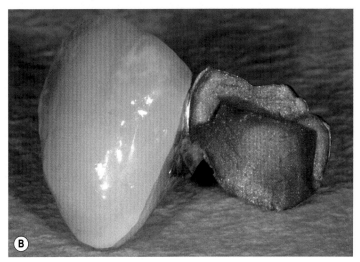

Fig. C8.2.14 (A) Split pontic design. (B) Assembled.

Restoration design and manufacture

Experienced laboratory support enabled the use of unusual split-pontic design comprising:

- A precious gold alloy framework made up of a wing and a pontic core

- A layer of laboratory composite to cover the pontic core

- A separate crown made up of esthetic porcelain to be cemented over the pontic core.

This design was selected because esthetic assessment was not possible until the primary tooth had been extracted. If the pontic had been deemed unsatisfactory at try-in, it could have been cemented temporarily and replaced with an improved version without having to disturb the cemented alloy retainer.

Materials

Alloy framework

Type IV gold alloy was selected in this example for the following reasons:

- Yellow/gold in colour for enhanced esthetics

- Less abrasive to opposing dentition

- Good casting properties

- Compatible with veneering porcelain

- Biocompatible

- Polishable

- Corrosion resistant

- Nickel and beryllium free (hypo-allergenic).

The fit surface was sandblasted using alumina particles. This is the favoured contemporary technique for surface preparation as it:

- Increases the surface area for cement wetting

- Promotes chemical interaction with the luting resin

- Is a simple and predictable technique

- Does not require expensive equipment.

Composite

The alloy pontic core was also sandblasted and primed (Metal primer II, GC Corp., Japan) before application of a thin layer of laboratory composite (Gradia, GC Corp., Japan).

Porcelain

For strength and esthetics the pontic porcelain was lithium disilicate glass (E-max, Ivoclar Vivadent, Liechtenstein). Contemporary pontic designs may be bullet shaped or modified ridge lap forms. They should minimize soft tissue contact and be designed to:

- Resist food accumulation

- Minimize plaque retention

- Facilitate cleaning.

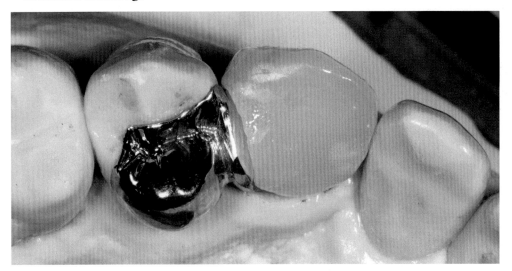

Fig. C8.2.15   Completed restoration on model.

Shade test

The porcelain shade was tested by comparing the pontic against the adjacent lateral incisor. This was done immediately before dehydration, which tends to lighten teeth until they rehydrate much later.

Extraction

Following removal of the temporary flowable composite (using a sharp hand instrument), the fractured primary canine was extracted carefully to minimize haemorrhage and post-operative swelling and resorption.

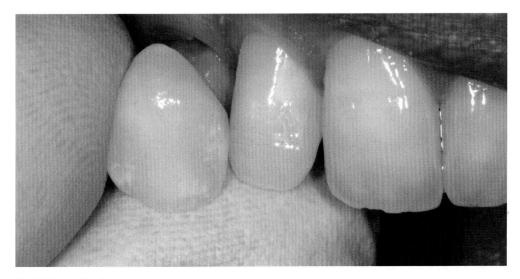

Fig. C8.2.16 Shade test.

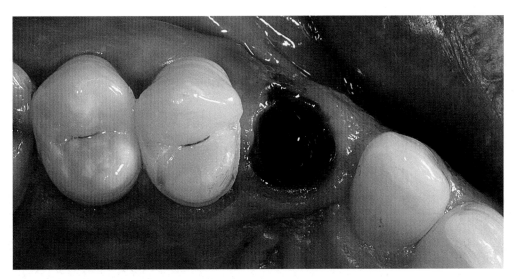

Fig. C8.2.17 Extraction of primary canine.

Isolation

Quality moisture control is one of the critical parameters governing the success of adhesive procedures in dentistry.

While the use of a rubber dam is not common in general dental practice, it is considered to be the optimum method for moisture control and conveys a number of important benefits:

- Ensures complete isolation for the entire duration of the cementation procedure
- Airway protection when delivering restorations coated in slippery adhesive
- Greater patient comfort
- Improved visibility.

CLINICAL TIPS FOR ISOLATING RBB PREPARATIONS WITH A RUBBER DAM

- Build confidence by practising with simple restorations first
- Minimize the number of rubber dam holes
- Minimize dam tension by leaving a space between holes in the pontic area
- Place clamp on a tooth distal to the prepared one
- Use specialized cord (Fig. C8.2.18) (or floss/sections of dam) to stabilize the dam

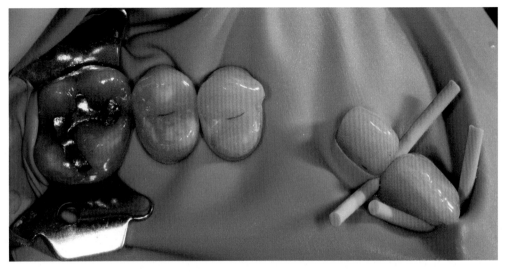

Fig. C8.2.18   Isolation with a rubber dam.

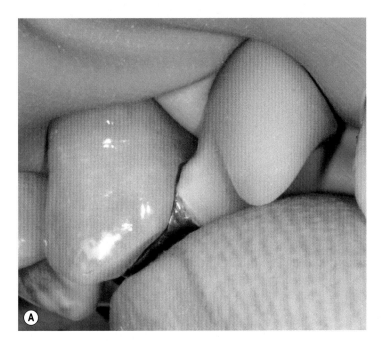
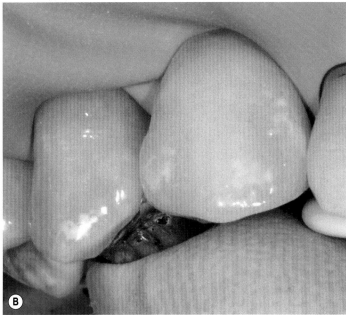

Fig. C8.2.19   (A) Try-in of retainer. (B) Try-in of pontic.

Try-in

Following isolation, the preparation was cleaned carefully to remove the acquired pellicle using dry (oil-free) pumice in a rubber cup. The retainer was then tried in place (Fig. C8.2.19A) and the 'split-pontic' porcelain crown tried onto the retainer (Fig. C8.2.19B).

> **CLINICAL TIP**
>
> Water soluble try-in pastes may be used to stabilize restorations when assessing the occlusion and esthetics prior to isolation (in non-immediate replacement cases) and before the decision is made for final cementation.

Restoration surface preparation

The fit surface was sandblasted to improve the bond strength with the luting resin. Alloy fitting surfaces should be clean and free of any saliva, blood, oil or plaque contaminants. (It is recommended to clean the restoration surface in an ultrasonic unit for 2 minutes.)

In this case, the fit surface of the retainer was painted with a specialized surface primer (Alloy Primer, Kuraray Dental, Japan) and left for a few seconds prior to cementation (Fig. C8.2.20A). This has been shown to increase bond strength to precious alloys (but is unnecessary when cementing the more conventional non-precious alloy RBBs). Silane primer was applied to the fitting surface of the pontic crown (Fig. C8.2.20B).

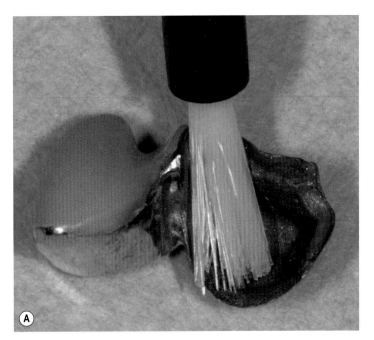
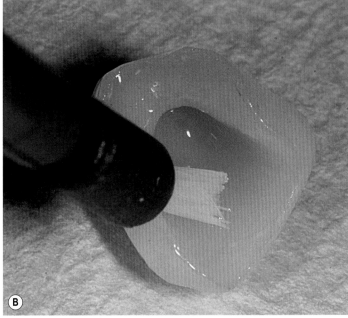

Fig. C8.2.20 (A) Surface preparation of metal retainer. (B) Surface preparation of ceramic pontic.

Tooth surface preparation

The prepared surfaces were etched with phosphoric acid gel (30–40%), which was gently agitated for 15 seconds to give a uniform etch pattern. Care was taken to avoid etching beyond preparation margins, where excess luting resin may bond and be difficult to accurately remove without risk of iatrogenic damage to the underlying enamel.

CLINICAL TIPS

When etching unprepared, young enamel, the surface is more acid resistant. This fluoridated, potentially aprismatic enamel surface layer requires longer etching times. (Etching times of 30–60 seconds have been advocated in various studies.)

Adjacent teeth may be protected from contamination with etch, adhesive or excess luting resin using polytetrafluoroethylene tape.

Washing and drying

The preparation was washed thoroughly to remove all traces of etchant and dried with gentle airflow. The 'frosty' appearance of well-etched enamel is a reassuring sign of the micro-porous, high-energy surface that will promote:

- Resin tag formation

- High bond strength

- Increased wettability by the (lower surface tension) cement.

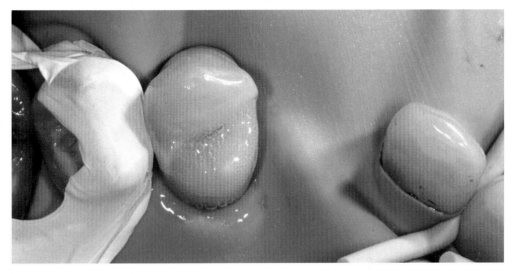

Fig. C8.2.21   Phosphoric acid etch.

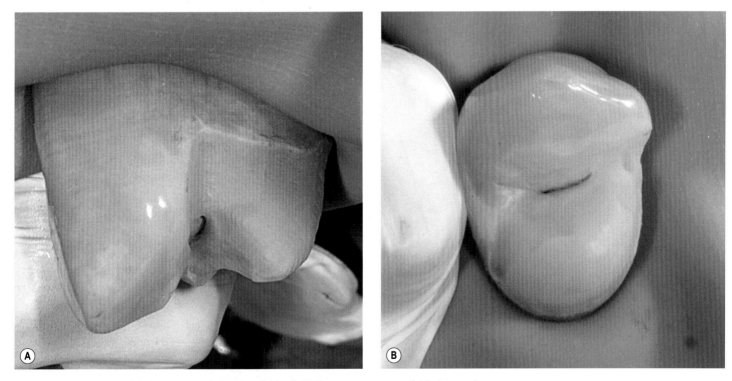

Fig. C8.2.22   (A) Etchant washed off. (B) Frosty appearance of dried enamel.

CLINICAL TIPS (DRYING)

- Blow air (onto the rubber dam) to test that the airflow is free from contaminants

- Regularly service triple-syringe seals and compressors to prevent water and/or oil contamination of the airstream

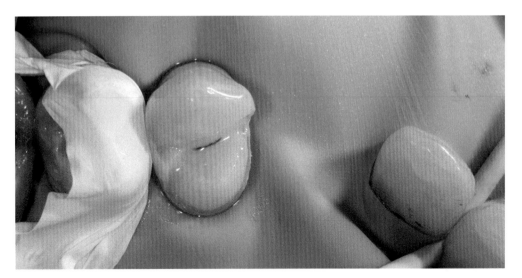

Fig. C8.2.23 Adhesive applied.

Adhesive

In this case, the Panavia F 2.0 dual cure adhesive system was used (Kuraray Co. Ltd, Japan). One drop each of Panavia adhesive (ED Primer II) liquid A and B were dispensed into a mixing well and mixed immediately before application to the etched tooth surface (not to the restoration surface) and left for 30 seconds. The adhesive solvent was then evaporated with gentle airflow.

CLINICAL TIPS

- The adhesive mixture must be used within 3 minutes after mixing

- Pooling of excess adhesive should be avoided as this may speed the polymerization reaction

- Panavia adhesive does not require light curing at this stage, as it may inhibit accurate seating of the restoration

Luting resin

Panavia F 2.0 dual-cure luting cement contains 10-methacryloyloxydecyl di-hydrogen phosphate (MDP) and forms high bond strengths with sandblasted alloy surfaces and adhesives. Other beneficial properties of Panavia are:

- High strength

- High rigidity

- Low solubility.

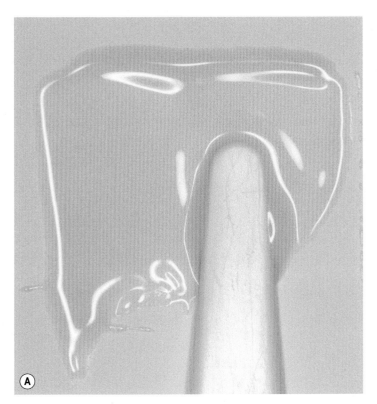 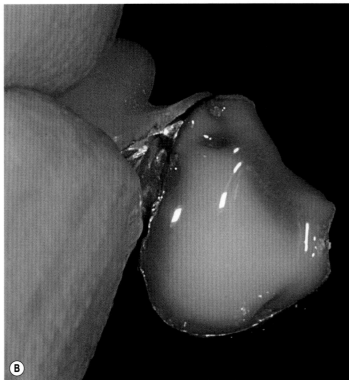

Fig. C8.2.24 (A) Luting resin mixed over a wide area. (B) Luting resin applied to retainer wing.

Equal amounts of paste A and B were mixed for 20 seconds (Fig. C8.2.24A) and applied to the wing of the restoration as soon as possible after dispensing and mixing (Fig. C8.2.24B).

CLINICAL TIPS

- Ensuring that there is no residual moisture on the mixing slab or spatula will also prevent reduction in working time

- Variable setting times will result if Panavia is mixed inadequately

- A timer may be used to measure the mixing time

- Opaque shades are available to mask grey 'shine through' in certain anterior situations

- While Panavia F 2.0 paste may also be applied to the tooth surface, working time will be reduced (to 60 seconds) as ED Primer II accelerates the set

Note: when using the chemically cured version (Panavia 21), working time may be lengthened by mixing the cement over a wide area, as its set requires anaerobic conditions and this will prevent polymerization of the deeper layers.

Cementation

The resin-coated retainer was seated and held in place while excess cement was removed using a disposable brush.

Accuracy of seating was confirmed immediately, before the anaerobic setting reaction was too far advanced. The excess was kept to a minimum as Panavia is difficult to remove once set without damaging adjacent hard and soft tissues, or the polished metal framework surface.

CLINICAL TIPS

- The presence of preparation features simplifies cementation in terms of speed and accuracy

- While cantilevers are easy to locate without accidently wiping off the luting resin, more complex fixed/fixed frameworks are more difficult to manipulate

- Fixed/movable designs may be considered to be the most difficult in this respect, especially when preparations have different paths of insertion and the danger of cement contamination of movable joints ensues

- For the inexperienced practitioner, practice and technique familiarization with simpler cases is highly recommended

- If a non-preparation technique has been employed, cementation can be challenging and uncomfortable. A very steady hand is required to accurately locate the casting wing and hold it firmly in place for the entire duration of the setting procedure

- To reduce this difficulty, castings may be made with incisal/occlusal extensions to confirm seating precision and stabilize the casting during setting. These extensions are cut off later, although vibrations to the new cement luting layer may have a negative effect

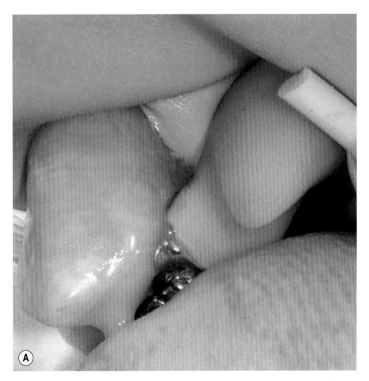 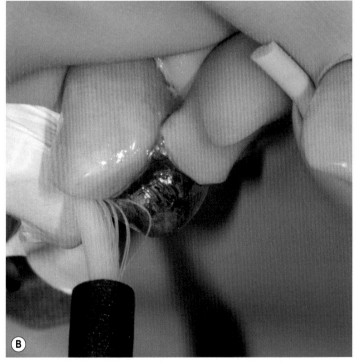

Fig. C8.2.25 (A) Retainer seated. (B) Removal of excess luting resin.

Dual curing

Marginal luting cement was light cured following the manufacturer's instructions before application of oxygen inhibiting paste (Oxyguard II, Kuraray Co. Ltd, Japan) around the restoration margins. As well as creating anaerobic conditions that promote the chemical cure, the latest version of the material contains a catalyst to enhance the setting reaction. It was applied using a disposable brush tip and removed with a cotton wool roll and water spray after 3 minutes.

Crown cementation

A thin layer of unfilled resin composite was applied to the pontic core following manufacturer's instructions. The crown was then filled with a translucent luting resin cement (NX3 Nexus, Kerr).

Light curing

The luting resin was partially light cured for 10 seconds (Fig. C8.2.28A) and the excess cement removed using sharp hand instruments. Polymerization was completed with a further 60 second light cure from all angles.

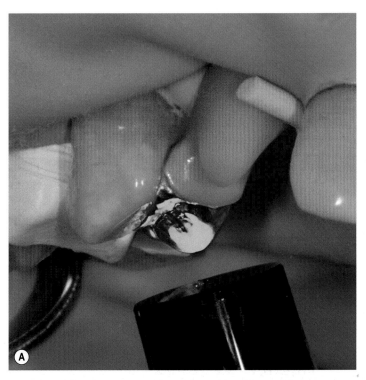 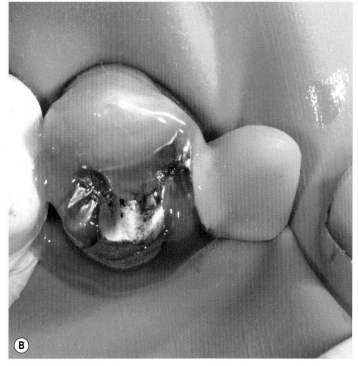

Fig. C8.2.26   (A) Marginal luting resin light cured. (B) Oxygen inhibiting paste.

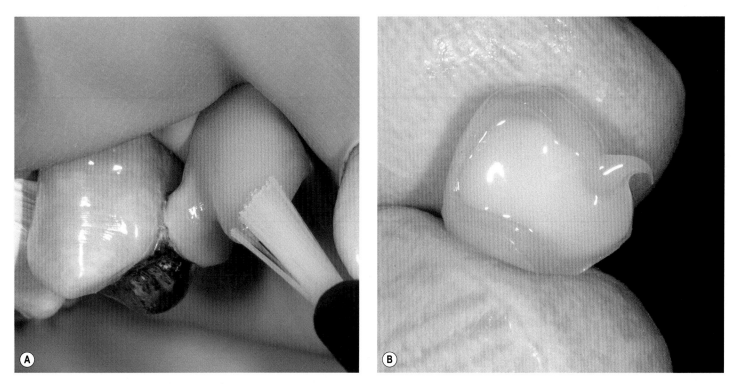

Fig. C8.2.27   (A) Adhesive applied to pontic core. (B) Luting resin applied to pontic crown.

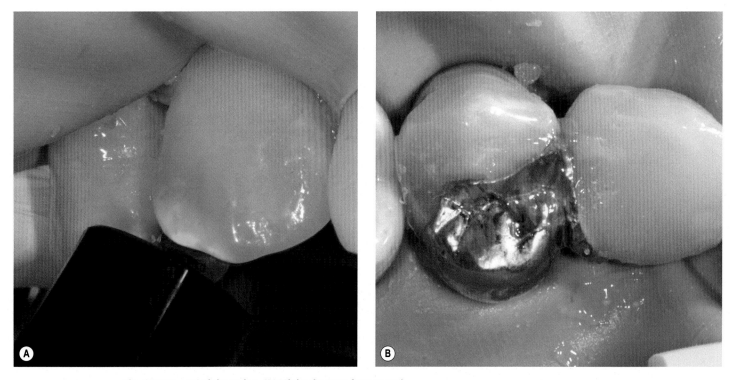

Fig. C8.2.28   (A) Light curing. (B) Minimal excess for removal.

CLINICAL TIPS

Excess set cement may also be removed using diamond (or tungsten carbide) burs or polishing tips. Light pressure and copious water spray must be employed to prevent heating of the metal framework and softening of the adhesive layer.

Rubber dam removal

Rubber dam was removed from under the pontic by stretching it buccally and cutting with scissors. Following rubber dam removal, it was possible to confirm that complete haemostasis had been achieved.

Esthetic assessment

One disadvantage of this immediate replacement technique is that it was impossible to confirm that the restoration meets esthetic requirements until after cementation is complete. Careful assessment and planning at the outset are essential to reduce the risk of sub-optimal appearance.

Furthermore, isolation during the operative procedure causes dehydration of adjacent teeth, resulting in their lighter appearance. Therefore, the accuracy of shade matching cannot be assessed fully until rehydration has occurred at the review appointment.

Occlusal assessment

The prescribed occlusal design was assessed using articulating paper and shim-stock. Minor adjustments were made using burs and polishers with care not to overheat the restoration. Tungsten carbide burs were favoured over diamond

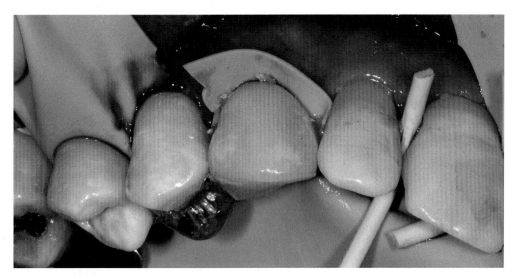

Fig. C8.2.29   Rubber dam removal technique.

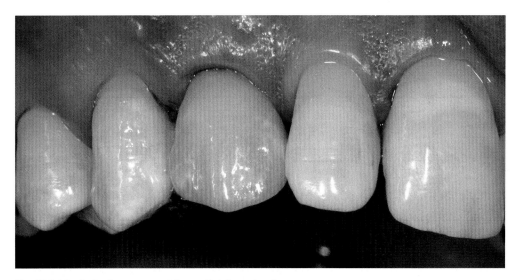

Fig. C8.2.30   Esthetic assessment (immediately post-op).

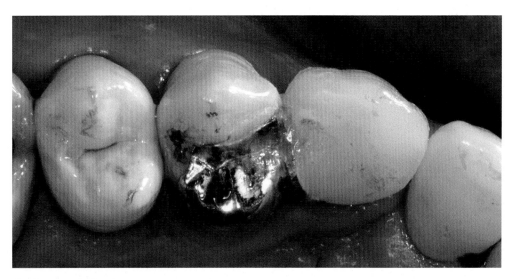

Fig. C8.2.31   Occlusal assessment.

burs, which may have put deep scratches into the alloy surface and been difficult to polish out.

The final occlusal scheme should have:

- Normal contacts on all other teeth

- Stable contact between the retainer and the opposing teeth in the intercuspal position

- No contacts on the restoration during excursions

- No contacts on restoration margins.

Oral hygiene

Careful oral hygiene instructions and demonstrations were given on the use of:

- Specialized powered brush heads
- Interdental brushes
- Specialized dental floss.

The patient was warned of the danger of biting hard foods directly on bridge and advised to wear a protective mouthguard for impact sports.

Review

The importance of regular reviews was stressed at the outset. The recommended guidelines for review intervals for adhesive bridgework are 2 weeks (Fig. C8.2.33) and monthly recalls during the first 6 months, as most adhesive and other failures are seen in this period.

At the review appointment, minor refinements (and final excess cement removal) were carried out and the restoration was assessed with regard to the following:

- Esthetics
- Occlusion in intercuspal position and all excursions
- Presence of wear facets in the restoration and adjacent teeth
- Presence of plaque (directly or using disclosing agents) to assess caries risk
- Periodontal condition, measured by conventional methods and compared to baseline records
- Abutment mobility
- Pulp tests
- Radiographic assessment at prescribed intervals (with written reports).

In this case, soft tissue healing following extraction of the fractured primary tooth was assessed in the short term and post-extraction resorption in the longer. This case describes a minimally invasive indirect esthetic technique for immediate tooth replacement that was rewarding for both patient and operator.

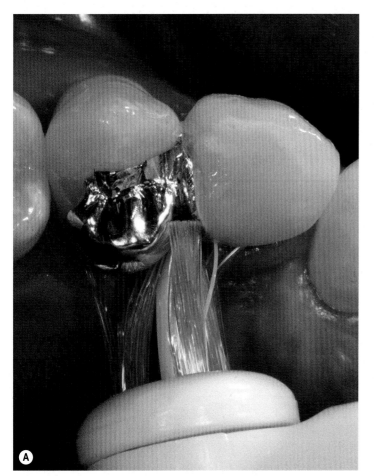

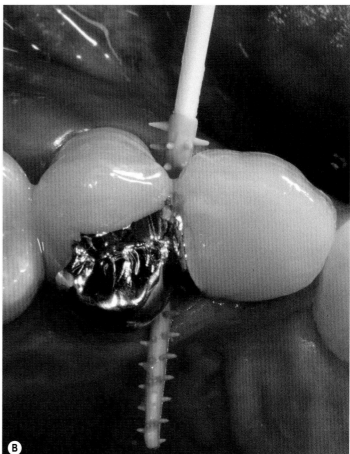

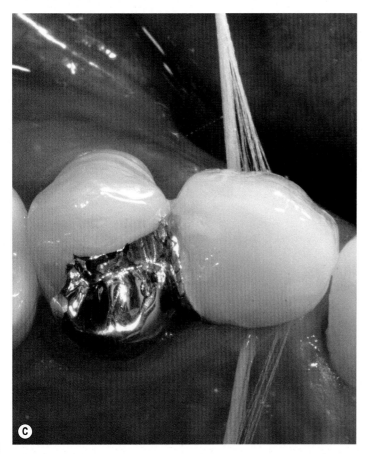

Fig. C8.2.32 Oral hygiene instruction. (A) Specialized brush. (B) Interdental brush. (C) Floss.

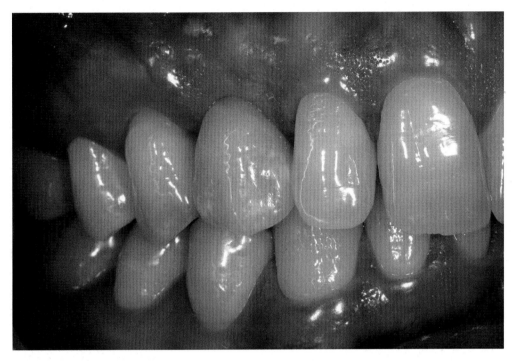

Fig. C8.2.33   Restoration complete.

ACKNOWLEDGEMENTS

The author would like to thank his technicians Adrian and Jacque Rollings (and Mark Bladen, who assisted with the design and framework construction for Clinical Case 8.2), his mentors Dr Adrian Shortall and Dr Jim McCubbin, for their enduring support and friendship, and Professor Richard Verdi, for reviewing the manuscript.

Further reading

Burke FJT. Resin-retained bridges: fibre-reinforced versus metal. Dent Update 2008;35: 521–6.

Chan AW, Barnes IE. A prospective study of cantilever resin-bonded bridges: an initial report. Aust Dent J 2000;45(1):31–6.

Department of health. Adult Dental Health Survey. United Kingdom, <http://www.hscic.gov.uk/pubs/dentalsurveyfullreport09>; 2009.

Djemal S, Setchell D, King P, Wickens JJ. Long-term survival characteristics of 832 resin-retained bridges and splints provided in a post-graduate teaching hospital between 1978 and 1993. Oral Rehabil 1999;26(4):302–20.

Gilmour AS. Resin-bonded bridges: a note of caution. Br Dent J 1989;167(4):140–1.

Goldstein RE. Esthetics in Dentistry, vol. 2. 2nd ed. Hamilton, ON: BC Decker Inc; 2002.

Hood JA, Farah JW, Craig RG. Modification of stresses in alveolar bone induced by a tilted molar. J Prosthet Dent 1975;34(4):415–21.

Hussey DL, Linden GJ. The clinical performance of cantilevered resin-bonded bridgework. J Dent 1996;24(4):251–6.

Hussey DL, Pagni C, Linden GJ. Performance of 400 adhesive bridges fitted in a restorative dentistry department. J Dent 1991;19(4):221–5.

Ibbetson R. Clinical considerations for adhesive bridgework. Dent Update 2004;31(5):254–6, 258, 260.

Johnsen DC. A review of orthodontic sequelae to early first permanent molar extraction. Some promise – many pitfalls. W V Dent J 1976;50(2):9–12.

Livaditis GJ. Cast metal resin-bonded retainers for posterior teeth. J Am Dent Assoc 1980;110:926–9.

Olin PS, Hill EM, Donahue JL. Clinical evaluation of resin-bonded bridges: a retrospective study. Quintessence Int 1991;22(11):873–7.

Rochette AL. Attachment of a splint to enamel of lower anterior teeth. J Prosthet Dent 1973;30:418–23.

Shillingburg HT Jr, Grace CS. Thickness of enamel and dentine. J South Calif Dent Assoc 1973;33–52.

Shillingburg HT, Sather DA, Wilson EL. Fundamentals of Fixed Prosthodontics. Chapter 28. Kent, UK: Quintessence Publishing; 2012.

Shillingburg HT, Sather DA, Wilson EL. Fundamentals of Fixed Prosthodontics. Chapter 17. Kent, UK: Quintessence Publishing; 2012.

Steele JG, Jepson NJ, McColl E, Swift B. Finding Ways to Improve the Effectiveness of Resin-Bonded Bridges in Primary Dental Care. Centre for Health Services Research. University of Newcastle upon Tyne. Report number 107; 2001.

Tay WM. Resin Bonded Bridges: A Practitioners Guide. New York: Martin Dunitz Ltd; 1992.

Van Dalen A, Feilzer AJ, Kleverlaan CJ. A literature review of two-unit cantilevered FPDs. Int J Prosthodont 2004;17:281–4.

REFERENCES

1. The NHS Information Centre. Adult dental health survey 2009. Available from: <www.ic.nhs.uk>; 2010.

2. Priest GF. Failure rates of restorations for single-tooth replacement. Int J Prosthodont 1996;9(1):38–45.

3. Goodacre CJ, Bernal G, Rungcharassaeng K, Kan JY. Clinical complications in fixed prosthodontics. J Prosthet Dent 2003;90:31–41.

4. Tay WM. Resin Bonded Bridges: A Practitioner's Guide. New York: Martin Dunitz Ltd; 1992.

5.   Goldstein RE. Esthetics in Dentistry, vol. 2. 2nd ed. Hamilton, ON: BC Decker Inc; 2002.

6.   Aukes JN, Käyser AF, Felling AJ. The subjective experience of mastication in subjects with shortened dental arches. J Oral Rehabil 1998;15(4):321–4.

7.   Love WD, Adams RL. Tooth movement into edentulous areas. JPD 1971;25:271–7.

8.   Kiliaridis S, Lyka I, Friede H, et al. Vertical position, rotation, and tipping of molars without antagonists. Int J Prosthodont 2000;13(6):480–6.

9.   University Hospital of Copenhagen. The Dental Trauma Guide. <http://dentaltraumaguide.org>; 2010.

10. Nelson JN, Ash MM. Wheeler's Dental Anatomy, Physiology and Occlusion. 9th ed. Philadelphia: WB Saunders; 2009.

11. Morgan C, Djemal S, Gilmour G. Predictable resin-bonded bridges in general dental practice. Dent Update 2001;28:501–8.

12. Rochette AL. Attachment of a splint to enamel of lower anterior teeth. J Prosthet Dent 1973;30:418–23.

13. Djemal S, Setchell D, King P, Wickens J. Long-term survival characteristics of 832 resin-retained bridges and splints provided in a post-graduate teaching hospital between 1978 and 1993. J Oral Rehab 1999;26(4):302–20.

14. Imbery TA, Eshelman EG. Resin-bonded fixed partial dentures: a review of three decades of progress. J Am Dent Assoc 1996;127(12):1751–60.

15. El-Mowafy O, Rubo MH. Resin-bonded fixed partial dentures – a literature review with presentation of a novel approach. Int J Prosthodont 2000;13(6):460–7.

16. Tredwin CJ, Setchell DJ, George GS, Weisbloom M. Resin-retained bridges as predictable and successful restorations. Alpha Omegan 2007;100(2):89–96.

17. Livaditis GJ. Cast metal resin-bonded retainers for posterior teeth. J Am Dent Assoc 1980;110:926–9.

18. Hussey DL, Pagni C, Linden GJ. Performance of 400 adhesive bridges fitted in a restorative dentistry department. J Dent 1991;19(4):221–5.

19. Steele JG, Jepson NJ, McColl E, Swift B. Finding Ways to Improve the Effectiveness of Resin-Bonded Bridges in Primary Dental Care. Centre for Health Services Research. University of Newcastle upon Tyne. Report number 107; 2001.

20. Creugers NH, Van 't Hof MA. An analysis of clinical studies on resin-bonded bridges. J Dent Res 1991;70(2):146–9.

21. Van Dalen A, Feilzer AJ, Kleverlaan CJ. A literature review of two-unit cantilervered FPDs. Int J Prosthodont 2004;17:281–4.

22. Goodacre CJ, Campagni WV, Aquilino SA. Tooth preparations for complete crowns: an art form based on scientific principles. J Prosthet Dent 2001;85(4):363–76.

CHAPTER 9

Minimally Invasive Replacement of Missing Teeth:
Part 2 – Tooth-Coloured Materials

L. MACKENZIE

INTRODUCTION

In response to patient and professional demands for more esthetic dental materials, the future of restorative dentistry is likely to consist entirely of tooth-coloured, metal-free restorations. Rigorous research and development is being carried out worldwide to engineer and test dental materials that have equivalent physical properties to metal restorations and, ultimately, natural tooth structure, allowing them to resist the complex functional forces of the oral environment and also match the esthetics of the patient's natural dentition.

In addition to esthetic demands and as a result of a well-documented history of poor longevity rates for the majority of dental restorations, the dental profession is increasingly searching for operative techniques that preserve the maximum amount of tooth tissue and do not have catastrophic results for the supporting teeth when failure eventually occurs.

This chapter continues the theme of the preceding one, but describes the latest innovative methods of tooth replacement that employ resin composite materials and high-strength ceramics.

MINIMALLY INVASIVE TOOTH REPLACEMENT WITH RESIN COMPOSITE MATERIALS

Since its advent, use of resin composites has revolutionized many restorative procedures and promoted the use of minimally invasive techniques.[1] The latest method employs resin composite restorations containing fibres to enhance their physical properties[1,2] and is currently the only technique that allows dentists to fabricate esthetic adhesive bridges of sufficient strength directly within the mouth.[2]

While these techniques are still considered to be at an experimental stage[3] and there are only a limited number of long-term clinical studies, experienced clinicians are now reporting reasonable longevity rates from these restorations[4,5] (Fig. 9.1), particularly with those fabricated intra-orally.[4] These encouraging statistics are likely to improve as design parameters and the materials continue to be investigated and optimized.

Since their introduction, one of the earliest applications for resin composites was to treat tooth loss by bonding recently extracted or prosthetic teeth to adjacent abutments[6] (Figs 9.2 and 9.3). While these techniques remain useful as an immediate temporary option, they cannot be expected to have much clinical longevity as a result of the poor bond between acrylic and enamel and the brittle nature of the resin composite connector.[1] Figure 9.4 demonstrates an innovative

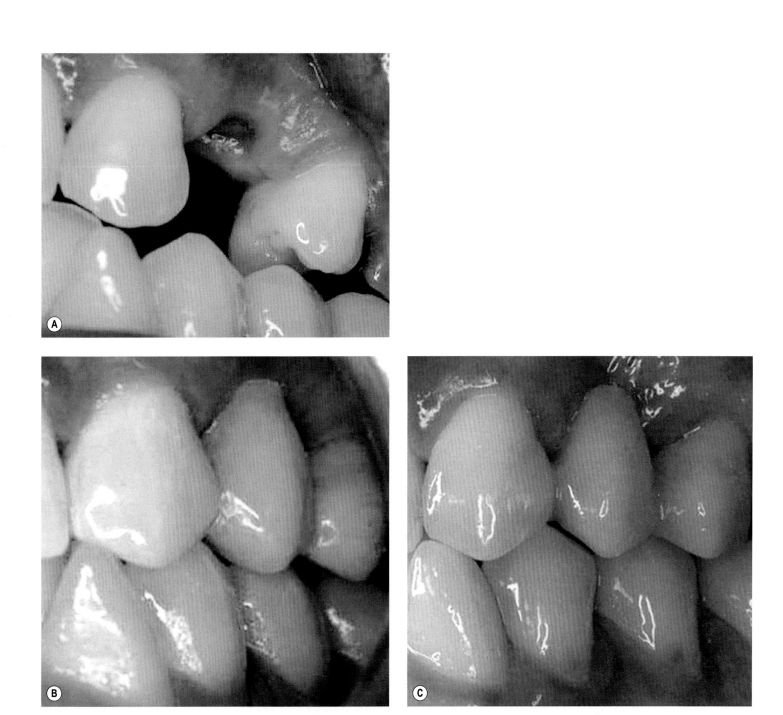

Fig. 9.1 Minimally invasive fibre-reinforced composite FRC-RBB by one of the world's most experienced clinicians in this area. (A) Pre-op, (B) post-op, (C) restoration at 10 years. Courtesy of Professor P. Vallittu.

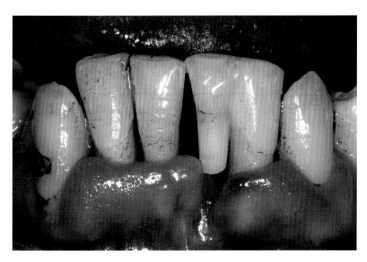

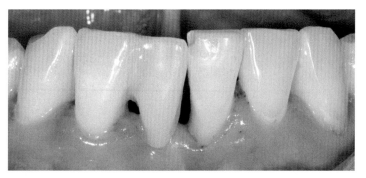

Fig. 9.3 Composite resins may be used to temporarily attach acrylic prosthetic teeth. Courtesy of Professor D.G. Perryer.

Fig. 9.2 Recently extracted teeth may be temporarily bonded to adjacent teeth.

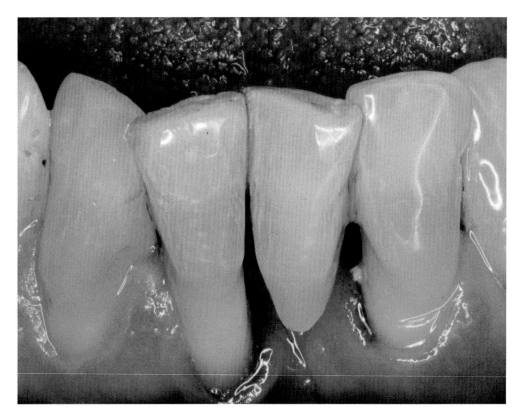

Fig. 9.4 Appearance at 27 years of an extracted lower incisor bonded to both (unprepared) adjacent abutment teeth via a non-precious fixed/fixed lingual retainer. Courtesy of Dr J. McCubbin.

technique that has been used to overcome these drawbacks. This involves supporting a recently extracted tooth with a lingual metal framework bonded to it and to the adjacent teeth with a composite.

FIBRE-REINFORCED COMPOSITE RESIN-BONDED BRIDGES

Since the 1960s, various manufacturing industries have used fibres with the strength of metal alloys[1] to reinforce composite materials. Fibre-reinforced dental restorations were introduced in the 1990s[7] to treat of a number of common dental problems including replacement of missing teeth.

Methods for tooth replacement using fibre-reinforced composite resin-bonded bridges (FRC-RBBs) may be divided into those fabricated directly in the mouth (direct FRC-RBBs) and those that involve the more familiar indirect approach (indirect FRC-RBBs). Semi-direct techniques may also be employed where partial construction on bridge frameworks may be carried out chairside or in a laboratory with the aim of simplifying intra-oral fabrication. Both techniques share common advantages and disadvantages and have the same general clinical indications.

Indications for FRC-RBBs

FRC-RBBs are versatile restorations that may be used to restore esthetics provisionally or in the longer term; they may be constructed using minimally invasive techniques and are particularly useful in situations where alternative treatment options are biologically or financially precluded (Fig. 9.5). FRC-RBBs may be used to restore esthetics in the following situations:

- Where abutment teeth are unrestored or minimally restored.

- For the immediate restoration of esthetics following extraction or traumatic loss of an anterior tooth.

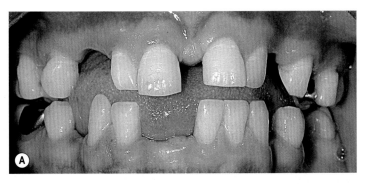 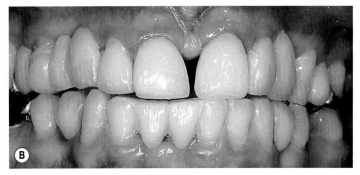

Fig. 9.5A,B   Minimally invasive FRC-RBBs restoring multiple edentulous areas. Courtesy of Dr A.C. Shortall.

- Where metal display may compromise esthetics, e.g. where metal wings of traditional RBBs may cause grey 'shine-through' on thin anterior abutments.[1]

- To maintain space in the developing dentition to simplify future orthodontic or esthetic restorative interventions.[9]

FRC-RBBs may be used for provisional restorations in the following situations:

- As inexpensive, long-term temporary restorations while stabilizing oral health.

- To postpone more invasive treatments such as implants.[9]

- As conservative transitional restorations during the healing period following implant placement.[9]

CLINICAL TIPS

The use of FRC-RBBs usually leaves all other future restorative options open.

FRC-RBBs may be used in clinical situations where other restorative options are compromised, such as where:

- Adhesive restorations may compensate for sub-optimal retention and resistance form in abutment teeth.

- Abutment of teeth has unfavourable angulations, and to minimize tooth preparation.

- Mobile abutment teeth may lead to inaccuracies in impression taking and cementation or limit the prognosis of more rigid restorations.[9]

- Implants are biologically or financially precluded.

FRC-RBBs may also be used where patient demand excludes metal restorations for hypersensitivity or psychological reasons.

Contra-indications for FRC-RBBs

Moisture control

As with all adhesive techniques, the inability to maintain isolation throughout the entire procedure will almost certainly guarantee early failure.

Functional contra-indications

These methods should also be avoided in clinical situations where:

- There is insufficient room for an adequate volume of supporting substructure fibres.

- Tooth loss/movement has resulted in a long span.

- Posterior use carries a higher risk of early failure because of the higher functional loads involved.

- The less rigid framework will be subjected to forces of higher magnitude, e.g. severe parafunction.[9]

In clinical situations where FRC-RBB is an option, it is also important to consider the potential advantages and disadvantages relative to other techniques (see Box 9.1 and the following text).

Technique sensitivity

Direct FRC–RBB is currently the only method of delivering a functional and esthetic replacement tooth with minimal or no abutment preparation and in a single appointment.[2,9]

It has been suggested that this approach may be too technique sensitive for the average practitioner. However, Clinical Case 9.1 (later in this chapter) describes how specialized materials, equipment and a simplified placement technique may be used to promote the quick, efficient and predictable replacement of a missing tooth and Clinical Case 9.2 describes the indirect alternative technique carried out by a final year dental undergraduate at a UK dental school.

How does fibre-reinforcement work?

Fibre-reinforcement enhances physical properties by stopping crack formation and propagation that may lead to restoration failure;[1] this fibre framework may be considered somewhat analogous to that of the alloy in a metal–ceramic bridge.

Various clinically significant factors have been identified as influences on the ability of glass fibres to reinforce composite bridges (see Box 9.2 and the following text).

Fibre type

Materials promoted for FRC-RBBs vary in constitution, diameter and the way that the individual fibres are arranged into bundles. The main materials used are:

- Glass fibres

- Ultra-high molecular weight polyethylene

- Kevlar fibres.

The most widely accepted design in Europe employs a substructure comprising continuous unidirectional glass fibre bundles imbedded in a dimethylacrylate/polymethylmethacrylate resin matrix.[10]

**BOX 9.1
ADVANTAGES AND
DISADVANTAGES OF
FRC-RBBS**

Advantages of FRC-RBBs[1,2]

- Allows the immediate replacement of missing teeth in a single visit

- Often minimal (or no) tooth preparation required

- Improved esthetics derived from use of entirely tooth-coloured materials

- Better adhesion of luting resins to bridge framework[4]

- Less expensive (no laboratory fee, impression required)

- Suitable for young patients with large immature pulp chambers and more translucent teeth

- Suitable for older patients who may not tolerate alternatives operatively or financially

- Frequently obviates the need for local anaesthetic

- Restoration failure may be readily repaired[4]

- Versatile design allows fibres to be orientated to respond to physical requirements

- More flexible restorations allow abutment movement without stressing the tooth/restoration interface[4]

- Less abrasive properties will reduce wear on opposing teeth

- FRC-RBBs have high reported patient satisfaction rates

Disadvantages of FRC-RBBs[1,2]

- Direct placement is technique-sensitive and requires training

- Laboratory construction requires technicians to learn a new technique

- Compared to porcelain, loss of surface lustre may compromise esthetics

- Inferior reported longevity rates (to date) versus metal ceramic (although survival rate statistics are improving)

- Optimum designs and clinical limits have yet to be established

- Water absorption may reduce fatigue limits of restoration over time[9]

- Restorations may be more plaque-retentive than alternatives

- Lower cost may perhaps reduce the likelihood of patients optimizing home care of restorations[4]

BOX 9.2 **FACTORS INFLUENCING REINFORCEMENT OF FRC-RBBS**[1,2,9]	• Fibre type
	• Fibre volume within the restoration
	• Adhesion at the fibre–resin interface
	• Fibre orientation
	• Fibre position within the restoration
	• Veneering composite

Fibre volume

Fracture of the less rigid veneering composite overlying the fibres is the most common mode of failure observed and has been attributed to insufficient framework support.

Optimum framework rigidity is achieved by increasing the diameter of the cross section. The greater the number of fibres within the restoration, the greater its resistance will be to fracture.[5,8] Care must be taken, however, not to incorporate too many fibres and risk their exposure during shaping and finishing procedures as this will result in degradation of the fibre–resin interface and reduce restoration longevity.

Bonding of fibres to the matrix

Ideally the reinforcing fibres should be bonded to the more flexible overlying resin composite.[1] Adhesion at the fibre–resin interface allows loads to be transferred to the fibres and increases their resistance to being pulled out. Poorly bonded fibres to which little load is transferred may be described as equivalent to having voids within the material.

It is therefore important that the fibre framework is infiltrated (wetted) by adhesive resin efficiently.[1,4] This is influenced by the fibre architecture and whether wetting agents are pre-impregnated* during manufacture,[8] e.g. StickTech (GC, Japan) (Fig. 9.6A), or require manual impregnation with adhesive by the dentist or technician, e.g. Ribbond (WA, USA) (Fig. 9.6B).

Fibre orientation

The direction of the glass fibre bundles influences the reinforcement of the veneering composite. While woven fibres offer multi-directional reinforcement, unidirectional fibres can be orientated in the direction in which the highest stress is predicted in the areas subject to the greatest loads.[1]

---

* As these resins are sensitive to light, they are kept in a lightproof foil to maintain their flexible non-polymerized state until they are required.

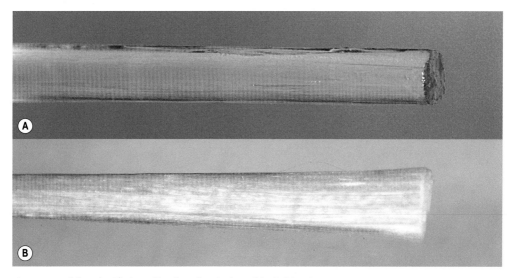

Fig. 9.6 Unidirectional glass-fibre bundles designed for bridge framework construction. (A) Pre-impregnated with resin. (B) Dry.

Position of the fibres in the framework

Fibres should be positioned within the prosthesis in the location and direction most likely to inhibit crack propagation. Load resistance research[11–13] into the magnitude and direction of stresses occurring within FRC specimens (Fig. 9.7) has demonstrated that for fixed/fixed designs:

- Fibres within the pontic should be positioned where the restoration is subject to greatest tension.[1,9,11–13] The tensile aspect of a bridge pontic is that closest to the gingivae and so the bulk of fibres should be positioned here, leaving just enough space for veneering composite gingivally.

- Fibres should also be positioned to reinforce the interproximal connector areas, which is another area of high stress.[5,12]

Veneering resin composite

Composition of the veneering resin composite has a significant effect on the rigidity and therefore the longevity of the final restoration.[13] Studies using hybrid or micro-filled resin composites have demonstrated that compatibility of fibres to the bonding agent and to the veneering composite is essential for maximum efficiency.

When using direct techniques, a variety of resin composite shades and stains may be used to help match the esthetics of adjacent natural teeth (Fig. 9.8).

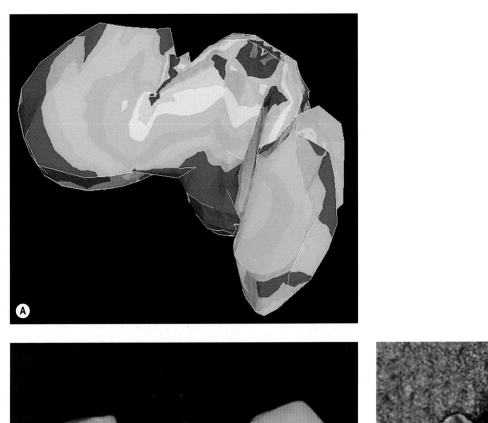

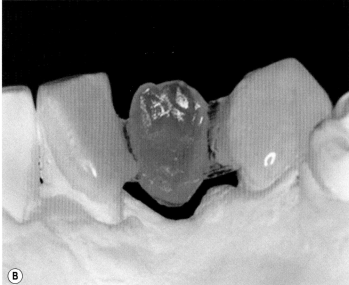
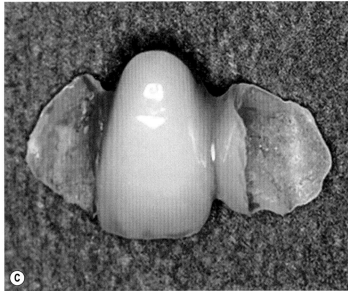

Fig. 9.7A–C (A) Laboratory testing of fibre-reinforced composites helps practitioners optimize restoration design (B,C). Courtesy of Professor A. Shinya.

For indirect FRC-RBBs the quality of adhesion to the composite luting cement is also vital. The veneering composite should be optimized with regard to:

- Resistance to fracture from fibre framework
- Co-polymerization of fibre framework and veneering composite
- Physical properties

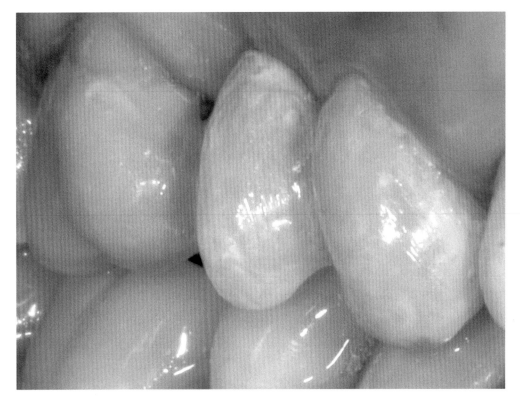

Fig. 9.8 FRC-RBB is the only technique that allows the fabrication of esthetic definitive bridges directly within the mouth. Courtesy of Dr P. Sands.

- Wear properties

- Esthetic properties.

Designing FRC-RBBs

Results from ongoing clinical and laboratory studies now provide practitioners with a range of guidelines for optimization of FRC-RBBs. When designing a restoration, the following parameters should be considered.

Tooth preparation

These techniques frequently require little or no tooth preparation. As with other forms of bridgework, abutments should be ideally unrestored or minimally restored. Where existing restorations are present, they may be removed to:

- Provide sufficient room for the fibre framework

- Improve retention and resistance form

- Prevent over-contouring of the adhesive retainers.

Framework design

Fixed/fixed designs are recommended for both direct and indirect FRC-RBBs. As it is a critical determinant of success, designs should allow a high volume of substructure fibres to be incorporated within the restoration.

Retainer design

Retainer design is the subject of considerable research[14–18] and is often based on the condition and restorative state of abutment teeth. Practitioners should choose the type(s) that promote the maximum preservation of tooth tissue. They can be:

- Extra-coronal (full/partial coverage)

- Surface retained

- Inlay retained

- Hybrid/combination designs.

Extra-coronal

Promising survival rates of up to 5 years have been described for partial and full coverage retainers, although tooth preparation is more invasive.

Surface-retained

Surface-retained restorations (Fig. 9.9) are the most conservative option and may be considered in favourable occlusions that allow sufficient room for material. If occlusal interferences are likely to be introduced, shallow preparations (ideally confined to enamel) may be made to optimize fibre volume. Survival probability has been shown to be lower for surface-retained restorations,[2] which have a higher risk of de-bonding.[5] Care is required to ensure the patient

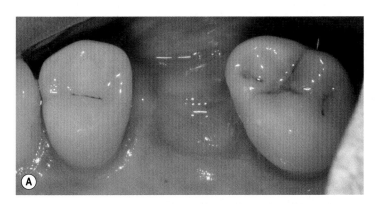
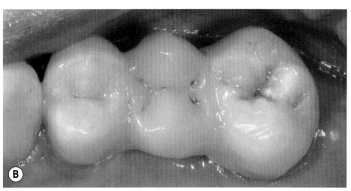

Fig. 9.9A,B A surface-retained FRC-RBB restoring a missing upper premolar preserves all of the natural tooth tissue of both abutments. Courtesy of Dr P. Sands.

receiving this type of restoration is capable of maintaining adequate oral health and oral hygiene methods.

Inlay-retained

Inlay-type cavities have been shown to be useful at resisting rotational forces.[5] There is no agreement on specific dimensions, but cavities that are 2 mm × 2 mm × 2 mm are considered adequate.[5] For molar teeth at least two fibre bundles are recommended and space for this may often be created by the removal of existing restorations.

Hybrid design

One of the benefits of these techniques is that they are versatile and may be adapted to each clinical situation, enabling the most conservative, minimally invasive design (see Clinical Case 9.1).

Longevity of FRC-RBBs

Whilst FRC RBBs are still regarded as experimental restorations,[3] clinical evaluations at a number of centres worldwide have demonstrated encouraging results for four or more years, using a range of restorations incorporating high fibre-volume framework designs. Even though relatively short-term clinical data is currently available, these techniques show promise and survival rates can be expected to improve as designs are refined and practitioners' skills for handling resin composites develop with experience.[4]

Failure

While it is difficult to simulate complex clinical loading situations in the laboratory, in vitro load testing can help predict the likely mode of failure by investigating:

- Fatigue resistance over time when specimens are subjected to repeated loads.

- Long-term effect of water absorption.

- Areas where restorations are subject to the greatest stresses.

When reviewing failed restorations using a new technique, it is important to diagnose the cause of failure. This will inform improvements to replacement or repaired restorations and may increase their longevity.

The most prevalent mode of failure reported is restoration fracture.[5] This initiates within the more brittle veneering composite material and propagates through to the fibres,[9] with resultant chipping or loss of considerable portions of the veneering resin composite.

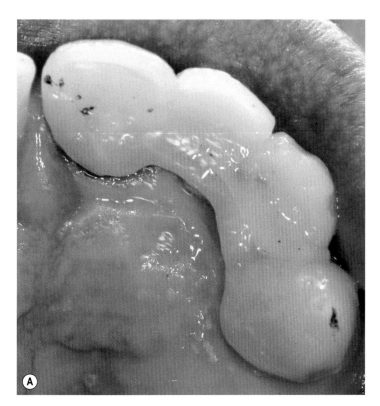 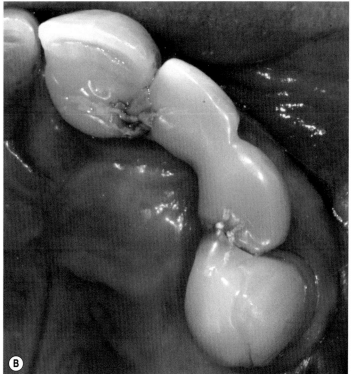

Fig. 9.10A,B   A FRC-RBB replacing two anterior teeth (A) has failed after several years due to fracture of the veneering resin composite (B).

Ultra-high molecular weight woven-fibre frameworks are less likely to fracture than those fabricated from glass fibres. Fracture of veneering composite is the predominant form of failure seen with these restorations (Fig. 9.10). When it occurs, careful analysis and recording of the mode of failure will allow future restorations to be designed with frameworks that support the veneering composite more effectively.

One of the great benefits of composite materials over alloys and porcelain is that restoration defects are often amenable to repair and such techniques may be used to prolong the functional survival of the restoration.[4]

Patients with FRC-RBBs should be monitored regularly and assessed with regard to the following:[9]

• Fracture/chipping involving veneering composite

• Fracture involving composite and framework

• Marginal leakage

• Marginal stain

• Wear resistance

- Anatomical form

- Surface integrity/texture/lustre

- Shade/colour stability

- Plaque levels, gingival inflammation.

MINIMALLY INVASIVE TOOTH REPLACEMENT WITH ALL-CERAMIC MATERIALS

INTRODUCTION

Esthetics has been demonstrated as the primary influence on the patient's perception of success with regard to the replacement of missing teeth. Following the positive response to all-ceramic crowns there is now a range of all-ceramic restorative systems that may be adapted for bridgework, and these are considered to be the prospective replacements for metal–ceramic restorations.[19]

The use of all-ceramic bridges is currently still rather controversial and metal–ceramic equivalents are still considered optimal in terms of predictability.[20] Ongoing clinical and laboratory testing of a range of ceramic materials is one of the fastest advancing areas in dental materials research; ultimately, long-term clinical data will result in more specific guidelines for case selection in order to deliver predictable, functional and esthetic success.

MATERIALS FOR ALL-CERAMIC RBBS

A variety of dental ceramics have been advocated for use in dental bridgework and are now approaching the properties required for the esthetic and minimally invasive replacement of missing teeth. The most recent developments involve the use of zirconia–yttria ceramics for the fabrication of high performance bridge frameworks and are the focus of the following text.

Zirconia–yttria bridges

Zirconia is a ceramic with a fine grained polycrystalline micro-structure that confers strength.[19] As a result it has been in considerable demand for esthetic, load-bearing restorations since its introduction to dentistry in 2002.

Some contemporary zirconia-based restorative systems contain an additional stabilizing oxide, based most commonly on the chemical element yttria.[19] The resultant material is known as yttrium tetragonal zirconia polycrystal (Y-TZP). It has the highest reported ceramic fracture resistance and enables restorations to withstand loads, in thin section, many times higher than those created in the mouth.[19]

While long span bridges may be fabricated entirely from high strength Y-TZP, this may compromise esthetics as pure zirconia is white. Most contemporary restorations are therefore comprised of a high strength zirconia framework covered with an overlying veneer of conventional esthetic porcelain.

When selecting all-ceramic materials for the indirect fixed replacement of missing teeth, it is important to inform the patient fully, both verbally and in written form, of their advantages and disadvantages (see the following text).

ADVANTAGES OF ALL-CERAMIC BRIDGES[19–21]

Strength

A bridge's resistance to mechanical stresses (flexural strength) is dependent upon the type of ceramic used in the framework and on the esthetic veneering porcelain used to cover it. The relative thicknesses of each layer are also important, as is the bond strength between the veneer and the significantly stronger Y-TZP core.[19]

Rigidity

Y-TZP frameworks have a high modulus of elasticity. This reduces stress on the weaker veneer layer and increases the load-bearing capacity of the restoration as a whole. Compatible feldspathic veneering porcelains are designed to match the modulus of elasticity and coefficient of thermal expansion of the underlying framework.

Fracture resistance

The mode of failure observed most commonly in all-ceramic bridges is chipping or fracture of the brittle veneering porcelain, which may extend to the framework and often involves the pontic/framework connector area. This is a result of tensile forces on the gingival aspect propagating pre-existing micro-cracks within the material.[20]

Micro-cracks mainly originate at the core/veneer interface[20] and the thickness ratio of these layers is a dominant factor in controlling the crack initiation site and potential for failure. Therefore, it is essential to optimize the thickness of these layers to ensure that the ceramic veneer is under compressive stress and the core framework is under tensile stress.

Transformation toughening

Y-TZP frameworks have increased ability to limit crack propagation (fracture toughness) as the material possesses a unique property known as transformation toughening. When tensile stress forces are applied to Y-TZP, it reacts by localized volumetric expansion (in the range of 3–5%). The resultant localized compressive forces squeeze fracture tips to counteract and arrest propagating cracks.[20]

Thermal conductivity

As ceramics are insulators, an all-ceramic bridge may be selected to offer greater pulp protection in certain clinical situations, compared to the metal–ceramic alternatives.

Biocompatibility

Zirconia-based materials were originally used for hip replacements and extensive evaluations have demonstrated that they are well tolerated by biological tissues and they are a good alternative in patients with proven hypersensitivity to metal alloys, e.g. nickel, palladium.

Zirconia frameworks also exhibit better chemical and dimensional stability compared to other high strength ceramics, as they are free of the glass component that has been shown to be more susceptible to corrosion in saliva over the long term.[20] In addition, the veneering porcelain may also be glazed to reduce the abrasion potential on opposing natural antagonists.

Radiopacity

Zirconia has a similar radiopacity to metals, enabling improved long-term radiographic monitoring compared to other tooth-coloured materials.

Esthetics

All-ceramic materials deliver increased depth of translucency allowing a more natural light transmission through the entire restoration. This eliminates the need for an excessively white opaque layer to mask the grey metal substructure.

The veneering ceramic should also match the optical properties of the core material and imitate the polychromatic appearance of adjacent natural teeth with respect to hue, chroma and value and translucency (Fig. 9.11).

While additional tooth tissue may need to be sacrificed to make room for the additional thickness required for ceramic strength and esthetics, supra-ginigival finishing lines often can be employed without compromising overall esthetics.[19]

All-ceramic bridges are useful in clinical situations where metal frameworks may compromise esthetics, including:

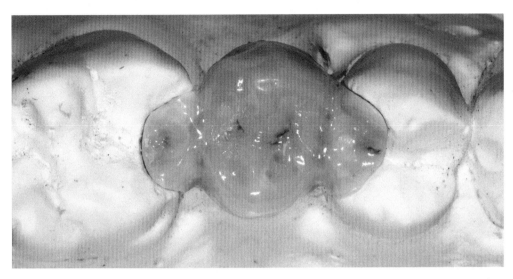

Fig. 9.11 A minimally invasive ceramic bridge replacing a missing premolar (see Clinical Case 9.3) and incorporating a Y-TZP framework supporting an esthetic veneering porcelain.

- Thin/translucent anterior teeth

- Cases where occlusal coverage is required.

As there is no need to mask metal substructures, all-ceramic bridges may promote an even more conservative approach in certain areas where there is minimal/no contact on the retainers, e.g. the replacement of missing lower incisors.

Marginal fit

Good marginal adaptation is essential to prevent:

- Cement dissolution

- Micro-leakage

- Increased plaque retention

- Increased risk of secondary caries.

CAD/CAM technology (Fig. 9.12) is employed increasingly in the fabrication of all-ceramic restorations,[20] and currently there are over 20 milling systems capable of delivering restorations whose marginal fit is within the clinically acceptable range (Fig. 9.13).

While available software, hardware, camera, scanning and milling machines all have inherent limitations,[19] technological advances will improve precision with regard to marginal and internal fit.

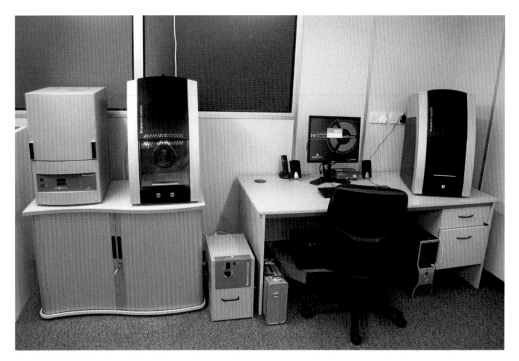

Fig. 9.12 CAD/CAM laboratory equipment for the design and manufacture of indirect restorations. (A & J Rollings Dental Laboratories, England.)

DISADVANTAGES OF ALL-CERAMIC BRIDGES

Despite their advantages, currently available bridges are contra-indicated in clinical situations where:

- There is insufficient room for the required connector dimensions (e.g. Class II Division II malocclusions).[20]

- There are heavy localized stresses on contact areas.[20]

- Moisture control cannot be optimized for the entire cementation procedure.

Ceramic resin-bonded bridges share many of the same disadvantages with their metal–ceramic counterparts; in addition they have the following disadvantages:

- Natural white colour of zirconia frameworks may compromise esthetics in certain situations.

- Chairside adjustments are difficult to polish effectively.

- Restorations cannot be sectioned and soldered if major modifications are necessary.[20]

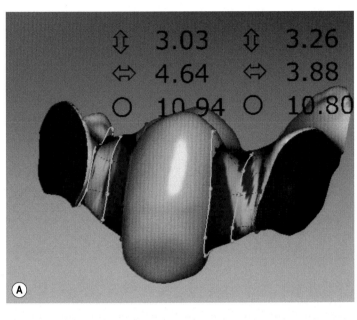

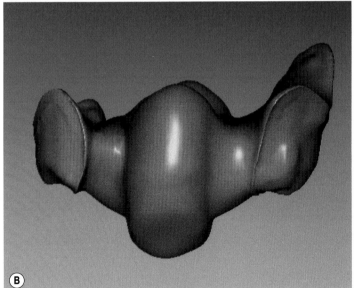

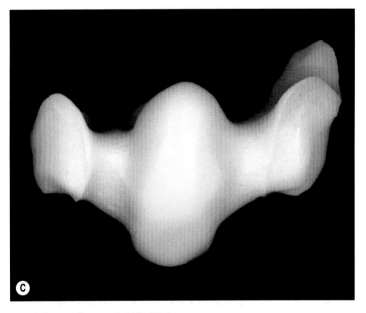

Fig. 9.13A–C   Design and manufacture of a Y-TZP framework for an all-ceramic RBB. (A) Connector design. (B) Digital framework design. (C) Completed framework. Courtesy of A & J Rollings.

- Failed restorations may be difficult to remove.

- Lack of definitive design guidelines.

- Lack of long-term clinical studies.[20]

Longevity

While reported survival rates for all-ceramic bridges are variable, data from ongoing clinical studies shows promise.[20] Continuing trials are likely to optimize case selection further with regard to choice of materials, manufacturing techniques, design considerations and support for esthetic veneering porcelains.[20]

Failure

In common with other forms of bridgework, failure may occur due to partial or total de-cementation, secondary caries and/or periodontal disease. However, the predominant modes of failure for ceramic RBBs in general have been demonstrated as:

- Fracture at the connector[26] between the pontic and the retainer.

- Chipping fractures where veneering porcelains have been used.

CAD/CAM technology is useful in this respect as it allows framework and connector designs to be optimized for specific materials and clinical situations. (Fig. 9.14)

While Y-TZP frameworks may reduce the likelihood of irretrievable fracture, older restorations exhibit commonly small chipping fractures of the veneering porcelain.[19]

When ceramic restorations are tested in laboratory experiments that simulate clinical conditions (e.g. use of intermittent dynamic cyclic forces, artificial saliva, temperature fluctuations and humidity control),[19] results tend to indicate lower failure loads compared to conventional in vitro fracture toughness tests. This more clinically relevant data will help to inform practitioners in the design and manufacture of all-ceramic bridges of the future.

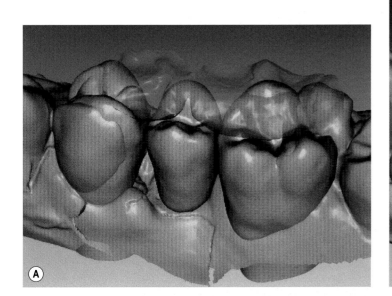

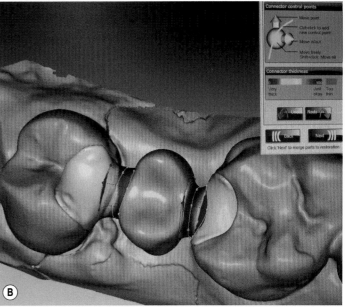

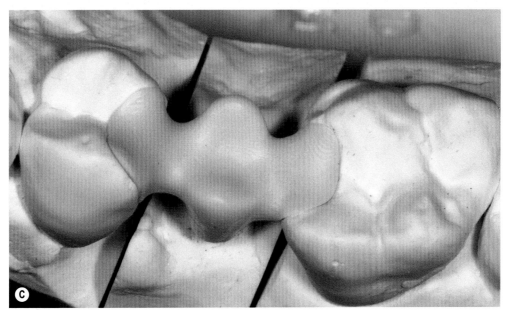

Fig. 9.14A–C Design and manufacture stages to optimize connector strength for an all-ceramic bridge.
Courtesy of A & J Rollings.

CLINICAL CASE 9.1: DIRECT FIBRE-REINFORCED COMPOSITE RESIN-BONDED BRIDGE

Key reference: an excellent clinical guide[19] to fibre reinforcements for minimally invasive bridges is available from StickTech (GC, Japan).

Case history

An 80-year-old female patient presented having fractured a crowned upper lateral incisor, leaving a root with a sub-gingival carious lesion. All treatment options were presented including an implant-retained restoration or endodontics followed by a post-retained indirect restoration, but these were rejected on financial grounds.

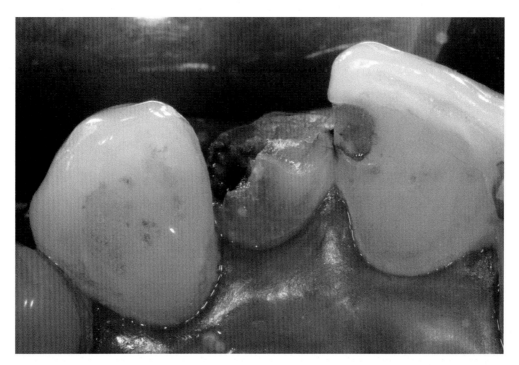

Fig. C9.1.1   Fractured, carious lateral incisor.

Care plan

As immediate restoration of the space was necessary for esthetic reasons, the decision was made to extract the carious root and employ a direct FRC-RBB by virtue of the following favourable clinical conditions:

• Remaining dentition relatively intact

• Favourable occlusal stability with no evidence of parafunction

- Edge-to-edge occlusion provides ample room for high-volume fibre framework

- Healthy periodontal condition

- Presence of sufficient enamel for adhesion to minimally restored abutment teeth

- Removal of distal Class III restoration on upper right central incisor allowed use of an inlay retainer at negligible biological expense.

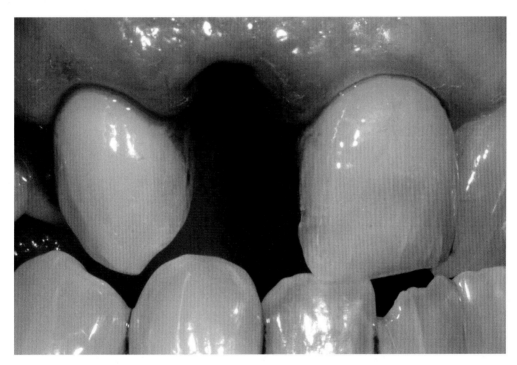

Fig. C9.1.2   Treatment plan: direct FRC-RBB.

Design

As bridge design is a key ingredient to successful clinical performance, the following design features were selected.

Fixed/fixed design

This is recommended for all FRC bridges whether direct or indirect, as it delivers increased support for retainers and offers greater surface area for bonding. Cantilever FRC-RBBs exhibit poorer longevity and should be reserved for temporary restorations or where unsuitable mobility characteristics of potential abutment teeth prevail.

Retainer design

The prescription comprised a non-invasive surface retainer on the canine and an inlay retainer on the central incisor requiring minimal tooth preparation.

CLINICAL TIPS

Hybrid veneering resin composite was chosen for strength and esthetics. A shade test was carried out by light curing a sample of the material on the labial surface of the adjacent tooth. This was done prior to isolation as teeth will dehydrate and lighten during the operative procedure and without etching or bonding procedures.

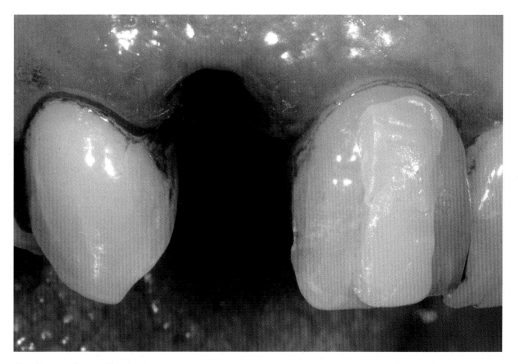

Fig. C9.1.3 Composite shade test.

Technique tips

- Resorbable cellulose gauze was packed into the extraction socket to reduce the risk of haemorrhagic moisture contamination during the procedure.

- A pre-formed cellulose acetate crown form was measured and adjusted to fit the space, for use later in the controlled application of the direct composite pontic.

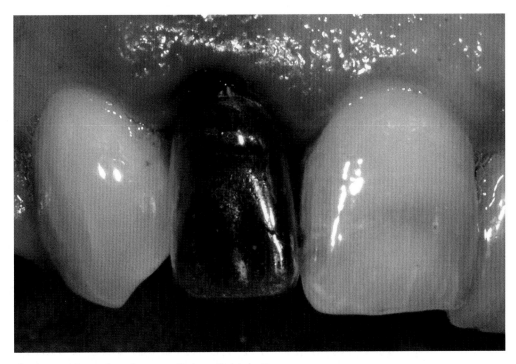

Fig. C9.1.4   Crown form for controlled pontic fabrication.

Isolation

Moisture control was achieved using a rubber dam that was secured with a clamp on a distal tooth and the use of dam stabilizing cord. The dam was reflected into the gingival sulcus and a floss ligature used to further improve isolation. The Class III proximal restoration was then removed from the central incisor.

CLINICAL TIPS

As well as guaranteeing isolation, the dam also acts as a gingival matrix to control composite adaptation gingivally. In this respect, it is important that rubber dam holes are positioned to allow flexibility during placement.

Measuring the fibre

Measuring precisely simplifies fibre placement and avoids wastage. A piece of dam stabilizing cord* was used to measure fibre bundles accurately (Fig. C9.1.6A) before cutting the required amount, together with its silicone bedding (Fig. C9.1.6B). The remaining fibres were replaced immediately in the lightproof packet.

---

*   Periodontal probes or dental floss are suggested alternatives, but may be harder to control or bend around corners.

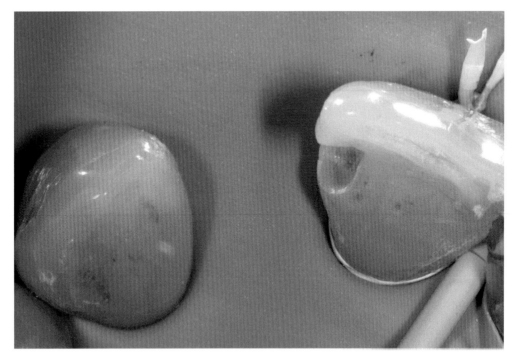

Fig. C9.1.5 Isolation.

Pre-impregnated unidirectional glass fibres were used (everStick, GC, Japan) containing light-sensitive monomers that cross-link during polymerization to form a multi-phase polymer network with the overlying resin composite.

Once cut, fibres should be shielded from the light and protected from contamination as this may impair the oxygen inhibited surface layer that is essential to optimize bonding with the veneering resin composite.

Storage recommendation: everStick products should be refrigerated (+2° to +8°) but direct contact with refrigerator walls should be avoided.

Tooth surface preparation

The areas to be bonded were:

• Cleaned using a pumice and water mix in a rubber cup

• Rinsed with water and air-dried

• Etched with 37% ortho-phosphoric acid

• Rinsed with water and air-dried again.

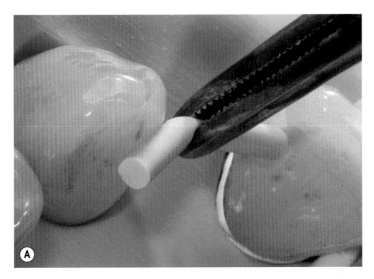 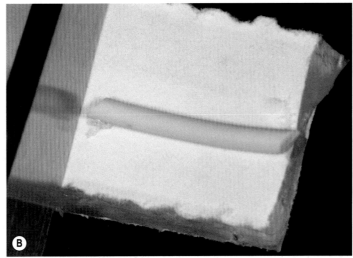

Fig. C9.1.6   (A) Precise measurement. (B) Cutting of glass fibres.

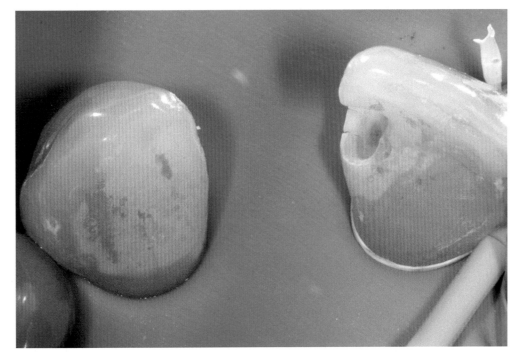

Fig. C9.1.7   Tooth surface preparation.

Adhesive

Adhesive resin was applied to the entire bonding area and light cured as per manufacturer's instructions. A thin layer of flowable resin composite was then applied to the retainer surfaces but was not light cured at this stage.

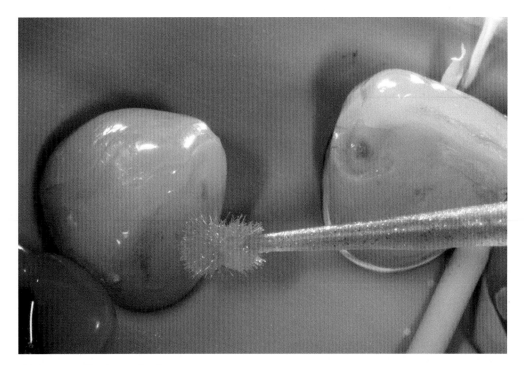

Fig. C9.1.8   Adhesive application.

Fibre placement

One end of the fibre bundle was placed into the uncured lining of flowable resin composite in the inlay cavity and the other end pressed tightly onto the palatal surface of the canine using a specialized instrument (StickSTEPPER, LM instruments, Finland). The retainers were light cured individually for 5–10 seconds, while shielding the rest of the fibre bundle from the light using the same instrument.

When placing the fibres it is important to spread them as widely as possible on the bonding areas and position the pontic framework in a form that curves towards the gingiva to optimize reinforcement.

Flowable composite

A second thin layer of flowable resin composite was then applied to provide a seal with subsequent fibre bundles.

Increasing fibre volume

Additional fibre bundles were added to increase the cross-sectional diameter of the framework. This increases the rigidity and resistance to occlusal loading of the final restoration. Approximately 2 mm of space was left between the fibres and the gingiva.

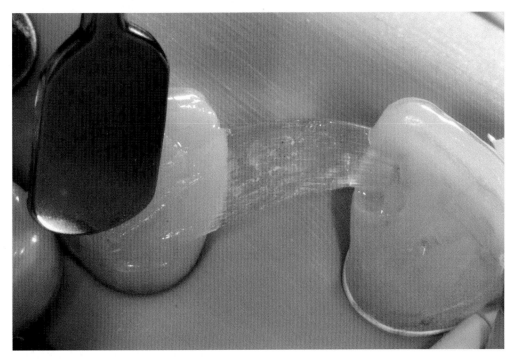

Fig. C9.1.9   Fibre placement.

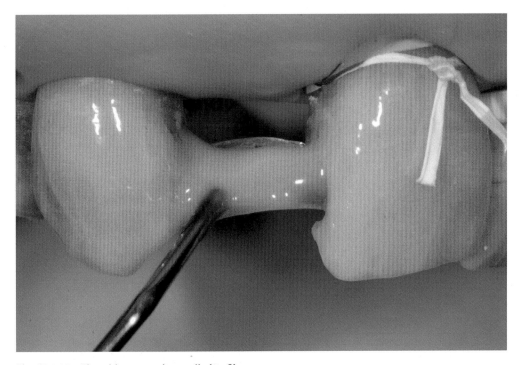

Fig. C9.1.10   Flowable composite applied to fibres.

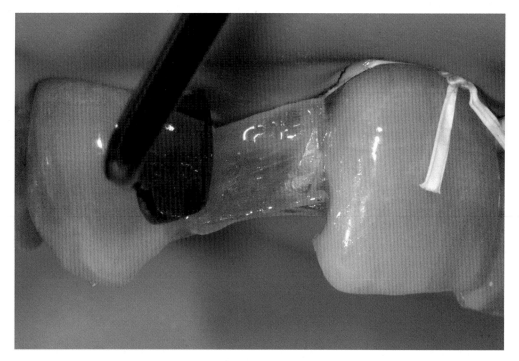

Fig. C9.1.11   Maximizing volume of bridge framework.

Light-cure framework

The entire fibre frame was then covered with a thin layer of flowable resin composite and light cured for 40 seconds from all directions.

Composite placement

An initial increment of hybrid resin composite was applied gingivally, while depressing the rubber dam to create a 'socket-fit' pontic. Care was taken to avoid blocking the embrasure areas, which would have increased the risk of fibre exposure or iatrogenic tooth damage during finishing.

Crown form preparation

The crown form was modified to fit over the framework (Fig. C9.1.14A) and pierced with a probe to allow composite venting (Fig. C9.1.14B). This reduced the risk of voids, which have been implicated as a possible cause of premature failure.

Pontic construction

The crown form was filled with hybrid resin composite of the pre-determined shade (Fig. C9.1.15A) and applied also over the fibre framework (Fig. C9.1.15B). Excess was removed with a suitable hand instrument.

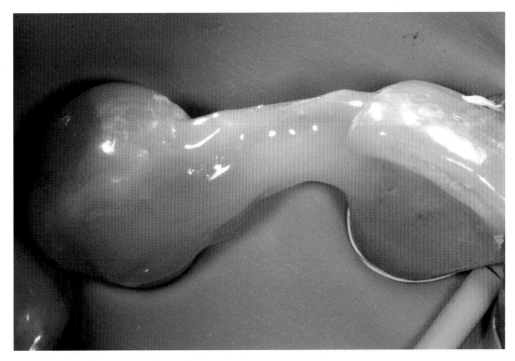

Fig. C9.1.12   Framework covered with flowable composite and light cured.

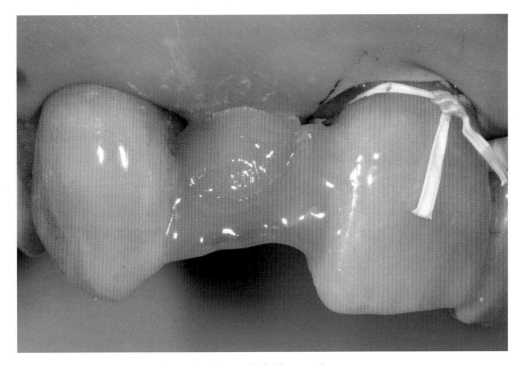

Fig. C9.1.13   Application of gingival increment of hybrid composite.

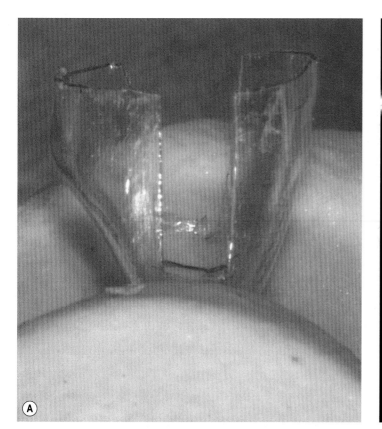

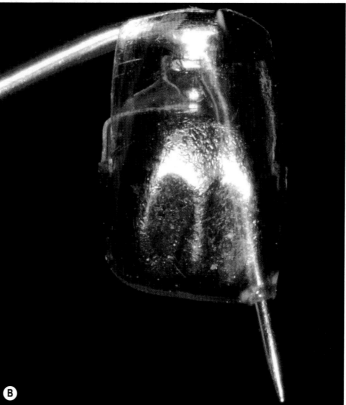

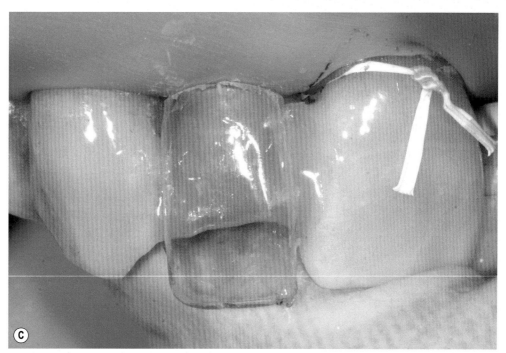

Fig. C9.1.14   Crown form. (A) Cut. (B) Perforated. (C) Tried in over framework.

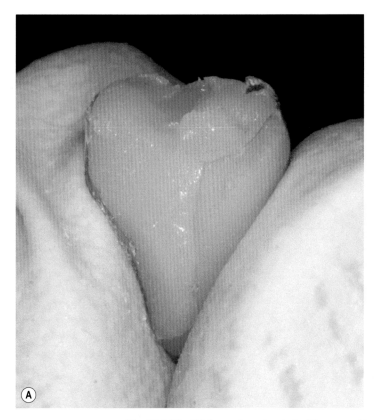
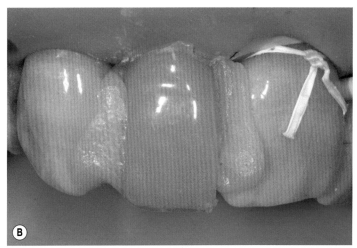

Fig. C9.1.15 (A) Crown form loaded with composite. (B) Crown form applied to fibre framework.

Gingival contour

Finger pressure was applied to improve adaptation to the framework and to the initial gingival increment. Forcing the pontic into the socket also reduces the potential risk of space under the final restoration following post-extraction resorption.

Light curing

Following removal of further excess material, the restoration was light cured from all directions. As well as controlling the shape of the pontic, the crown former eliminated oxygen during polymerization. This should result in improved physical and stain-resistance properties.

Crown form removal

Careful placement technique should minimize finishing time following crown form removal.

Finishing

Adjustments were made using suitable burs, with care not to damage the glass fibres.

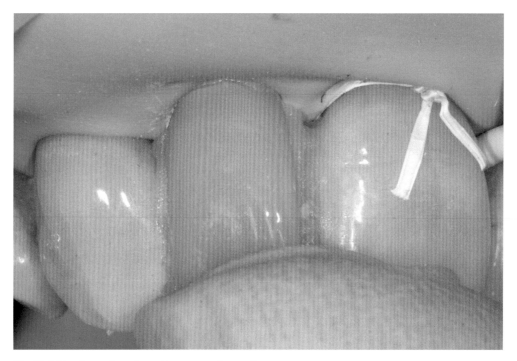

Fig. C9.1.16 Crown from forced into extraction socket.

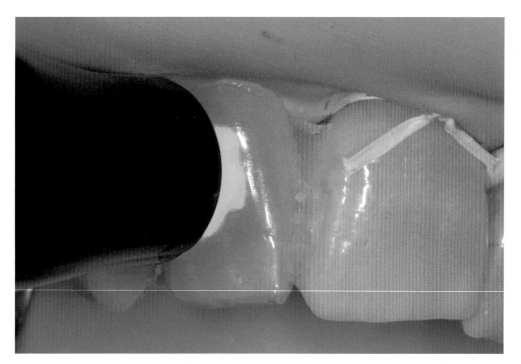

Fig. C9.1.17 Pontic light cured.

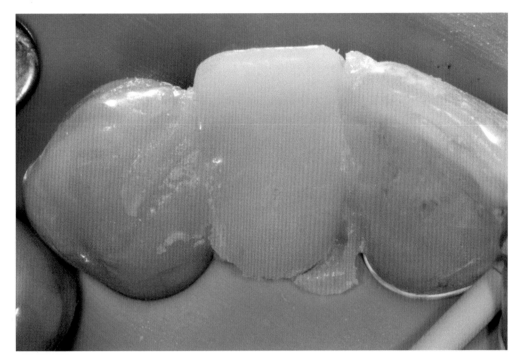

Fig. C9.1.18 Crown form removal.

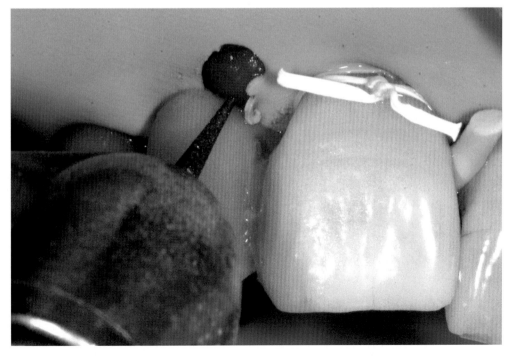

Fig. C9.1.19 Pontic adjustment.

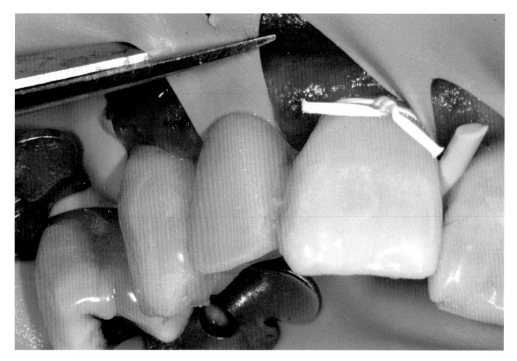

Fig. C9.1.20 Rubber dam removal technique.

Rubber dam removal

Removal of the rubber dam was simplified by pulling from under the pontic and cutting with scissors.

Embrasure contour

The connector area was adjusted to allow effective oral hygiene measures and the patient was informed in the use of suitable interdental cleaning aids.

Occlusal adjustment

As fracture of the veneering resin composite is the mode of failure observed most commonly, careful adjustments were made to eliminate occlusal interferences in all excursions.

Restoration assessment

All aspects of the completed restoration were examined. The patient had been warned previously of the apparent initial colour mismatch due to the dehydration of the natural adjacent teeth. This will rebound in the next few days.

Review

At the outset, the patient was informed of the importance of regular examinations to assess oral hygiene, function and esthetics. Careful technical notes were made at all stages to optimize future direct FRC-RBB procedures.

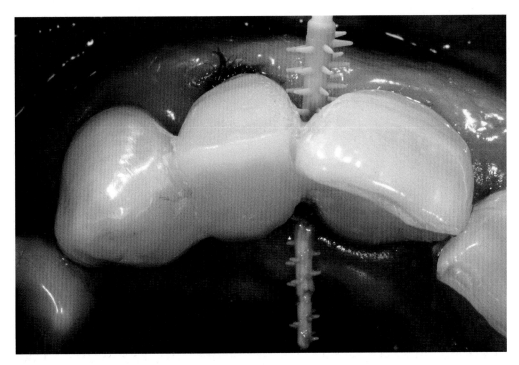

Fig. C9.1.21 Pontic shaped to allow cleaning.

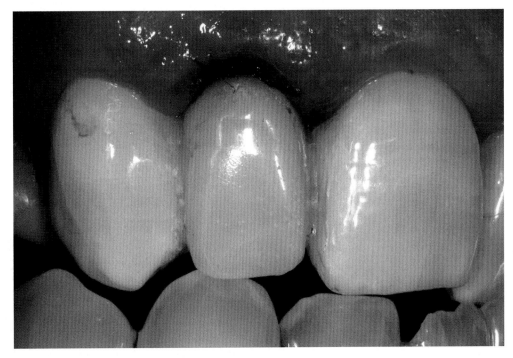

Fig. C9.1.22 Pontic prior to occlusal adjustment.

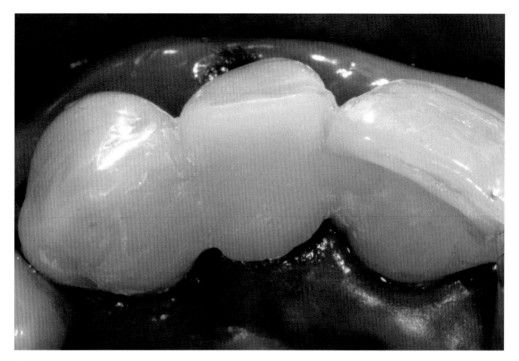

Fig. C9.1.23 Restoration assessment.

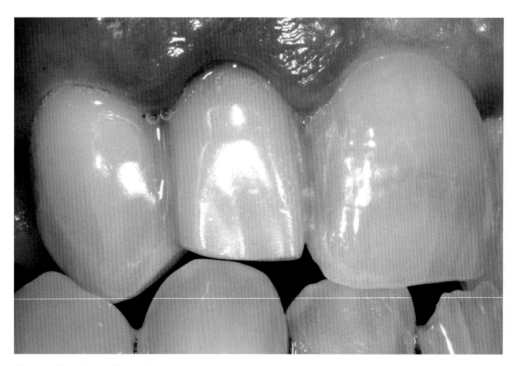

Fig. C9.1.24 Restoration review.

CLINICAL CASE 9.2: INDIRECT FIBRE-REINFORCED COMPOSITE RESIN-BONDED BRIDGE

Indications

Indirect FRC-RBBs are indicated for the same clinical situations as direct, as in this example where carious lesions required restoration on proximal surfaces adjacent to a space left following loss of an upper second premolar.

Indirect fabrication is less technique sensitive as:

- Moisture control is simplified.

- Enhanced polymerization of composite resins is possible with use of heat, pressure or vacuum. This may improve flexure and wear resistance and colour stability.[8]

- Laboratory polishing may also reduce the tendency for plaque accumulation.[20]

While technicians will need to learn a new technique of RBB construction, this fabrication method is a straightforward laboratory resin composite application. There are no time-consuming stages, where errors may occur during waxing, investing and casting procedures.

Indirect FRC-RBBs may be used also for more complex clinical cases that would be challenging for intra-oral manufacture. Research continues in their use for restoring implant abutments, where they may be conventionally luted or screw retained.[8]

Minimally invasive preparation

The bridge was designed to optimize fibre volume within the restoration, whilst preserving the maximum amount of residual tooth tissue. Initial preparation was confined to accessing and excavating the proximal carious lesions using suitable small burs.

Preparation complete

Following minimally invasive caries removal, abutments were prepared to receive inlay retainers. No attempt was made to remove all undercuts as this would have involved unnecessary destruction of strong, healthy tooth tissue and luting resin composite will be able to fill them during cementation.

An occlusal cavity was prepared to treat a secondary carious lesion, but its restoration was postponed until the fit appointment where the rubber dam isolation would optimize placement.

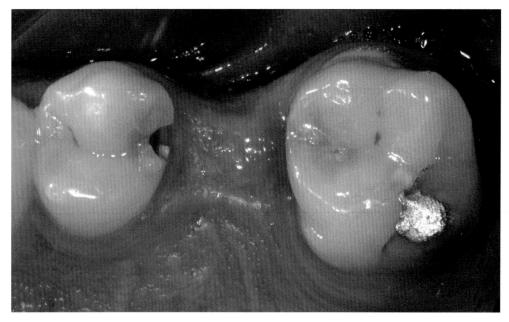

Fig. C9.2.1   Treatment plan: minimally invasive indirect FRC-RBB.

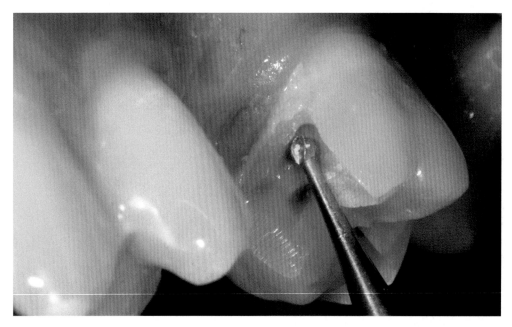

Fig. C9.2.2   Caries excavation.

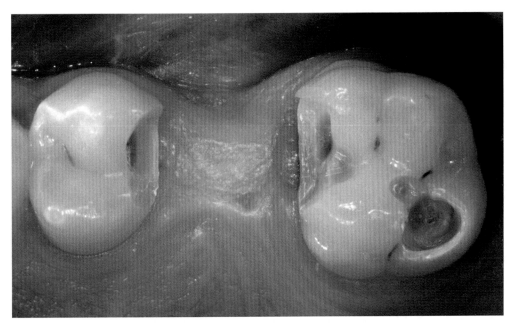

Fig. C9.2.3   Preparation complete.

Silicone and alginate impressions were taken to record the upper and lower arches, respectively, and all three cavities were temporized using a flexible light-cured resin designed for this purpose.

Model construction

Die stone models were cast and articulated. Accurate occlusal registration and articulation were essential to minimize the need for adjustment that may have:

- Exposed the fibres and resulted in premature degradation of the fibre/resin interface

- Left a thin layer of veneering composite that would be prone to fracture.

Wax was applied to block out undercuts and to modify the gingival embrasure shape, allowing fabrication of connectors with hygienic emergence profiles. The altered cast was then duplicated to fabricate a working model.

Framework construction

The fibre framework was fabricated to maximize the volume of pre-impregnated unidirectional glass fibre bundles (GC, Japan) and minimize concomitantly the volume of the less fracture resistant veneering resin composite.

Additional fibres were orientated perpendicular to the initial layers as this has been shown to increase restoration strength.[5]

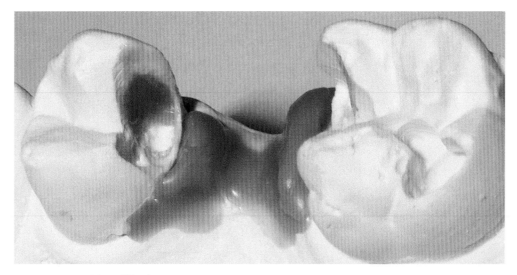

Fig. C9.2.4 Model modification.

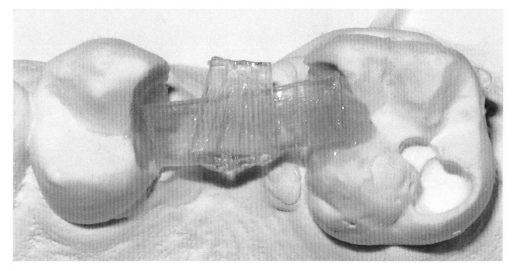

Fig. C9.2.5 Framework construction.

Veneering composite placement

Fabrication was completed by incremental placement and light curing of a laboratory composite (Sinfony, 3M ESPE, Seefeld, Germany) to form a ridge lap pontic, with a reduced occlusal table, to minimize occlusal forces. Appropriate composite stains were applied to improve esthetics using tinted flowable resin composites designed for this purpose.

During construction it has been demonstrated that it is crucial to minimize voids. To maintain the oxygen-inhibited surface layer that maximizes bond strength between fibres and composite increments, specialized resin (Stick-RESIN, GC, Japan) was applied in thin layers.

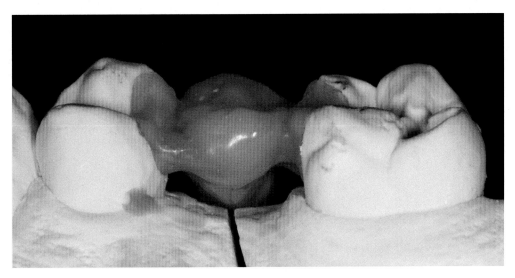

Fig. C9.2.6   Veneering composite applied.

Try-in/fit surface preparation

Following isolation, removal of temporary restorations and try-in, the fit surfaces were roughened lightly with a diamond bur (and not sandblasting, which is contraindicated for this purpose) to expose fibres on the cementing surfaces. This is especially important when using surface-retained FRC-RBBs.

The restoration was then washed with water to remove debris and air-dried before application of a specialized solvent-free adhesive resin (StickRESIN, Stick-Tech, Finland), which is designed to activate the polymer network within the fibres and create a reliable bond.

The restoration was stored in dark conditions until required for cementation and for at least 3–5 minutes to allow resin/fibre interaction.

Immediately prior to cementation, gentle airflow was used to remove excess adhesive agent which may affect the fit. The restoration was then light cured for 10 seconds.

Tooth surface preparation

Tooth surfaces were prepared for cementation by:

- Cleaning inlay preparations using a pumice and water mix in a rubber cup

- Etching with 37% ortho-phosphoric acid for 15 seconds. Note: the recommended enamel etching time for surface-retained FRC-RBBs is longer (45–60 seconds)

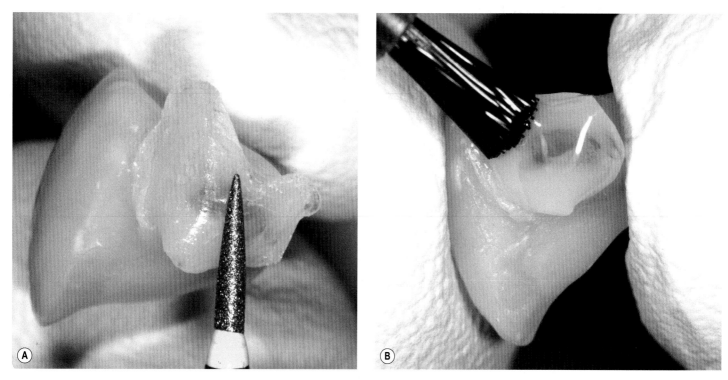

Fig. C9.2.7   Fit surface preparation. (A) Roughening. (B) Application of solvent free resin.

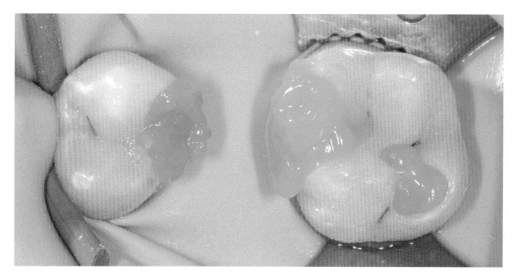

Fig. C9.2.8   Phosphoric acid etchant applied.

- Rinsing with water and gentle air-drying

- Application of adhesive resin as per the manufacturer's instructions.

Cementation

Dual-cure luting resin was then applied to the fit surfaces of the restoration and to the inlay preparations. Note: chemically cured composite luting resins may

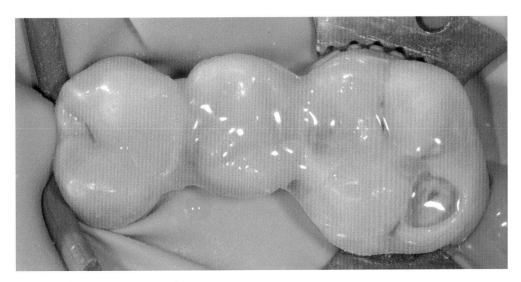

Fig. C9.2.9   Restoration cementation.

also be used, but phosphate and glass ionomer cements are not suitable for cementing indirect fibre-reinforced restorations. The restoration was seated and excess cement removed carefully using a suitable brush.

Glycerine gel (or suitable translucent alternative) was applied to cover marginal areas. This excludes oxygen and improves the polymerization reaction during light curing.

The Class I cavity was then restored using conventional resin materials and techniques.

Finishing

The occlusion was checked using articulating paper and refined using suitable composite finishing burs and discs. It was important to avoid any exposure of framework fibres during finishing procedures, especially in the connector areas.

Restoration check

As the patient presented with active carious lesions and was considered to be at high risk of further disease, fastidious care was taken to remove any plaque retentive factors and to reinforce the necessity for the patient to carry out effective, standard care preventive measures.

Review

The importance of regular reviews was established at the outset. These reviews were then scheduled for suitable intervals to allow monitoring and reinforcement of plaque control, as well as the assessment of functional and esthetic factors.

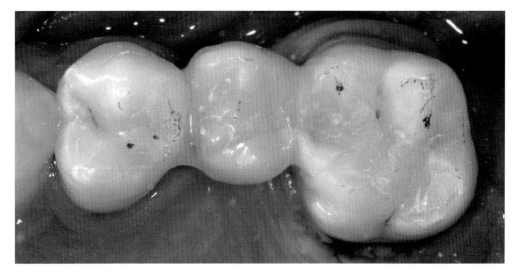

Fig. C9.2.10   Occlusal assessment.

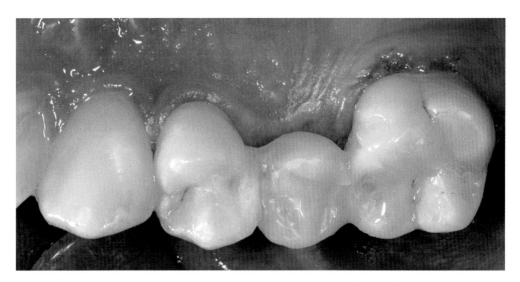

Fig. C9.2.11   Removal of plaque retention factors.

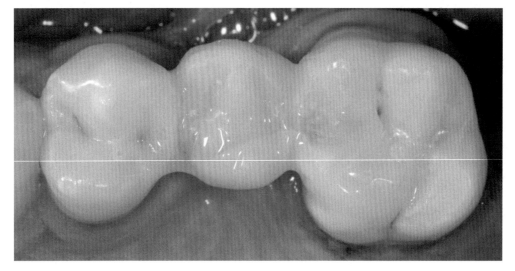

Fig. C9.2.12   Restoration review.

CLINICAL CASE 9.3: ALL-CERAMIC RESIN-BONDED BRIDGE

Case history

Extraction of an upper second premolar was the unfortunate end to a cycle of repeated restoration failures and replacements in a 35-year-old male patient.

Care plan

Following a suitable period of healing, and as oral hygiene, occlusal and periodontal conditions were favourable, the full range of treatment alternatives was outlined to the patient. The risk/benefit ratio of each option was presented in detail including the non-treatment option, which was ruled out in this case, for esthetic reasons.

The option selected with informed consent was a resin-bonded zirconia framework ceramic bridge. Bridge design was based on esthetics and the anticipated occlusal, functional forces on the restoration. Fixed/fixed designs are generally favourable rather than cantilevers that suffer increased stress at the connector due to leverage on the pontic.[20] Minimally invasive inlay retainers were prescribed for abutment teeth[22] adjacent to the space and were designed to minimize occlusal contacts on the restoration.[23]

The decision was also made to investigate and restore an incipient carious lesion in the central pit of the molar abutment.

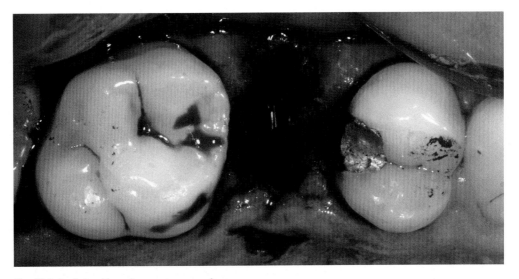

Fig. C9.3.1   Extraction of an upper premolar.

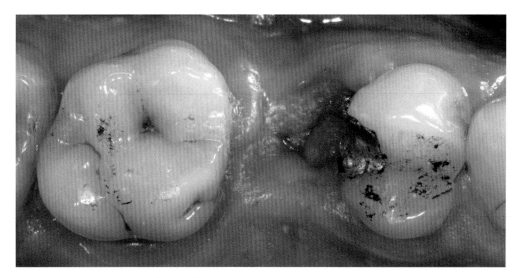

Fig. C9.3.2   Treatment plan: all-ceramic RBB.

Preparation

Following shade selection and local anaesthesia, abutment preparation was carried out to optimize space requirements for the selected materials, whilst preserving the maximum amount of tooth tissue. General recommended preparation guidelines for all-ceramic bridges include:[24]

- While ceramic wing thickness may be only 0.6 mm in certain clinical situations, occlusally no areas of the preparation should allow less than 2 mm of material to optimize strength.[21]

- Internal line angles should be rounded to minimize stress on the residual tooth tissue and the restoration.[20]

- Proximal box wall preparations should diverge, avoid undermining enamel and optimize the surface area available for adhesion.

- Abutment preparations should be mutually parallel (although undercuts may be blocked out if paralleling would involve excessive hard tissue removal).

- No bevels should be placed as this will result in thin marginal ceramic prone to fracture.

- Floors should be smooth (but do not need to be flat).

- Margins should be supra-gingival and confined ideally to enamel.

- Cavo-surface angle should be well defined* and ideally with a 90° butt joint.

---

*   When intra-oral digital impressions are employed, distinct cavo-surface angles are essential to enable accurate recording of preparation margins.[19]

Connector design

This is a vital factor governing fracture resistance and is affected significantly by the size, shape and position of the connector.[20] The recommended connector height from interproximal papilla to marginal ridge is ≥4 mm for most systems.[19] These requirements must be balanced against the risk of closing embrasures and complicating plaque control procedures for the patient.

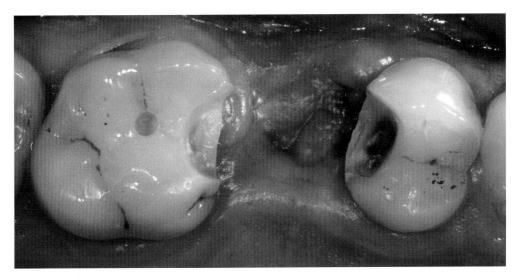

Fig. C9.3.3   Abutment preparation complete.

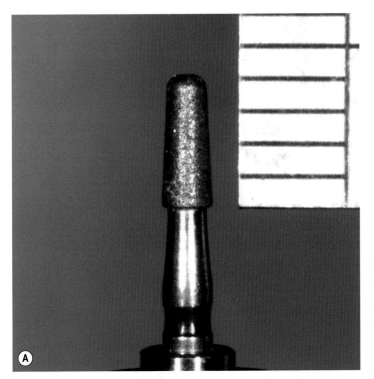

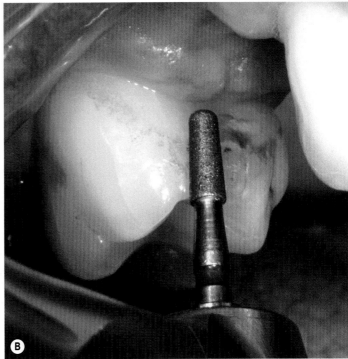

Fig. C9.3.4   (A) Bur measurement. (B) Enables minimally invasive retainer design.

CLINICAL TIPS

- Pre-operatively measuring burs will enhance precision in meeting the connector dimension requirements for each material

- Use of tapered burs will reduce the risk of undercutting and automatically creating divergent preparations

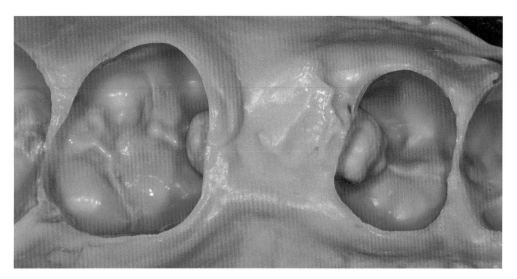

Fig. C9.3.5   Impression.

Impression

Ceramic bridges may be manufactured using traditional impression and waxing techniques or from digital impressions captured intra-orally or, as in this case, by scanning a model cast from a conventional silicone impression. An opposing alginate impression was used for construction of a model that was also processed digitally using the same non-contact photo-optical white light and laser scanner to provide a 3D digital occlusal record.

Provisional restoration

Inlay preparations were restored temporarily with a flexible light-cured resin material designed for this purpose. This allows easy removal with no risk of altering the prepared surfaces.

Computer aided design[25]

A virtual model of the preparation created by 3D software (Fig. C9.3.7A) on which the bridge framework was designed. The framework is designed 20–25% larger than the actual restoration to account for shrinkage during the final sintering stage. The pontic was selected from a range of options (Fig. C9.3.7B)

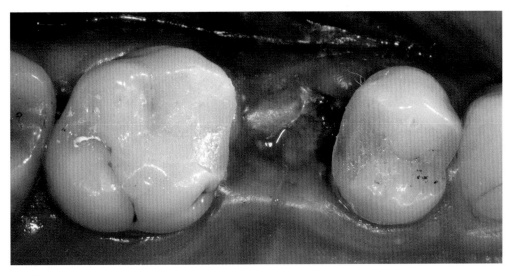

Fig. C9.3.6   Temporary restorations.

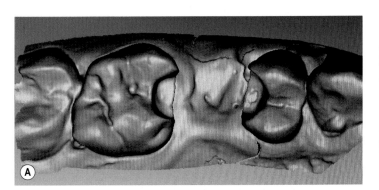

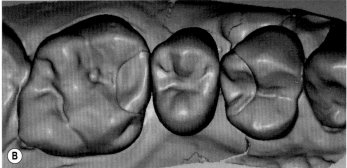

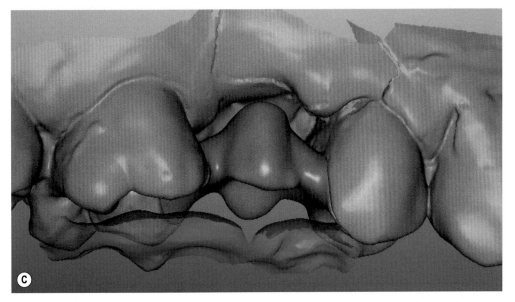

Fig. C9.3.7   Computer aided bridge design. (A) Virtual model. (B) Pontic design. (C) Occlusal design.

and was modified to fit the photo-optically scanned functional impression of the opposing arch (Fig. C9.3.7C).

The machine then shrank the pontic digitally, to account for the desired thickness of veneering porcelain, and designed the connectors to match the requirements of each material. The ceramicist then modified the framework digitally to maximize strength and support for the overlying porcelain and create smooth embrasure contours to minimize stress concentration.[19]

Framework manufacture

A separate unit milled the framework from a prefabricated blank of partially sintered zirconia (Fig. C9.3.8A). The material has a chalk-like consistency (Fig. C9.3.8B) that is easily machinable and with less wear and tear on milling hardware;[19] this reduced the risk of micro-cracks that may be associated with the milling of fully sintered blanks.[19] The framework was heated slowly and sintered to full density, precisely following manufacturer's instructions (Fig. C9.3.8C).

Veneering porcelain

A very thin wash of layering ceramic was applied to wet the surface of the framework (Fig. C9.3.9A) and maximize support for the subsequent layers of veneering porcelain, which was then added to optimize esthetics and match the polychromatic appearance of natural teeth (Fig. C9.3.9B).

Porcelains with high fusing temperatures were used as they are the most compatible with zirconia. As reinforcement of the veneering feldspathic porcelain is critical to success, the manufacturer's instructions should be followed carefully with regard to magnitude and rate of increase and decrease of firing temperatures.

Surface preparation

The full contour restoration was painted with a glaze (Fig. C9.3.10A) and fired to produce fit surfaces that may be sandblasted and then etched with hydrofluoric acid to allow adhesive cementation. Etching of pure zirconia is impossible, as its crystalline structure is too dense. Adhesion was enhanced by painting the fit surfaces with a silane primer (Fig. C9.3.10B), and this was carried out chairside at the cementation appointment.

Try-in

Following removal of the temporary dressing and isolation, the restoration was tried in. Although no surface fit adjustments were necessary in this case, corrections if required may be carried out using appropriate burs.

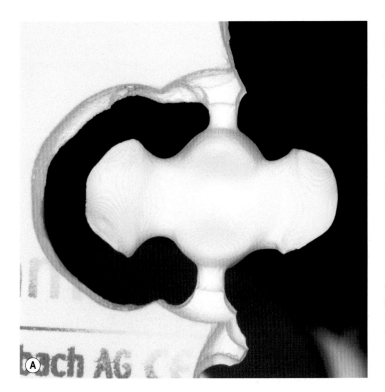

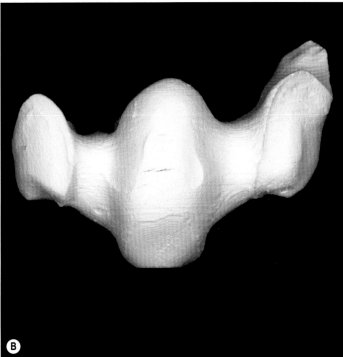

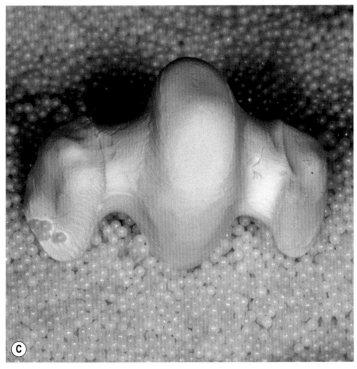

Fig. C9.3.8   Framework manufacture. (A) Milled framework.
(B) Pre-sintered framework. (C) Sintered framework.

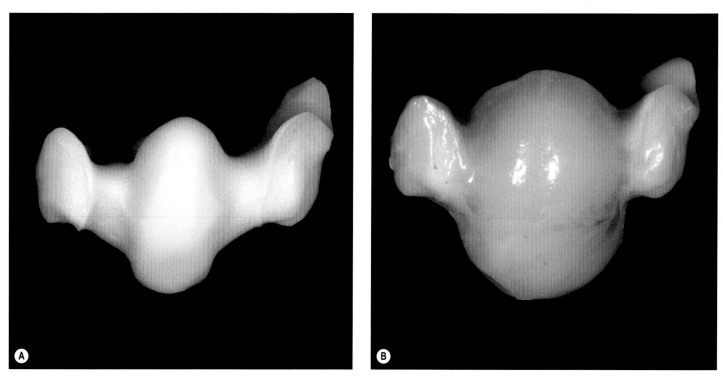

Fig. C9.3.9 (A) Framework complete. (B) Veneering porcelain.

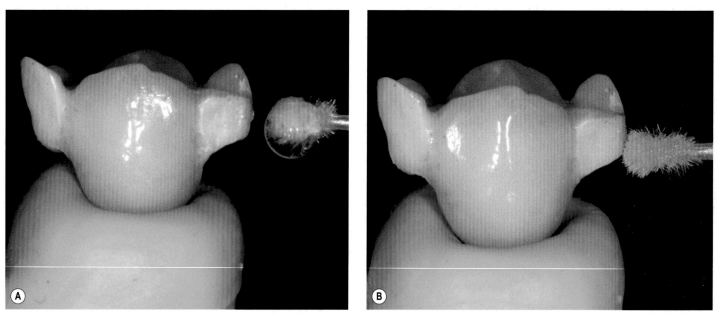

Fig. C9.3.10 Fit surface preparation. (A) Etching of glazed surface. (B) Silane primer.

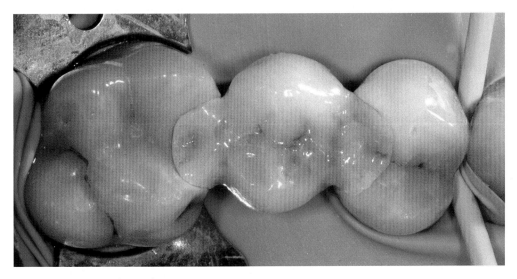

Fig. C9.3.11   Restoration try-in.

Tooth surface preparation

The inlay preparations were etched using 37% ortho-phosphoric acid for 15 seconds. Etchant was then thoroughly washed off the preparations and dried with gentle airflow to prevent dentine dehydration.

CLINICAL TIPS: ETCHING

- Viscous etching gel enhanced control of placement

- Coloured gels reduced the risk of etching too far beyond restoration margins, which would have allowed excess luting resin to stick

- The etchant was agitated gently with a suitable instrument to burst air bubbles and optimize the etch pattern

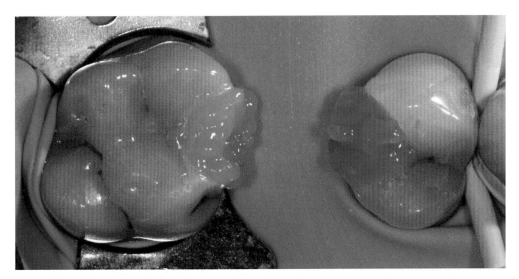

Fig. C9.3.12   Abutment teeth etched.

Adhesive

While (less technique-sensitive) self-etching cements may be used, optimum adhesion is considered to be gained by etch and rinse systems. A strong durable bond is required for all adhesively cemented restorations to:

- Improve retention
- Reduce risk of micro-leakage
- Increase the restorations' resistance to fracture initiation and propagation
- Allow transfer of occlusal forces to the abutment teeth.

Note: low film thickness adhesive resins should be used and pooling eliminated to allow accurate seating of the prosthesis.

Luting cement

Resin-based or resin-modified glass ionomer cements are considered appropriate for the cementation of adhesive all-ceramic restorations. In this example NX3 Nexus resin-based luting cement (Kerr, Switzerland) was chosen as it offered the following benefits:

- Dual-cure ensured polymerization in areas that light would not reach.
- Good esthetic properties.
- Try-in gels were available to stabilize the restoration during assessment.
- Different shade luting resins offered flexibility in esthetic achievement.

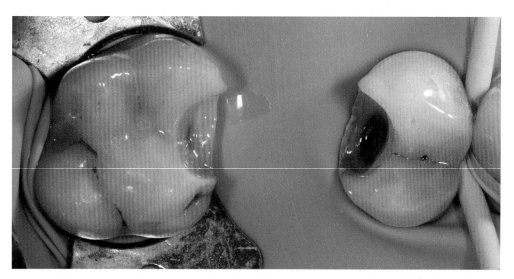

Fig. C9.3.13   Adhesive applied.

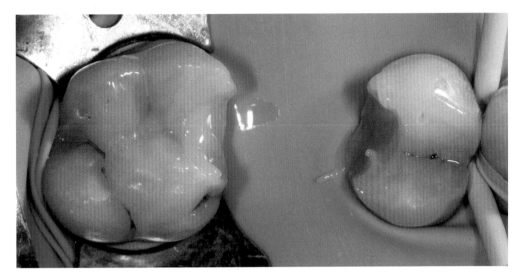

Fig. C9.3.14   Luting resin applied.

The cement was mixed and applied to the abutment preparations using a suitable brush. The restoration was then seated.

Note: traditional non-adhesive luting techniques may be used for full or partial-coverage restorations and are useful in clinical situations where moisture control is difficult.

Cementation

The restoration was seated and excess cement removed with a different (dry) brush. Remaining marginal excess was light cured for 10 seconds and removed with a sharp instrument. The restoration was then polymerized so that all surfaces received at least a 60-second light cure. It has been suggested that flow of luting resins into porcelain flaws on the fit surface and subsequent shrinkage on polymerization may seal defects and reduce fracture propagation further.

Finishing and polishing

Following rubber dam removal, the occlusion was checked in the intercuspal position and in all excursions using articulating paper. Adjustments were made using appropriate finishing burs, abrasive discs and with pastes designed for polishing porcelain. Copious coolant and gentle pressure were used to reduce the risk of introducing flaws into the restoration.

The patient was instructed in the necessary protocols for home care of the bridge and advised on specific oral hygiene products suitable in this respect.

CLINICAL TIPS

Prior to cementation, the buccal surface of the pontic was marked with a felt pen to reduce the risk of incorrect orientation. It is particularly important to avoid such time-consuming errors when chemically cured cements are used.

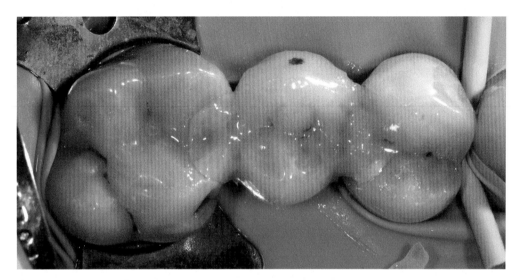

Fig. C9.3.15   Cementation.

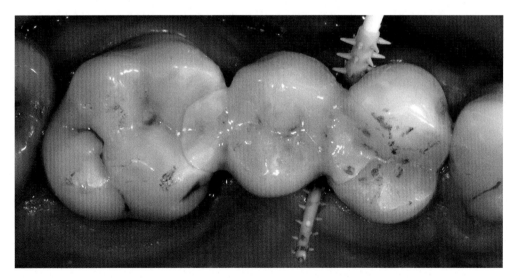

Fig. C9.3.16   Oral hygiene instruction.

Restoration assessment

The restoration was given a final inspection to check for any excess cement and the patient was then given a mirror to confirm that esthetic expectations had been met.

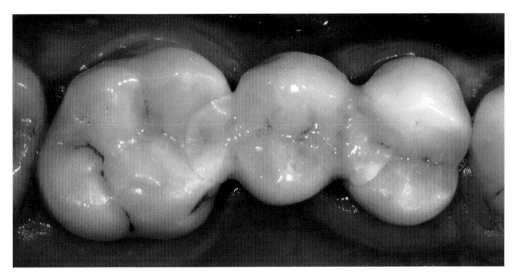

Fig. C9.3.17   Restoration assessment.

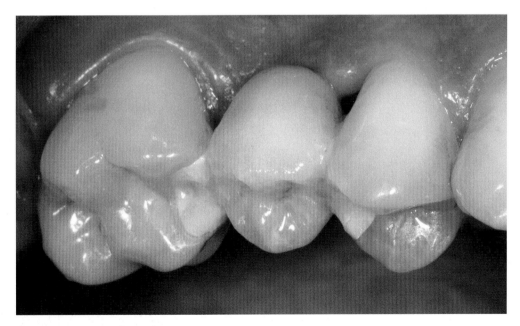

Fig. C9.3.18   Restoration review.

Review

Regular reviews were scheduled and are essential to monitor for the common modes of failure seen with all-ceramic bridges.[26] Long-term evaluation of successful (and unsuccessful) restorations will help to inform future minimally invasive esthetic restorative procedures.

ACKNOWLEDGEMENTS

The author would like to thank Professor P. Vallittu, Professor A. Shinya, Dr Peter Sands, Professor Giles Perryer, Dr Luke Greenwood, Mr Glyn Thomas (Clinical Case 9.2), Adrian and Jacque Rollings (Clinical Case 9.3), Dr Adrian Shortall, Dr Jim McCubbin, Professor Richard Verdi, and all the patients who were kind enough to allow the preceding operative procedures to be photographed and used to illustrate Chapters 8 and 9.

Further reading

Aida N, Shinya A, Yokoyama D, et al. Three-dimensional finite element analysis of posterior fiber-reinforced composite fixed partial denture, Part 2: influence of fiber reinforcement on mesial and distal connectors. Dent Mater J 2011;30(1):29–37.

Bachhav VC, Aras MA. Zirconia-based fixed partial dentures: a clinical review. Quintessence Int 2011;42:173–82.

Burke FJT. Resin-retained bridges: fibre-reinforced versus metal. Dent Update 2008;35:521–6.

Burke FJT, Ali A, Palin W. Zirconia-based all-ceramic crowns and bridges: three case reports. Dent Update 2006;33:401–10.

Butterworth C, Ellakwa AE, Shortall ACC. Fibre-reinforced composites in restorative dentistry. Dent Update 2003;30:300–6.

Clinical Guide. Fibre Reinforcements for Minimally Invasive Bridges. Turku, Finland: StickTech Ltd. Available from: <www.sticktech.com>; 2011.

Ellakwa AE, Shortall ACC, Shehata MK, Marquis PM. The influence of fibre placement and position on the efficiency of reinforcement of fibre reinforced composite bridgework. J Oral Rehabil 2001;28:785–91.

Freilich MA, Meiers JC. Fiber-reinforced composite prosthese. Dent Clin N Am 2004;48:545–62.

Freilich MA, Meiers JC, Duncan JP, et al. Clinical evaluation of fiber-reinforced fixed bridges. JADA 2002;133:1524–34.

Garoushi S, Lassila L, Vallittu PK. Resin-bonded fiber-reinforced composite for direct replacement of missing anterior teeth: a clinical report. Int J Dent 2011;20:42–5.

Göncü Başaran E, Ayna E, Uçtaşli S, et al. Load-bearing capacity of fiber reinforced fixed composite bridges. Acta Odontol Scand 2013;71(1):65–71.

Kara HB, Aykent F. Single tooth replacement using a ceramic resin bonded fixed partial denture: a case report. Eur J Dent 2012;6:101–4.

Karaarslan ES, Ertas E, Ozsevik S, Usumez A. Conservative approach for restoring posterior missing tooth with fiber reinforcement materials: four clinical reports. Eur J Dent 2011;5(4):465–71.

Keulemans F, De Jager N, Kleverlaan CJ, Feilzer AJ. Influence of retainer design on two-unit cantilever resin-bonded glass fiber reinforced composite fixed dental prostheses: an in vitro and finite element analysis study. J Adhes Dent 2008;10(5):355–64.

Keulemans F, Lassila LV, Garoushi S, et al. The influence of framework design on the load-bearing capacity of laboratory-made inlay-retained fibre-reinforced composite fixed dental prostheses. J Biomech 2009;42(7):844–9.

Lassila LV, Garoushi S, Tanner J, et al. Adherence of *Streptococcus mutans* to fiber-reinforced filling composite and conventional restorative materials. Open Dent J 2009;3:227–32.

Ozcan M, Breuklander MH, Vallittu PK. The effect of box preparation on the strength of glass fiber-reinforced composite inlay-retained fixed partial dentures. J Prosthet Dent 2005;93(4):337–45.

Ozyesil AG, Usumez A. Replacement of missing posterior teeth with an all-ceramic inlay-retained fixed partial denture: a case report. J Adhes Dent 2006;8(1):59–61.

Song HY, Yi YJ, Cho LR, Park DY. Effects of two preparation designs and pontic distance on bending and fracture strength of fiber-reinforced composite inlay fixed partial dentures. J Prosthet Dent 2003;90(4):347–53.

Vallittu PK. Survival rates of resin-bonded, glass fiber-reinforced composite fixed partial dentures with a mean follow-up of 42 months: a pilot study. J Prosthet Dent 2004;91(3):241–6.

van Heumen CC, Tanner J, van Dijken JW, et al. Five-year survival of 3-unit fiber-reinforced composite fixed partial dentures in the posterior area. Dent Mater 2010;26(10):954–60.

van Heumen CC, van Dijken JW, Tanner J, et al. Five-year survival of 3-unit fiber-reinforced composite fixed partial dentures in the anterior area. Dent Mater 2009;25(6):820–7.

Xie Q, Lassila LV, Vallittu PK. Comparison of load-bearing capacity of direct resin-bonded fiber-reinforced composite FPDs with four framework designs. J Dent 2007;35(7):578–82.

Yokoyama D, Shinya A, Gomi H, et al. Effects of mechanical properties of adhesive resin cements on stress distribution in fiber-reinforced composite adhesive fixed partial dentures. Dent Mater J 2012;31(2):189–96.

REFERENCES

1. Butterworth C, Ellakwa AE, Shortall ACC. Fibre-reinforced composites in restorative dentistry. Dent Update 2003;30:300–6.

2. Burke FJT. Resin-retained bridges: fibre-reinforced versus metal. Dent Update 2008;35:521–6.

3. Jokstad A, Gökçe M, Hjortsjö C. A systematic review of the scientific documentation of fixed partial dentures made from fiber-reinforced polymer to replace missing teeth. Int J Prosthodont 2005;18(6):489–96.

4. Vallittu PK. Survival rates of resin-bonded, glass fiber-reinforced composite fixed partial dentures with a mean follow-up of 42 months: a pilot study. J Prosthet Dent 2004;91(3):241–6.

5. van Heumen CC, Tanner J, van Dijken JW, et al. Five-year survival of 3-unit fiber-reinforced composite fixed partial dentures in the posterior area. Dent Mater 2010;26(10):954–60.

6. Ibsen RL. One appointment technique using an adhesive composite. Dent Surv 1973; 49:30–2.

7. Altieri JV, Burstone CJ, Goldberg AJ, Patel AP. Longitudinal clinical evaluation of fiber-reinforced composite fixed partial dentures: a pilot study. J Prosthet Dent 1994;71(1):16–22.

8. Frielich MA, Meiers JC. Fiber-reinforced composite prostheses. Dent Clin N Am 2004;48: 545–62.

9. Karaarslan ES, Ertas E, Ozsevik S, Usumez A. Conservative approach for restoring posterior missing teeth with fiber reinforcement materials: four clinical reports. Eur J Dent 2011; 5(4):465–71.

10. Garoushi S1, Vallittu P, Lassila L. Fiber-reinforced composite for chairside replacement of anterior teeth: a case report. Libyan J Med 2008;3(4):195–6.

11. Aida N, Shinya A, Yokoyama D, et al. Three-dimensional finite element analysis of posterior fiber-reinforced composite fixed partial denture Part 2: influence of fiber reinforcement on mesial and distal connectors. Dent Mater J 2011;30(1):29–37.

12. Yokoyama D, Shinya A, Gomi H, et al. Effects of mechanical properties of adhesive resin cements on stress distribution in fiber-reinforced composite adhesive fixed partial dentures. Dent Mater J 2012;31(2):189–96.

13. Ellakwa AE, Shortall ACC, Shehata MK, Marquis PM. The influence of fibre placement and position on the efficiency of reinforcement of fibre reinforced composite bridgework. J Oral Rehabil 2001;28:785–91.

14. Keulemans F, De Jager N, Kleverlaan CJ, Feilzer AJ. Influence of retainer design on two-unit cantilever resin-bonded glass fiber reinforced composite fixed dental prostheses: an in vitro and finite element analysis study. J Adhes Dent 2008;10(5):355–64.

15. Keulemans F, Lassila LV, Garoushi S, et al. The influence of framework design on the load-bearing capacity of laboratory-made inlay-retained fibre-reinforced composite fixed dental prostheses. J Biomech 2009;42(7):844–9.

16. Ozcan M, Breuklander MH, Vallittu PK. The effect of box preparation on the strength of glass fiber-reinforced composite inlay-retained fixed partial dentures. J Prosthet Dent 2005; 93(4):337–45.

17. Song HY, Yi YJ, Cho LR, Park DY. Effects of two preparation designs and pontic distance on bending and fracture strength of fiber-reinforced composite inlay fixed partial dentures. J Prosthet Dent 2003;90(4):347–53.

18. Xie Q, Lassila LV, Vallittu PK. Comparison of load-bearing capacity of direct resin-bonded fiber-reinforced composite FPDs with four framework designs. J Dent 2007;35(7):578–82.

19. Bachhav VC, Aras MA. Zirconia-based fixed partial dentures: a clinical review. Quintessence Int 2011;42:173–82.

20. Raigrodski AJ. Contemporary all-ceramic fixed partial dentures: a review. Dent Clin North Am 2004;48(2):viii, 531–44.

21. Williams S, Albadri S, Jarad F. The use of zirconium, single retainer, resin-bonded bridges in adolescents. Dent Update 2001;38:706–10.

22. Ozyesil AG, Usumez A. Replacement of missing posterior teeth with an all-ceramic inlay-retained fixed partial denture: a case report. J Adhes Dent 2006;8(1):59–61.

23. Kara HB, Aykent F. Single tooth replacement using a ceramic resin bonded fixed partial denture: a case report. Eur J Dent 2012;6(1):101–4.

24. Hilton TJ, Ferracane JL, Broome JC. Summitt's Fundamentals of Operative Dentistry: a Contemporary Approach. 4th ed. London: Quintessence Publishing Ltd; 2013.

25. Burke FJT, Ali A, Palin W. Zirconia-based all-ceramic crowns and bridges: three case reports. Dent Update 2006;33:401–10.

26. Kelly JR, Tesk JA, Sorensen JA. Failure of all-ceramic fixed partial dentures in vitro and in vivo: analysis and modeling. J Dent Res 1995;74(6):1253–8.

INDEX

Page numbers followed by "f" indicate figures, "t" indicate tables, and "b" indicate boxes.